Innovative Concepts in Inflammatory Bowel Diseases

Innovative Concepts in Inflammatory Bowel Diseases

EDITED BY

J. Emmrich and S. Liebe

Abteilung für Gastroenterologie
Medizinische Klinik
Klinikum der Universität Rostock
D-18057 Rostock
Germany

E. F. Stange

Bereich für Gastroenterologie
Klinik für Innere Medizin
Medizinische Universität zu Lübeck
D-23538 Lübeck
Germany

Proceedings of the Falk Symposium 105 (Baltic Sea Symposium) held in
Rostock, Germany, April 30–May 2, 1998

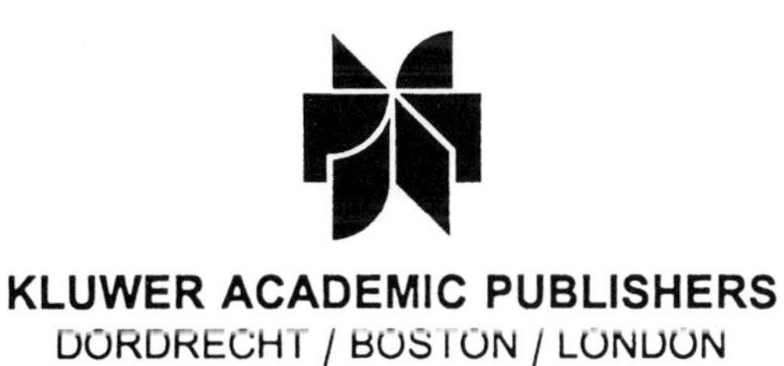

KLUWER ACADEMIC PUBLISHERS
DORDRECHT / BOSTON / LONDON

Library of Congress Cataloging in-Publication Data is available.

ISBN 0–7923–8749–X

Published by Kluwer Academic Publishers,
P. O. Box 17, 3300 AA Dordrecht, The Netherlands

Sold and distributed in North, Central and South America
by Kluwer Academic Publishers
101 Philip Drive, Norwell, MA 02061, U.S.A.

In all other countries, sold and distributed
by Kluwer Academic Publishers,
P. O. Box 322, 3300 AH Dordrecht, The Netherlands

Printed on acid-free paper

Printed and bound in Great Britain by MPG Books, Bodmin, Cornwall.

Contents

CONTENTS

Section V: Epithelial Barrier in IBD

Section VI: Endotoxin and IBD

Section VII: Diagnosis of IBD

Section VIII: IBD and Malignancy

List of Principal Authors

T. Andus
Klinik und Poliklinik für Innere Medizin I
Klinikum der Universität Regensberg
D-93042 Regensburg
Germany

S. C. Bischoff
Department of Gastroenterology and
    Hepatology
Medical School of Hannover
D-30623 Hannover
Germany

R. S. Blumberg
Gastroenterology Division
Harvard Medical School
Brigham and Women's Hospital
75 Francis Street
Boston
MA 02115-6195
USA

J.-F. Colombel
Department of Hepatogastroenterology
Hôpital Huriez
CH et U Lille
F-59037 Lille
France

A. Dignass
Charité-Campus Virchow
Medizinische Klinik m.S.
Hepatologie u. Gastroenterologie
Augustenberger Platz 1
D-13353 Berlin
Germany

R. Duchmann
Innere Medizin II.
Medizinische Klinik und Poliklinik
Universitätklinikum des Saarlandes
Kirrberger Str.
D-66421 Homburg/Saar
Germany

A. Ekbom
Department of Medical Epidemiology
Karolinska Institutet
P.O. Box 281
S-17177 Stockholm
Sweden

C. O. Elson
Division of Gastroenterology and
    Hepatology
The University of Alabama at
    Birmingham
UAB Station
Birmingham
AL 35294-0007
USA

J. Emmrich
Abteilung Gastroenterologie
Klinik und Poliklinik für Innere Medizin
Klinikum der Universität Rostock
Ernst-Heydeman-Str 6
D-18057 Rostock
Germany

C. Folwaczny
Medizinische Klinik
Klinikum Innenstadt der LMU
    München
Ziemssenstr. 1
D-80336 München
Germany

K. R. Gardiner
Department of Surgery
The Queens University of Belfast
Institute of Clinical Science
Grosvenor Road
Belfast
BT12 6BJ
UK

V. Gross
Medizinische Klinik II
Klinikum St Marien
Mariahilfbergweg 7
D-92224 Amberg
Germany

K. Hauenstein
Radiologische Klinik
Klinikum der Universität Rostock
Gertrudenplatz 1
D-18057 Rostock
Germany

U. T. Hopt
Chirurgische Klinik
Klinikum der Universität Rostock
Schillingallee 35
D-18055 Rostock
Germany

A. Kantele
Central Hospital of Central Finland
Keskussairaalantie 19
FIN-40620 Jyväskylä
Finland

W. Kruis
Innere Abteilung
Evangelisches Krankenhaus Kalk
Buchforststr. 2
D-51103 Köln
Germany

P. Layer
Innere Abteilung
Israelitisches Krankenhaus
Orchideenstieg 14
D-22297 Hamburg
Germany

H. Lochs
IV. Medizinische Klinik
Schwerpunkt Gastroenterologie
Medizinische Fakultät (Charité)
Humboldt-Universität zu Berlin
Schumannstr. 20-21
D-10117 Berlin
Germany

K. Loeschke
Medizinische Klinik
Klinikum Innenstadt der LMU
  München
Ziemssenstr. 1
D-80336 München
Germany

J.-M. Löhr
Abteilung Gastroenterologie
Klinik und Poliklinik für Innere Medizin
Klinikum der Universität Rostock
Ernst-Heydemann-Str. 6
D-18057 Rostock
Germany

D. Ludwig
Bereich Gastroenterologie
Klinik für Innere Medizin
Medizinische Universität zu Lübeck
Ratzburger Allee 160
D-23538 Lübeck
Germany

J. Mestecky
Department of Microbiology – Box 1
The University of Alabama at
  Birmingham
757 BBRB, 845 19th Street South
Birmingham
AL 35294-2170
USA

M. F. Neurath
Laboratory of Immunology
I Medizinische Klinik
Klinikum der Universität
Langenbeckstr. 1
D-55131 Mainz
Germany

A. S. Peña
Free University Hospital
Department of Gastroenterology
PO Box 7057
NL-1007 MB Amsterdam
The Netherlands

R. Porschen
Abteilung Innere Medizin I
Medizinische Klinik und Poliklinik
Eberhard-Karls-Universität
Otfried-Müller-Str.10
D-72076 Tübingen
Germany

P. Pozarowski
Department of Clinical Immunology
Medical School of Lublin
ul. Jaczewskiego 8
PL-20-950 Lublin
Poland

C. Prantera
Gastroenterologia
Ospedale Nuovo Regina Margherita
Via Morosini 30
I-00153 Roma
Italy

D. H. Present
Mount Sinai Medical Center
12 East 86th Street
New York
NY 10028-0517
USA

A. Raedler
Medizinische Abteilung
Krankenhaus Tabea
Kösterbergstr. 32
D-22587 Hamburg
Germany

H. C. Rath
Klinik und Poliklinik für Innere Medizin I
Klinikum der Universität Regensburg
D-93042 Regensburg
Germany

M. Reinshagen
Abteilung Innere Medizin I
Medizinische Klinik und Poliklinik
Klinikum der Universität Ulm
Robert-Koch-Str. 8
D-89081 Ulm
Germany

E.-O. Riecken
Abteilung für Gastroenterologie
Medizinische Klinik und Poliklinik
Universitätsklinikum Benjamin Franklin
 der Freien Universität Berlin
Hindenburgdamm 30
D-12200 Berlin
Germany

N. Runkel
Chirurgische Klinik I
Universitätsklinikum Benjamin Franklin
 der Frein Universität Berlin
Hindenburgdamm 30
D-12200 Berlin
Germany

F. Schier
Department of Paediatric Surgery
University Medical Center Jena
Bachstr. 18
D-07740 Jena
Germany

J. Schölmerich
Klinik und Poliklinik für Innere Medizin I
Klinikum der Universität Regensburg
D-93042 Regensburg
Germany

F. Seibold
Medizinische Poliklinik
Universität Würzburg
Klinikstrasse 6
D-97070 Würzburg
Germany

A. Stallmach
Innere Medizin II
Medizinische Klinik und Poliklinik
Universitätskliniken des Saarlandes
Kirrberger Strasse
D-66421 Homburg/Saar
Germany

E. F. Stange
Bereich für Gastroenterologie
Klinik für Innere Medizin
Medizinische Universität zu Lübeck
D-23538 Lübeck
Germany

H. Tlaskalová-Hogenová
Division of Immunology and
 Gnotobiology
Institute of Microbiology CSAS
Videnska 1083
CZ-142 20 Prague
Czech Republic

J. H. Zivny
1 LF UK
Department of Pathophysiology
U nemocnice 5
CZ-128 53 Prague 2
Czech Republic

Preface

Chronic inflammatory bowel disease, ulcerative colitis and Crohn's disease represent an important medical problem, since they have a devastating impact on the quality of life and require longstanding medical care. The causes of these diseases are unknown, and therapy is often unsatisfactory. Many medical disciplines are involved in tackling the immensely complex studies on aetiology, pathogenesis, clinical course and treatment protocols. Therefore, meetings are necesssary to bring together experts from different fields of science to find a unified view on clinical and basic research.

This book presents the papers from an international conference that took place in May 1998 in Rostock on the basic and clinical aspects of inflammatory bowel diseases. This Falk symposium on the coast of the Baltic Sea allowed scientists and clinicians coming especially from the countries around the Baltic Sea to talk together and form new collaborations. The conference included seven sessions that provided forums for in-depth discussions of several aspects of chronic inflammatory bowel diseases.

The main themes of the meeting were genetics, animal models, immunology, epithelial cells, endotoxin, diagnostic procedures, malignancy, medical therapies, and surgery. In each session, in state-of-the-art-lectures, top experts presented the very latest developments in their respective research areas followed by special lectures on defined aspects of inflammatory bowel diseases. A poster session was organized to encourage investigators in these fields, particularly younger workers, to present their recent data and actively participate in the meeting. There were intensive discussions between basic scientists and clinicians providing suggestions concerning future research and clinical management of patients with inflammatory bowel diseases. Readers of this book will therefore find a 'state-of-the-art' overview of the exciting developments in the pathogenesis, diagnosis and clinical management of inflammatory bowel diseases.

J. Emmrich
S. Liebe
E.F. Stange

Section I
IBD and Genetics

1
Relevant genes in IBD

J.-F. COLOMBEL, D. HERESBACH, A. CORTOT and
J.-P. HUGOT

INTRODUCTION

Epidemiological evidence suggests that the cause of inflammatory bowel disease
(IBD) is multifactorial with a strong genetic component. Identification of the relevant susceptibility genes would be a critical step in the understanding of the
pathogenesis of these diseases and for the development of new targeted therapies.
The genetic model of IBD is complex and encompasses the concept of polygenic
inheritance, genetic heterogeneity and environmental contribution[1]. Pointers to
the chromosomal location of susceptibility genes might be provided by the association of IBD with particular known genetic disorders (such as Turner's syndrome)[2] and by observing the effect of targeted genetic manipulations in animal
models[3]. However, the most profitable strategies for the identification of IBD susceptibility loci have, to date, relied on either the investigation of candidate genes
or genome-wide searches using large numbers of families.

CANDIDATE GENE APPROACHES

In the candidate gene approach, considering the central role of the immune
system in IBD, most studies have examined genes that participate in the development and regulation of the immune and inflammatory response. Even molecular genotyping has produced conflicting results and no definitive conclusions can
be drawn so far when considering all patients irrespective of phenotypes.
However, studies of the contribution of a number of potentially important genes
have provided insight into heterogeneity in particular within ulcerative colitis
(UC).

HLA genes

The contribution of major histocompatibility complex genes has received considerable attention in IBD. In Japanese and Jewish patients, HLADRB1*1502
is associated with susceptibility to UC[4,5]. Studies in other ethnic groups have

revealed conflicting results[6,7]. The explanation for these discrepancies could be provided by the documented ethnic variabilities in HLA class II frequencies: in Japanese and Jewish populations, DRB1*1502 is the most common allele, but this allele is rare in non-Jewish Caucasians and appears to play little role in IBD pathogenesis in this group[1]. More consistent results suggest that HLA plays an important role in determining UC phenotype. Data from Oxford showed that HLADRB1*0103 was strongly predictive of need for surgery[7]. This association was greatest in patients with extensive disease, extraintestinal manifestations (EIM), particularly aphthous stomatitis, arthritis and uveitis. In contrast, the frequency of DRB1*04 allele was reduced in patients with distal colitis and EIM[8] (Table 1). The DRB1*0301–DQB*201 haplotype was predictive of extensive colitis particularly in female patients[7]. The results on HLA associations in Crohn's disease (CD) are even more conflicting than in UC. A highly significant association with the allele DRB3*03 was observed in a small group of patients and controls[9]. A significant association with the DRB1*01 allele was found in two studies from the United States and France[5,10]. In the former, the association was strongest with the HLADRB1*01–DQB1*0501 haplotype. Two studies in large populations from northern Europe have shown positive association with HLADRB1*07[10,11]. Interestingly, the DRB1*07 allele was also associated with psoriasis[12] and the concurrence of psoriasis and CD in both subjects and families has been described[13]. The most impressive result that was observed in the French study was an important decrease in HLADRB1*03 in CD[10] (Figure 1). The estimated strength of the negative association between carrying these alleles and CD was OR:0.46. This variation has also been described in Germany[11] and in the Netherlands[14], although in the latter study the result was only significant in a subgroup of patients with perianal disease. It might even be a wider characteristic of IBD, since it was also observed in UC[15]. This suggests that HLADRB1*03 alleles mediate resistance to IBD. The mechanisms underlying this protective effect are still speculative and require functional studies. It may be consecutive to a high affinity of the putative antigenic peptide of IBD to the DRB1*03 molecule. This affinity may competitively inhibit the effective presentation by another adequate molecule to immunocompetent cells.

Table 1 Allelic variations in susceptibility genes may influence the clinical pattern of UC. HLA-DRB1 allele frequency in patients and controls: genotype–phenotype analysis (from ref. 8).

	*DRB1*0103(%)*	*DRB1*04(%)*
Controls ($n = 472$)	3.2	35.8
Extensive colitis ($n = 76$)	15.8*	26.3
Distal colitis ($n = 23$)	8.7	4.3*
EIM ($n = 57$)	22.8*	22.8
No EIM ($n = 42$)	2.4[†]	19*

EIM, extra-intestinal manifestation.
* Significant vs controls.
[†] Significant vs EIM.

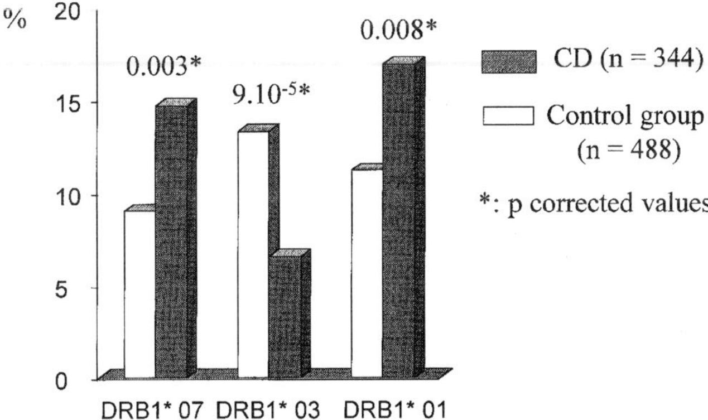

Figure 1 Association of HLA class genes with Crohn's disease in a French population[10]. Alleles DRB1*01 and DRB1*07 were associated with CD. There was a strong negative association between DRB1*03 and CD

TNF genes

Alteration in the production of tumour necrosis factor α (TNF-α) is well described in IBD, and recently two anti-TNF-α monoclonal antibodies have proved to be effective in comparison with placebo in chronic active CD[16,17]. The genes for TNF-α and TNF-β referred to as TNF locus are located on chromosome 6. Two different approaches have been used to study the association between TNF locus and IBD. A group from Los Angeles, using five microsatellite sequences within the TNF locus, determined TNF microsatellites allele frequencies at five loci. There were no differences in individual TNF microsatellites allele frequencies between IBD and controls. However, there was a CD-associated allelic combination TNF a2b1c2d4e1[18]. This haplotype was associated with the previously described HLA-DR1/DQ5 combination. Several groups studied the polymorphism at position −308 in the promoter region of the TNF-α gene. The results were discordant: the frequency of the TNF2 allele (associated with a higher level of TNF-α transcription) was found to be decreased in patients with UC in the Netherlands[19] and decreased in CD and in females with distal colitis in England[20]. No significant results were observed in other studies[8,21]. It is so far difficult to reconcile these results and it appears unlikely that these loci are important overall determinants of disease susceptibility. However, two promising aspects should be further tested: (1) a group from Amsterdam recently described specific combinations of four alleles in the TNF-α and LT-α genes which may be markers for altered TNF-α production in IBD subgroups[22]; (2) there is recent evidence that TNF microsatellites identify CD patients with poor response to anti-TNF (cA2) therapy[23].

Interleukin- 1 (IL-1) and the interleukin-1 receptor antagonist (IL-1ra)

Clinical studies and animal models provided evidence that the balance between proinflammatory cytokines IL-1α and IL-1β and their endogenous inhibitor IL-1ra is an important factor in the regulation of intestinal inflammation[24]. A

Table 2   IL-1ra allele 2 carriage in UC vs controls (overall and phenotype associations)

Ref.	Year	Country	Overall association	Particular phenotype
28	1994	USA	+	Pancolitis
29	1995	USA	+	
30	1995	USA	+	
20	1996	GB	−	
31	1996	Netherlands	−	Total or left-sided colitis
32	1997	France	−	Need for surgery
27	1997	Germany	−	

decrease in IL-1ra/IL-1α+β ratio has been found in inflamed colonic mucosa from patients with IBD but also from inflammatory controls[25-27]. The genes for IL-1α and IL-1β are located on the long arm of chromosome 2, in close linkage with the gene encoding IL-1ra. Mansfield *et al.* reported that, in a UK population, IL-1ra allele 2 was more frequent in UC patients than in controls (35% vs 24%)[28]. They found an odds ratio of 2.0 for UC in carriers of at least one copy of this allele when compared with healthy controls. This finding suggests that the allele 2 of IL-1ra is a marker for genetic susceptibility to UC. Moderate overrepresentation of IL-1ra genotype 2 was confirmed in some but not all subsequent studies (Table 2)[21,27,29-32]. The explanation for the differences between studies is not clear. It may be due to the small number of patients. Bioque *et al.* were able to show a significant difference in allele 2 carriage rates between CD, UC and controls only by combining their data in a Dutch population with data from Mansfield's study[31]. Disease heterogeneity may be most pertinent. Allele 2 of the IL-1ra may be associated exclusively with a particular subgroup of UC patients with extensive colitis and need for surgery[28]. However, this classification remains controversial, since disease extent in UC may vary considerably over time. A polymorphism has been described within the IL-1β gene, a Taq1 RFLP in exon 5. We and others have shown that the IL-1β allele frequencies of IBD patients did not differ from controls[31,32]. However, IL-1β allele 2 was significantly increased in non-carriers of IL-1ra allele 2[31,32] and IL-1ra allcle 2-IL-1β (Taq1) allcle 2 association was significantly decreased in CD and UC patients compared with controls[31].

The mucosal imbalance of the IL-1 system in IBD may thus be genetically determined: allele 2 of the IL-1ra has been associated with an impaired increase in IL-1ra in the colonic mucosa[27] and IL-1β allele 2 represents an IL-1β high secretor phenotype[33]. In conclusion, the current evidence that IL-1 system genes are important in overall susceptibility to IBD is unconvincing. However, functional studies of cytokine production in different subgroups of patients defined by the IL-1ra/IL-1β genotypes may be of importance to further clarify disease heterogeneity and in the treatment of these patients[31,32].

ICAM-1

ICAM-1 serves multiple functions in the propagation of inflammatory processes, the best characterized being facilitation of leukocyte migration from the intervascular space in response to inflammatory stimuli. Preliminary studies suggest that ICAM-1 monoclonal antibodies may be useful in CD[34]. ICAM-1 gene polymorphisms at codon 241 and at codon 469 (chromosome 19) have been studied by Yang *et al.*[35]. These two polymorphisms were not associated with CD or UC, but after stratification for pANCA status, some weak associations were found which might suggest that this polymorphism is associated with some subsets of IBD.

Other candidate genes

Studies involving T-cell receptor, IL-10, IL-2 and mucin genes have given inconsistent results or are still preliminary. Two genes encoding the transporter associated with antigen processing (TAP) proteins, TAP1 and TAP2, are located between HLA-DP and HLA-DQ. These molecules are involved in endogenous antigen processing. In CD no association was found with overall disease, but a significant decrease of TAP2AA genotype was found in patients who did not respond to steroid therapy[36]. A provocative association has recently been put forward between IBD and the DNA mismatch repair gene MLH1 on 3p which is associated with hereditary non-polyposis rectal cancer (HNPCC)[37]. Polymerase chain reaction products were analysed by single-strand conformation polymorphisms (MLH1 exons 9, 11, 14, 15 and 16) and polyacrylamide gel electrophoresis (markers D3S1611 and D3S1768). CD, UC and familial IBD were significantly associated with different MLH1 exon 15/D3S1611 haplotypes. D3S1611/D3S1678 haplotype was associated with CD whereas MLH1 exon 15/D3S1611 haplotype AA was protective. This study raises the question of whether family members of HNPCC kindreds are at risk for IBD. Interestingly, some pathological patterns (reduction in the colonic crypt in the presence of an excess of macrophages) observed in the colonic biopsies of HNPCC family members are reminiscent of IBD[38] and a member of one family, considered not at risk for HNPCC by genetic analysis, developed UC[39]. However, it must be stressed that the number of patients in Pokorny *et al.*'s study[37] was small, and their findings need to be reproduced by other centres. Meanwhile, clinicians should further explore the possibility of familial associations between IBD and HNPCC[40].

Refining association studies using serological markers

Emerging evidence points to distinct clinical patterns and heterogeneity within CD and UC[41]. As illustrated above, the power to detect susceptibility genes might be magnified considerably by studying disease subgroups: different susceptibility genes may underlie phenotypic differences in IBD. Identification of a particular phenotype will help the search for a corresponding gene. However, clinical classification of IBD is not yet standardized and there is a great interest in the hypothesis that pANCA and anti-*Saccharomyces cerevisiae* antibodies (ASCA) may help to stratify patients and to define homogeneous subgroups. Vasiliauskas *et al.* have suggested that, in patients with CD, serum pANCA expression characterizes a UC-like clinical phenotype[42]. We could not confirm this important finding in our own population[43], but the technique used to identify ANCA was different. An increased prevalence of pANCA was noted in unaffected UC family members in some[44] but not all studies[45] and consistent with genetic heterogeneity, a relationship between ANCA status and genotype has recently been confirmed: 92.7% of patients with the DR3 DQ2 TNF2 were ANCA positive vs 73.9% of the DR3 DQ2 TNF2 negative patients[46]. Data concerning ASCA are still preliminary[47]. Their presence in 20% of healthy relatives of patients with CD suggests that they may also represent a serological marker of genetic heterogeneity[48]. ASCA have been associated with a younger age at onset of CD and small bowel location, and the TNF a2b1c2d4e1a haplotype has been associated with ASCA positivity[49].

GENOME SEARCHING

Systematic screening of the entire human genome provided a strategy for the identification of susceptibility genes in multifactorial complex disorders such as IBD. This approach, which makes no prior assumption about the nature of susceptibility genes, aims to identify in the genome specific regions which are more often shared by affected individuals than expected by chance. Recent studies have emphasized the importance of access to large numbers of multiply-affected families and rigorous statistical design and analysis.

Chromosome 16 locus

A collaborative European study (using the Identity By Descent method) enabled the assignment of linkage to the pericentromeric region of chromosome 16 of a first CD-susceptibility locus named IBD1[50]. This finding has been replicated in independent data sets from four groups – the most important test of validity for linkage analysis in complex traits[51–54]. The linkage does not appear pertinent in Jewish patients, which further indicates heterogeneity within CD patients[51]. Fine mapping has recently allowed narrowing of the linkage to an 22 cM segment

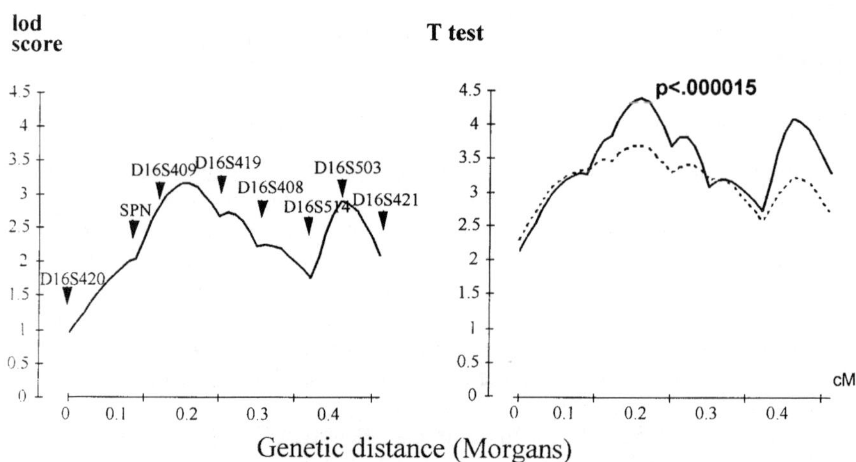

Figure 2 Multipoint interval analysis based on sib-pair allele sharing for loci in the pericentromeric region of chromosome 16. The largest lod score ($z = 3.17$) occurred between D16S409 and D16S419 (adapted from ref. 50)

Table 3 Positional candidate genes for IBD (adapted from ref. 1)

Chromosome	Gene product	Comments
16	CD11 integrin cluster	CR3 is involved in mycobacterial cell adhesion
	CD19	Involved in B lymphocyte function
	Sialophorin	Involved in leukocyte adhesion
	IL-4 receptor	IL-4-mediated regulation of macrophages is altered in IBD[56]; IL-4 is a critical mediator in the onset of early lesions in CD[57].
12	Interferon γ	Th1 cytokine with proinflammatory effects
	Integrin β7	Adhesion molecule involved in leukocyte migration in IBD
	Vitamin D receptor	Vitamin D has immune actions
7	EGFR	Growth factors regulate repair of damaged or ulcerated intestinal mucosa
	MUC3	Expression of this mucin gene is decreased in the ileal mucosa in CD[58]
3	Gαi2	Transgenic mice deficient in Gαi2 develop UC and adenocarcinoma of the colon[59]
	hMLH1	Positive association study reported[37]

EGFR, epidermal growth factor receptor; Gαi2, α subunit of inhibitory guanine nucleotide binding protein.

with a maximum lod score at D16S416 and D16S3117[55]. The region of the genome contains candidate genes which may be relevant to the pathogenesis of CD (Table 3). IBD1 contributed to a relative risk to siblings of 1.3 and therefore probably accounts for only a fraction of inherited susceptibility to CD. Whether this region also contributes to UC susceptibility is still debated[51,52,60]. Evidence of linkage was detected in the families affected only with UC but not in mixed (CD–UC) families. This suggests that the disease locus may be involved in both diseases but that the alleles predisposing to UC and CD are different.

Chromosome 12 locus

A second susceptibility locus to both UC and CD was mapped on the long arm of chromosome 12 in a 41cM region around D12S83 with a locus-specific relative risk to siblings of 2.0[61]. Promising positional candidate genes in the vicinity of tested markers include the genes encoding interferon γ, vitamin D receptor and integrin β7. This localization was further confirmed by two independent groups in Caucasian populations[62,63]. Several other groups were, however, unable to detect any linkage in family sets of comparable size (unpublished data). Several hypotheses may account for this discrepancy. First, the chromosome 12 locus may be more frequently involved in, or more penetrant for, UC than for CD. Second the sets of families may be heterogeneous so that linkage would not be detected in every series. The interaction between chromosomes 12 and 16 loci is not known and additional work is now necessary to understand if these genes act independently (genetic heterogeneity) or in interaction.

Other loci and future developments

In a UK data set of non-Jewish European Caucasians with UC, the sharing of alleles among affected sibling pairs provided strong evidence for linkage with DRB1 locus contrasting with the weakness of the overall associations noted[7]. However, negative results were subsequently reported in UC[64,65]. In the study by Hugot *et al.*[50], the initial screen identified a possible CD locus close to D1S236 on chromosome1, but the linkage result for this marker was not significant in the second family panel. In the study from Oxford, two further regions on chromosome 3 and 7 were identified; these provide a locus-specific relative risk of 1.8 and 1.9 respectively[61]. A further region on chromosome 2 and a marker within the HLA region on chromosome 6 showed positive linkage to UC[61]. Although these observations have not been replicated, it is likely that other genes may participate to the genetic susceptibility to IBD and are not yet identified. The loci mapped on chromosomes 12 or 16 are not involved in all families. Furthermore, in a genome-wide search, the high statistic threshold required for conclusion may contribute to false-negative results. In these conditions it is expected that other susceptibility loci may exist and future genome-wide or candidate gene studies will probably provide additional new susceptibility genes. The localization of susceptibility genes is the first step of a positional cloning approach. The next challenge is now to reduce the length of the genetic regions that contain the relevant genes. Several teams are working on this topic and the next months will probably see different results on the fine mapping of IBD1 or chromosome 12 loci.

An additional question which needs to be solved in the near future is the hypothesis of genetic anticipation in familial IBD. Several series have shown that IBD is diagnosed earlier in life among offspring than in an affected parent. This has been interpreted as evidence for genetic anticipation by the Johns Hopkins group in Baltimore, MD[66]. The term anticipation denotes an increase in severity or decrease in the age at onset as a disease is passed through generations. It has been described in monogenic neurological illnesses such as Huntington's disease and myotonic dystrophy[67]. In these diseases there is a firm evidence that anticipation reflects effects of genetic factors and has a true molecular basis. Amplification of DNA-triplet repeats within or adjacent to the disease gene occurs in successive generations. This instability of DNA is associated with increasing disease severity and earlier age at onset[67]. In Friedreich's ataxia the number of GAA repeats within the *frataxin* gene is strongly correlated with age at onset and with the rate of disease progression, suggesting that the expansion itself is the cause of the disease[68]. The list of conditions exhibiting anticipation is growing rapidly, and recognizing anticipation would be very important for a proper understanding of inherited susceptibility in CD. Recently, CAG repeat expansions have been observed in a subset of families with CD[69]. However, these findings have not yet been reproduced. Epidemiological data for genetic anticipation are subject to many biases, and other explanations such as an environmental cohort effect have been proposed for the age difference at diagnosis between parents and children[70,71]. Furthermore a recent study in a US population only found evidence for anticipation in Jewish families with CD, which further suggests genetic heterogeneity[72].

CONCLUSION

The candidate gene approach and genome-wide scanning are two complementary methods to discover the genes involved in the development of IBD. The number of candidate genes tested in association studies is growing rapidly. However, most of the data have so far been inconsistent. This may be due to methodological problems inherent to the case–control approach in heterogeneous populations. Recent studies suggest that the power of candidate gene studies is increased when disease heterogeneity is taken into account. Stratification of homogeneous subgroups of patients could first rely upon precise phenotypic characterization and potentially upon serological markers[41]. The results of the different genome searches in IBD, and CD in particular, are encouraging. Expansion of the data sets and methodological improvements in linkage analysis and association method with use of affected persons and their parents (transmission disequilibrium) may lead to definitive results in the future. Above all, the chance for future progress in identifying IBD-susceptibility genes is critically dependent on collaboration between groups.

Acknowledgements

This work was supported partly by the Association F. Aupetit, the Ministère de la Santé et de l'Action Humanitaire (Direction Générale de la Santé), INSERM (Grant 4T004C), CH et U de Lille, and the companies Ferring and Astra.

References

1. Parkes M, Satsangi J, Jewell DP. Mapping susceptibility loci in inflammatory bowel disease: why and how? Mol Med Today. 1997;3:546–53.
2. Hayward P, Satsangi J, Jewell DP. Inflammatory bowel disease and the X chromosome. Q J Med. 1996;89:713–18.
3. Elson CO, Sartor RB, Tennyson G, Riddell R. Experimental models of inflammatory bowel disease. Gastroenterology. 1995;109:1344–67.
4. Futami S, Aoyama N, Honsako Y et al. HLA-DRB1*1502 allele, subtype of DR15, is associated with susceptibility to ulcerative colitis and its progression. Dig Dis Sci. 1995;40:814–18.
5. Toyoda H, Wang SJ, Yang HY et al. Distinct associations of HLA class II genes with inflammatory bowel disease. Gastroenterology. 1993;104:741–8.
6. Duerr RH, Neigut DA. Molecularly defined HLA-DR2 alleles in ulcerative colitis and an antineutrophil cytoplasmic antibody-positive subgroup. Gastroenterology. 1995;108:423–7.
7. Satsangi J, Welsh KI, Bunce et al. Contribution of genes of the major histocompatibility complex to susceptibility and disease phenotype in inflammatory bowel disease. Lancet. 1996;347:1212–17.
8. Roussosmoustakaki M, Satsangi J, Welsh K et al. Genetic markers may predict disease behavior in patients with ulcerative colitis. Gastroenterology. 1997;112:1845–53.
9. Forcione DG, Sands B, Isselbacher KJ, Rutsgi A, Podolsky D, Pillai S. An increased risk of Crohn's disease in individuals who inherit the HLA class II DRB3*0301 allele. Proc Natl Acad Sci USA. 1996;93:5094–8.
10. Danzé PM, Colombel JF, Jacquot S et al. Association of HLA class II genes with susceptibility to Crohn's disease. Gut. 1996;38:69–72.
11. Reinshagen M, Loeliger C, Kuehnl P et al. HLA class II gene frequencies in Crohn's disease: a population based analysis in Germany. Gut. 1996;38:538–42.
12. Schmitt Egolnolf M, Boehncke WII, Ständer M, Biermann TII, Sterry W. Oligonucleotide typing reveals association of type I psoriasis with the HLA-DRB1*0701/2, -DQA1*0201, DQB1*0303 extended haplotype. J Invest Dermatol. 1993;100:749–52.

13. Hughes S, Wiliams SE, Turnberg LA. Crohn's disease and psoriasis. N Engl J Med. 1983;308:101.

14. Bouma G, Poen AC, Garcia-Gonzalez MA *et al.* HLA-DRB1*03, but not the TNFα-308 promoter gene polymorphism confers protection against fistulising Crohn's disease. Immunogenetics. 1998 (In press).

15. Heresbach D, Colombel JF, Danzé PM, Semana G. The HLADRB1*03016DQB1*0201 haplotype confers protection against inflammatory bowel disease. Am J Gastroenterol. 1996;5:1060.

16 Stack WA, Mann SD, Roy AJ *et al.* Randomised controlled trial of CDP 571 antibody to tumour necrosis factor-α in Crohn's disease. Lancet. 1997;349:521–4.

17. Targan SR, Hanauer SB, Van Deventer SJH *et al.* A short term study of chimeric monoclonal antibody cA2 to tumor necrosis factor-α for Crohn's disease. N Engl J Med. 1997;337:1029–35.

18. Plevy SE, Targan SR, Yang H, Fernandez D, Rotter JI, Toyoda H. Tumor necrosis factor microsatellites define a Crohn's disease-associated haplotype on chromosome 6. Gastroenterology. 1996;110:1053–60.

19. Bouma G, Xia B, Crusius JBA *et al.* Distribution of four polymorphisms in the tumour necrosis factor (TNF) genes in patients with inflammatory bowel disease (IBD). Clin Exp Immunol. 1996;103:391–6.

20. Louis E, Satsangi J, Rousosmoustakaki M *et al.* Cytokine gene polymorphisms in inflammatory bowel disease. Gut. 1996;39:705–10.

21. Heresbach D, Ababou A, Bourienne A *et al.* Etude du polymorphisme des microsatellites et des gènes du tumor necrosis factor (TNF) au cours des maladies inflammatoires chroniques de l'intestin. Gastroenterol Clin Biol. 1997;21:555–61.

22. Bouma G, Crusius JBA, Odkerk Pool M *et al.* Secretion of tumor necrosis factor α and lymphotoxin α in relation to polymorphism in the TNF genes and HLA-DR alleles. Relevance for inflammatory bowel disease. Scand J Immunol. 1996;43:456–63.

23. Plevy SE, Taylor K, DeWoody KL, Schaible TF, Shealy D, Targan SR. Tumor necrosis factor (TNF) microsatellite haplotypes and perinuclear anti-neutrophil cytoplasmic antibody (pANCA) identify Crohn's disease (CD) patients with poor clinical response to anti-TNF monoclonal antibody. Gastroenterology. 1997;112:1062A.

24. Cominelli F, Pizarro TT. Interleukin-1 and interleukin-1 receptor antagonist in inflammatory bowel disease. Aliment Pharmacol Ther. 1996;10:(Suppl. 2):49–53.

25. Nishiyama T, Misuyama K, Toyonaga A, Sasaki E, Tanikawa K. Colonic mucosal interleukin 1 receptor antagonist in inflammatory bowel disease. Digestion. 1994;55:368–73.

26. Casini-Raggi V, Kam L, Chong YJ, Fiocchi C, Pizarro TT, Cominelli F. Mucosal imbalance of IL-1 and IL-1 receptor antagonist in inflammatory bowel disease. J Immunol. 1995;154:2434–40.

27. Andus T, Daig R, Vogl D *et al.* Imbalance of the interleukin 1 system in colonic mucosa – association with intestinal inflammation and interleukin 1 receptor agonist genotype 2. Gut 1997;41:651–7.

28. Mansfield JC, Holden H, Tarlow JK *et al.* Novel genetic association between ulcerative colitis and the anti-inflammatory cytokine interleukin-1 receptor antagonist. Gastroenterology. 1994;106:637–42.

29. Duerr RH, Tran T. Association between ulcerative colitis and a polymorphism intron 2 of the interleukin-1 receptor antagonist. Gastroenterology. 1995;108:A812.

30. Tountas NA, Yang H, Coulter DI, Rotter JI. Increased carriage of allele 2 of IL-1 receptor antagonist (IL-1ra) in Jewish populations: the strongest known genetic association in ulcerative colitis. Gastroenterology. 1996;110:A1029.

31. Bioque G, Crusius JBA, Koutroubakis I *et al.* Allelic polymorphism in IL-1β and IL-1 receptor antagonist (IL-1Ra) genes in inflammatory bowel disease. Clin Exp Immunol. 1995;102:379–83.

32. Heresbach D, Alizadeh M, Dabadie A *et al.* Significance of interleukin-1β and interleukin-1 receptor antagonist genetic polymorphism in inflammatory bowel diseases. Am J Gastroenterol. 1997;92:1164–9.

33. Pociot F, Molvig J, Wogensen L. A Taq 1 polymorphism in the human interleukin-1β (IL-1b) gene correlated with IL-1b secretion *in vitro*. Eur J Clin Invest. 1992;22:396–402.

34. Yacyshyn B, Woloschuk B, Yacyshyn MB *et al.* Efficacy and safety of ISIS 2302 (ICAM-1 antisense oligonucleotide) treatment of steroid-dependent Crohn's disease. Gastroenterology. 1997;112:1123A.

35. Yang H, Vora DK, Targan SR, Toyoda H, Beaudet AL, Rotter JI. Intercellular adhesion molecule 1 gene associations with immunologic subsets of inflammatory bowel disease. Gastroenterology. 1995;109:440–8.

36. Heresbach D, Alizadeh M, Bretagne JF *et al.* TAP gene transporter polymorphism in inflammatory bowel disease. Scand J Gastroenterol. 1997;32:1022–7.

37. Pokorny RM, Hofmeister A, Galandiuk S, Dietz AB, Cohen ND, Neibergs HL. Crohn's disease and ulcerative colitis are associated with the DNA repair gene *MLH1*. Ann Surg. 1997;6:718–25.

38. Cristofaro G, Lynch HT, Caruso ML *et al.* New phenotypic aspects in a family with Lynch syndrome II. Cancer. 1987;60:51–8.

39. Caruso ML, Cristofaro G, Lynch HT. HNPCC-Lynch syndrome and idiopathic inflammatory disease. A hypothesis on sharing of genes. Anticancer Res. 1997;17:2647–50.

40. Sandborn WJ. Inflammatory bowel disease and hereditary nonpolyposis colorectal cancer: is there a genetic link? Gastroenterology. 1998;114:608–9.

41. Coche JC, Colombel JF. Heterogeneity of inflammatory bowel disease: clinical subgroups of patients. Research and Clinical Forums. IBD and Salicylates-3 1997;20:136–45.

42. Vasiliauskas EA, Plevy SE, Landers CJ *et al.* Perinuclear antineutrophil cytoplasmic antibodies in patients with Crohn's disease define a clinical subgroup. Gastroenterology. 1996;110:1810–19.

43. Jamar-Leclerc N, Reumaux D, Duthilleul P, Colombel JF. Do pANCA define a clinical subgroup in patients with Crohn's disease? Gastroenterology. 1997;112:316.

44. Shanahan F, Duerr RH, Rotter JI *et al.* Neutrophil autoantibodies in ulcerative colitis: familial aggregation and genetic heterogeneity. Gastroenterology. 1992;103:456–61.

45. Reumaux D, Delecourt L, Colombel JF, Noël LH, Duthilleul P, Cortot A. Anti-neutrophil cytoplasmic autoantibodies in relatives of patients with ulcerative colitis (letter). Gastroenterology. 1992;103:1706.

46. Satsangi J, Landers CJ, Welsh KI, Koss K, Targan SR, Jewell DP. The presence of antineutrophil antibodies reflects clinical and genetic heterogeneity within inflammatory bowel disease. Inflam Bowel Dis. 1998;4:18–26.

47. Quinton JF, Sendid B, Reumaux D *et al.* Anti-*Saccharomyces cerevisiae* mannan combined with antineutrophil antibodies in inflammatory bowel disease: prevalence and diagnostic role. Gut. 1998 (In press).

48. Sendid B, Quinton JF, Charrier G *et al.* Anti-*Saccharomyces cerevisiae* mannan antibodies (ASCA) in familial Crohn's disease. Am J Gastroenterol. 1998 (In press).

49. Vasiliauskas EA, Plevy SE, Targan SR. Stratification of Crohn's disease by antineutrophil cytoplasmic antibodies (ANCA) and anti-*Saccharomyces cerevisiae* antibody (ASCA) distinguishes phenotypic subgroups. Gastroenterology. 1997;112:1112A.

50. Hugot JP, Laurent-Puig P, Gower-Rousseau C *et al.* Mapping of a susceptibility locus for Crohn's disease on chromosome 16. Nature. 1996;379:821–3.

51. Ohmen JD, Yang HY, Yamamoto KK *et al.* Susceptibility locus for inflammatory bowel disease on chromosome 16 has a role in Crohn's disease, but not in ulcerative colitis. Hum Mol Genet. 1996;5:1679–83.

52. Parkes M, Satsangi J, Lathrop GM, Bell JI, Jewell DP. Susceptibility loci in inflammatory bowel disease. Lancet. 1996;348:1588.

53. Cho JH, Fu Y, Kirshner BS, Hanauer SB. Confirmation of a susceptibility locus for Crohn's disease on chromosome 16. Inflam Bowel Dis. 1997;3:186–90.

54. Cavanaugh J, Wilson S, Srami M *et al.* Affected sib-pair analysis of pericentromeric chromosome 16 markers in inflammatory bowel disease families. Gastroenterology. 1997;112:A946.

55. Hugot JP, Zouali H, Colombel JF *et al.* Fine mapping of the inflammatory bowel disease susceptibility locus 1 (IBD1) in the pericentromeric region of chromosome 16. Gastroenterology. 1998 (In press) (abstract).

56. Schreiber S, Heinig T, Panzer U *et al.* Impaired response of activated mononuclear phagocytes to interleukin 4 in inflammatory bowel disease. Gastroenterology. 1995;108:21–3.

57. Desreumaux P, Brandt E, Gambiez L *et al.* Distinct cytokine patterns in early and chronic ileal lesions of Chron's disease. Gastroenterology. 1997;113:118–26.

58. Buisine MP, Desreumaux P, Janin A *et al.* Complexity of mucin gene expression in Crohn's disease. Primary mucosal defect of MUC3 and MUC4 gene expression in Crohn's disease (Submitted).

59. Rudolph U, Finegold MJ, Rich SS *et al.* Ulcerative colitis and adenocarcinoma of the colon in Gαi2-deficient mice. Nature Genet. 1995;10:143–9.

60. Mirza MM, Lee J, Teare D *et al.* Evidence of linkage of the inflammatory bowel disease susceptibility locus on chromosome 16 (IBD1) to ulcerative colitis. J Med Genet. 1998;35:218–21.
61. Satsangi J, Parkes M, Louis E *et al.* Two stage genome wide search in inflammatory bowel disease provides evidence for susceptibility loci on chromosome 3, 7 and 12. Nature Genet. 1996;14:199–202.
62. Hampe J, Stokkers P, Nürnberg P *et al.* Linkage to a susceptibility region on chromosome 12 but not 16 in the north central European family sample by multipoint non-parametric linkage analysis. Gastroenterology. 1997;112:A990.
63. Duerr RH, Zhang L, Preston RA *et al.* Further evidence for an inflammatory bowel disease susceptibility locus on chromosome 12. Gastroenterology. 1997;112:A963.
64. Naom I, Lee J, Ford D *et al.* Analysis of the contribution of HLA genes to genetic predisposition in inflammatory bowel disease. Am J Hum Genet. 1996;59:226–33.
65. Mathew C, Easton D, Lennard-Jones J. HLA and inflammatory bowel disease. Lancet. 1996;348:68.
66. Polito II JM, Rees RC, Childs B, Mendeloff AI, Harris ML, Bayless TM. Preliminary evidence for genetic anticipation in Crohn's disease. Lancet. 1996;347:798–800.
67. McInnis MG. Anticipation: an old idea in new genes. Am J Hum Genet. 1996;59:973–9.
68. Dürr A, Cossee M, Agid Y *et al.* Clinical and genetic abnormalities in patients with Friedreich's ataxia. N Engl J Med. 1996;335:1169–75.
69. Cho JH, Fu Y, Pickles M, Kirschner B, Hanauer SB. CAG repeat expansion in subsets of families with Crohn's disease. Gastroenterology. 1997;112:948A.
70. Grandbastien B, Peeters M, Franchimont D *et al.* Anticipation in familial Crohn's disease. Gut. 1998;42:170–4.
71. Hugot JP, Colombel JF, Bélaïche J *et al.* Date of birth in familial Crohn's disease suggests environmental factors. Gastroenterology. 1998 (In press) (abstract).
72. Akolkar D, Heresbach D, Lesser M *et al.* Anticipation in Crohn's disease may be influenced by ethnicity of the transmitting parent. Gastroenterology. 1998 (In press).

2
Epidemiological aspects of IBD

A. EKBOM

Ulcerative colitis and Crohn's disease are diseases of the 20th century. They are, however, not entirely new entities. In the case of ulcerative colitis quite a few case-reports were presented in Great Britain as early as the 19th century. In 1909 a symposium took place at the Royal Society of Medicine in London, at which 317 cases from London hospitals were presented[1]. In 1932 Dr Burrill B. Crohn introduced the term 'regional ileitis' for the disease which was later named after him[2]. There were, however, earlier reports. In 1913 Kennedy Dalziel reported nine patients with a new entity described as 'chronic intestinal enteritis and not tuberculosis'[1]. Furthermore, in a retrospective study from Ireland, 29 cases of Crohn's disease were identified in the latter half of the 19th century[3].

No estimates exist of the annual incidence of ulcerative colitis or Crohn's disease until the 1930s. For ulcerative colitis, the average annual incidence rate per 10^5 for the period 1934 44 was estimated at 6.0 in Rochester, Minnesota[4]. For Crohn's disease there are two early studies: one from Olmsted County, Minnesota, in which the mean annual incidence per 10^5 for the period 1935–54 was 1.9[5] and one from Cardiff, United Kingdom, with an average annual incidence rate of 0.2 during the period 1935–45[6].

Since the 1960s there has been an increasing number of incidence studies of inflammatory bowel disease (IBD) published in an abundance of different journals. Those studies have often dealt with small populations or emanated from referral centres without a defined study base. Only a few studies have had a time-span exceeding 10 years and thus do not only provide cross-sectional data. Moreover, the estimates of incidence in different studies are often not comparable due to different methods in case ascertainment; some studies using only hospitalized patients; and the fact that, in many instances, the incidence figures have not been age-standardized. However, it is obvious from the studies with long duration and a consistent method of case ascertainment over time that there has been an increase in the annual incidence of both ulcerative colitis and Crohn's disease in western Europe and northern America since the Second World War[7–12]. There is also a strong correlation in incidence between ulcerative colitis and Crohn's disease. Areas or populations with a high incidence of mortality attributed to ulcerative colitis also have a high incidence of mortality rate attributed to Crohn's disease and vice-versa[13]. Although misclassification could be an issue (that is that in some instances Crohn's disease is misclassified as ulcerative colitis and vice-versa) it is unlikely that this could be the sole explanation for this correlation. Another interesting feature is the fact that in populations or areas where information exists about the temporal trends for the two diseases it is obvious that an increase in the incidence in ulcerative colitis precedes an increase in Crohn's disease. There also seems to be an almost consistent time lag of about 15–20 years between the shifts from low to high incidence areas in the two diseases[9,14–20]. The incidence of Crohn's disease in high-incidence areas seems to be levelling off at a rate of between 5 and 7 per 10^5 and per year[7,9] as opposed to ulcerative colitis in which recent studies, especially from Scandinavia, have shown a very high annual incidence of more than 20 per 10^5 and per year[21]. There are also some indications that this increase in ulcerative colitis is due to an increased frequency of patients with either ulcerative proctitis or distal colitis and the incidence of pancolitis has a pattern very similar to that of Crohn's disease[9].

Two separate Swedish studies have also found a birth cohort phenomenon for Crohn's disease showing that those born in the years immediately after the Second World War seem to have an especially high life-time risk for Crohn's disease[9,10]. However, studies from other centres, both in Scandinavia and elsewhere, have not been able to reproduce these results[6,7]. Another interesting feature with regard to descriptive epidemiology is that in low-incidence areas, high socioeconomic status seems to be associated with an increased risk with both ulcerative colitis and Crohn's disease[22], an association which is not present in high-incidence areas[23,24]. In high-incidence areas there is also an increased proportion of Crohn's colitis in patients with Crohn's disease and a decreased proportion of extensive colitis in patients with ulcerative colitis[9]. Moreover, there is also a male predominance in ulcerative colitis[8,9] and a female predominance in Crohn's disease[7,9] in high-incidence areas. Mortality data for Crohn's disease, as opposed to morbidity data, have also shown a similar gradient, with a male predominance in countries with low mortality rates for Crohn's disease and a female predominance in countries with high mortality rates[13].

The age-specific incidence rates for the two diseases vary substantially in different studies. However, in populations with high annual incidence rates the most prominent peak is in the age group 20–40 years, and in studies with low annual incidence rates the age-specific curves are flatter[7–9]. In periods of rising annual incidence rates the growth is mostly due to an increase in the age group 20–40 years[14,17,25]. There is a genetic component for both diseases and the two diseases are genetically linked. A family history of Crohn's disease is associated with both an increased risk of Crohn's disease and ulcerative colitis and vice-versa[26]. This genetic component has been used in order to explain the presumed increased susceptibility for IBD for those with a Jewish background. In Crohn's original description all 14 patients were Jewish[2] and an increased risk of ulcerative colitis among Jews was also reported in the 1950s from the Mayo Clinic[27] and additional studies in the 1950s and 1960s seem to give further credence to this hypothesis[28,29]. However, recent studies which have reported a positive association have some serious methodological flaws. The two Swedish studies[25,30] which have reported this association have in common that cases, the nominator, were defined by the investigators, and the population at risk were defined by other means, and without ensuring that the nominator and denominator emanated from the same study base. There are reasons to believe that the numbers in the nominators in both studies are exaggerated, thus giving a false-positive association. Similarly, in a study from South Africa[31] there was a lack of a denominator, and the authors used historical data instead, which probably constituted an underestimation of the persons at risk, also leading to a false-positive association. Other studies which have shown a positive association in most instances had low statistical power, or were performed in time periods or populations with a low incidence of IBD and the results could thus be confounded by socioeconomic status. Further credence to this theory is given by the fact that incidence data from Israel do not differ substantially from other comparable areas.

Another observation which was made in the 1960s and 1970s was the presence of differences in the incidence within Europe and northern America[32,33], indicating the existence of a north–south gradient. In a major undertaking in order to test the existence of such a gradient, 20 European centres during a 2-year period identified patients with either ulcerative colitis or Crohn's disease prospectively, using a uniform diagnostic approach which included regional case reviews[34]. This approach enabled the investigators to analyse differences in the annual incidence in different populations. For ulcerative colitis the authors found a wide variation but without a really consistent pattern. For ulcerative colitis the highest annual incidence was found in Iceland and the lowest in Almada in southern Portugal. However, Heraklion in Greece had one of the highest incidences. For Crohn's disease the highest incidence was reported from Maastricht in the Netherlands as well as Amiens in the northwest of France, and the lowest in Joannina in the northwest of Greece. There was no geographical gradient for Crohn's disease but a weak positive association was present for ulcerative colitis. Adjustment for tobacco consumption as well as education level diminished the differences between the north and south only marginally.

The validity of the results from collaborative European studies was further strengthened by results published from the different participating centres. Especially in Italy there were five participating centres from Milan in the north to Palermo in the south[35-37] and no north–south gradient could be found within this region. Another interesting feature of that study was that one centre from Israel also participated, and the incidence figures did not differ from the rest of the participating centres for either Crohn's disease or ulcerative colitis. This further strengthens the hypothesis of an absence of a special susceptibility among those with a Jewish ethnicity. One probable interpretation of the results is that the southern parts of Europe during the past 10 years have had a similar increase in the incidence of IBD which was present in northern Europe, especially in the United Kingdom and Scandinavia, during the 1950s and 1960s. One can only speculate as to the underlying reason for these trends in the annual incidence, but a special susceptibility for IBD among those with either a Jewish or northern European background seems less likely today than 20 years ago. There are indications that the 'window of opportunity' which will establish the future risk of IBD occurs very early in life[24]. Factors such as decreased perinatal mortality, better hygiene in childhood, compulsory vaccination programmes, and delayed exposures to infections in childhood are in accordance with the temporal trends we can see in IBD in different populations over time.

In conclusion, IBD is a disease of the 20th century in which the incidence in high-incidence areas has reached a plateau, and its clinical characteristics such as age and extent at diagnosis are subject to changes over time.

References

1. Hawkins C. Historical review. In: Allan RN, Keighley MRB, Alexander-Williams J, Hawkins C, editors. Inflammatory Bowel Disease. New York: Churchill-Livingstone;1983:1–7.
2. Crohn BB, Ginzburg L, Oppenheimer GD. Regional ileitis. A pathological and clinical entity. J Am Med Assoc. 1932;99:1323–9.
3. Walker JF, Fielding JF. Crohn's disease in Dublin in the latter half of the nineteenth century. Ir J Med Sci. 1988;157:235–7.
4. Sedlack RE, Nobrega FT, Kurland LT, Sauer WG. Inflammatory colon disease in Rochester, Minnesota, 1935–1964. Gastroenterology. 1972;62:935–41.
5. Sedlack RE, Whisnant J, Elveback RI, Kurland LT. Incidence of Crohn's disease in Olmsted County, Minnesota, 1935–1975. Am J Epidemiol. 1980;112:759–63.
6. Rose JDR, Roberts GM, Williams G, Mayberry JF, Rhodes J. Cardiff Crohn's disease jubilee: the incidence over 50 years. Gut. 1988;29:346–51.
7. Gollop JH, Phillips SF, Melton III LJ, Zinsmeister AR. Epidemiologic aspects of Crohn's disease: a populations-based study in Olmsted County, Minnesota, 1943–1982. Gut. 1988;29:49–56.
8. Stonnington CM, Phillips SF, Melton III LJ, Zinsmeister AR. Chronic ulcerative colitis: incidence and prevalence in a community. Gut. 1987;28:402–9.
9. Ekbom A, Helmick C, Zack M, Adami HO. The epidemiology of inflammatory bowel disease: a large, population-based study in Sweden. Gastroenterology. 1991;100:350–8.
10. Lapidus A, Bernell O, Hellers G, Persson PG, Löfberg R. Incidence of Crohn's disease in Stockholm County 1955–1989. Gut. 1997;41:480–6.
11. Thomas GA, Millar-Jones D, Rhodes J, Roberts GM, Williams GT, Mayberry JF. Incidence of Crohn's disease in Cardiff over 60 years: 1986–1990 an update. Eur J Gastroenterol Hepatol. 1995;7:401–5.
12. Langholz E, Munkholm P, Nielsen OH, Kreiner S, Binder V. Incidence and prevalence of ulcerative colitis in Copenhagen County from 1962 to 1987. Scand J Gastroenterol. 1991;26:1247–56.
13. Sonnenberg A. Geographic and temporal variations of sugar and margarine consumption in relation to Crohn's disease. Digestion. 1988;41:161–71.
14. Bergman L, Krause U. The incidence of Crohn's disease in central Sweden. Scand J Gastroenterol. 1975;10:725–9.
15. Samuelsson SM. Ulcerös colit och proctit. Uppsala: Department of Social Medicine. Thesis, University of Uppsala, 1976.
16. Björnsson S. Inflammatory bowel disease in Iceland during a 30-year period, 1950–1979. Scand J Gastroenterol. 1989;24(Suppl. 170):47–9.
17. Binder V, Both H, Hansen PK, Hendriksen C, Kreiner S, Torp-Pedersen K. Incidence and prevalence of ulcerative colitis and Crohn's disease in the County of Copenhagen 1962–1978. Gastroenterology. 1982;83:563–8.
18. Munkholm P, Langholz E, Haagen Nielsen O, Kreiner S, Binder V. Incidence and prevalence of Crohn's disease in the County of Copenhagen 1962–87. Scand J Gastroenterol. 1992;27:609–14.
19. Berner J, Kiaer T. Ulcerative colitis and Crohn's disease on the Faroe Islands 1964–1983. Scand J Gastroenterol. 1986;21:188–92.
20. Roin F, Roin J. Inflammatory bowel disease of the Faroe Islands, 1981–1988. Scand J Gastroenterol. 1989;24(Suppl. 170):44–6.
21. Moum B, Vatn MH, Ekbom A et al. Incidence of Crohn's disease in four counties in south-eastern Norway 1990–1993. Scand J Gastroenterol. 1996;31:355–61.
22. Acheson ED, Nefzger MD. Ulcerative colitis in the United States Army in 1944. Epidemiology: comparisons between patients and controls. Gastroenterology. 1963;44:7–19.
23. Gilat T, Hacohen D, Lilos P, Langman MJS. Childhood factors in ulcerative colitis and Crohn's disease. Scand J Gastroenterol. 1987;22:1009–24.
24. Ekbom A, Adami HO, Helmick C, Jonzon A, Zack M. Perinatal risk factors for inflammatory bowel disease: a case–control study. Am J Epidemiol. 1990;132:1111–19.

25. Hellers G. Crohn's disease in Stockholm County, 1955–1974. Acta Chir Scand. 1979; 490(Suppl.):1–84.
26. Orholm M, Munkholm P, Langholz E, Haagen Nielsen O, Sörensen TIA, Binder V. Familial occurrence of inflammatory bowel disease. N Engl J Med. 1991;324:84–8.
27. Sloan WP, Bargen JA, Gage RP. Life histories of patients with chronic ulcerative colitis: a review of 2000 cases. Gastroenterology. 1950;1:25–38.
28. Acheson ED. The distribution of ulcerative colitis and regional enteritis in United States veterans with particular reference to the Jewish religion. Gut. 1960;1:291–3.
29. Monk M, Mendeloff AI, Siegel CI, Lilienfeld A. An epidemiological study of ulcerative colitis and regional enteritis among adults in Baltimore. Gastroenterology. 1967;53:198–210.
30. Brahme F, Lindström C, Wenckert A. Crohn's disease in a defined population. An epidemiological study of incidence, prevalence, mortality, and secular trends in the city of Malmö. Gastroenterology. 1975;69:342–51.
31. Wright JP, Froggatt J, O'Keefe EA et al. The epidemiology of inflammatory bowel disease in Cape Town 1980–1984. S Afr Med J. 1986;70:10–15.
32. Kyle J. Crohn's disease in the northeastern and northern Isles of Scotland: an epidemiological review. Gastroenterology. 1992;103:392–9.
33. Sonnenberg A, McCarty DJ, Jacobsen SJ. Geographic variation in inflammatory bowel disease within the United States. Gastroenterology. 1991;100:143–9.
34. Shivananda S, Lennard-Jones J, Logan R et al. and the EC–IBD Study Group. Incidence of inflammatory bowel disease across Europe: is there a difference between north and south? Results of the European collaborative study on inflammatory bowel disease (EC-IBD). Gut. 1996;39:690–7.
35. Trallori G, Palli D, Saieva C et al. A population-based study on inflammatory bowel disease in Florence over 15 years (1978–92). Scand J Gastroenterol. 1996;31:892–9.
36. Ranzi T, Bodini P, Zambelli A et al. Epidemiological aspects of inflammatory bowel disease in a north Italian population: a 4-year prospective study. Eur J Gastroenterol Hepatol. 1996;8:657–61.
37. Tragnone A, Corrao G, Miglio F, Caprilli R, Lafranchi GA. Incidence of inflammatory bowel disease in Italy: A nationwide population-based study. Int J Epidemiol. 1996;25:1044–52.

3
HLA-antigens in IBD

A. S. PEÑA

INTRODUCTION

The major histocompatibility complex (MHC), in man called the human leuko-cyte antigen (HLA) complex, is located on the short arm of chromosome 6. More than 100 different genes are located in this region, and many of them are highly polymorphic, in other words, there are several allelic variants of each gene. Genes of the major histocompatibility complex (MHC) are excellent can-didate genes to study the genetics of IBD because of the role HLA antigens play in the immune response and the strong associations that exist in other immune-mediated diseases. There have been several studies of HLA associations in IBD but the different studies have yielded conflicting results.

Several authors have observed an increased prevalence of HLA-DR2 (DRB1*15) in ulcerative colitis (UC), especially in the Japanese population[1-5]. No conclusive data on this association in European Caucasian patients exist. We have studied HLA associations in a small group of Dutch patients and found that the DRB1*15 allele is more frequent in UC patients[6]. Moreover, Satsangi *et al.* of the United Kingdom, using non-parametric linkage-analysis in UC in 29 affected sib pairs, reported linkage of UC to the HLA-DRB1 locus, suggesting that this region is of importance for susceptibility to UC. No association with the DRB1*15 allele was observed in their patients[7,8]. However, when an analysis was made of the subgroup of patients who underwent a panproctocolectomy[9], there was an association with HLA-DRB*15. These results could not be confirmed in another family study from London in 43 families with multiple affected cases of UC or Crohn's disease (CD). Linkage analysis taking into account different models of transmission and the transmission disequilibrium test also gave a very low relative risk for HLA genes[10]. These last authors had two theories to explain the discrepant results: one is that HLA accounts for only a small component of the susceptibility and the other that the selection of fami-lies was different. The group in Oxford studied mainly affected sibling pairs whereas the group in London studied families with three or more cases of UC. Therefore, it is possible that these families have more highly penetrant genes distinct from those in sibling pairs[11]. Another explanation could be differences in the patients selected, e.g. in disease severity and extension within both groups.

Fistulizing CD has been proposed as a separate subgroup of patients with CD.

In recent years, advances have been made in disease classification[13,14]. An awareness of the importance of the long-term follow up of patients in assessing the natural course of the disease has contributed to better analysis between HLA and IBD. In addition, studies using molecular genotyping in combination with allele-specific oligonucleotide hybridization by polymerase chain reactions have contributed to understanding the association of HLA alleles and disease. The importance of the study of individual alleles within the HLA-DRB1 group has already been demonstrated in rheumatoid arthritis[15], type I diabetes mellitus[16,17] and, more recently, also in autoimmune hepatitis[18], and this approach is being applied to the association found between HLA, ulcerative colitis and Crohn's disease.

HLA AND ULCERATIVE COLITIS

Several authors have observed an increased prevalence of HLA-DR2 (DRB1*15) in UC, especially in the Japanese population[1,19]. Masuda *et al.*[2] reported an association with extensive colitis and intractability. Up until recently, there were no conclusive data on this association in European Caucasian patients. We have studied HLA associations in a group of Dutch patients and found that the DRB1*15 allele was more frequent in UC patients but the association was even stronger in patients with pancolitis[6]. Recent studies in Madrid, Spain have also confirmed the HLA-DR2 association in UC. HLA-DR2 was found in 33 of 107 patients with UC (33.6%) vs. 49 (24.5%) of 200 controls. The difference just fails to reach significance. However, the subtype HLA-DRB1*15 does reach significance: 31.8% vs. 20.0%; $p = 0.02$; OR = 1.9 (CI 1.05–3.29). The most significant association in Spain was a negative association with HLA-DR3: 11.2% in the UC group vs. 26.5% in the controls; $p = 0.001$; OR 0.3 (0.17–0.72)[20,21].

HLA-DRB1* SUBTYPES IN UC

The first studies of UC were performed in Japan. In Japanese[1,22], Jewish[23] and Turkish[24] patients, UC is associated with the allele, HLA-DRB1*1502; in Holland[6], Spain[20] and North America[4], UC is associated with the allele, HLA-DRB1*1501. Table 1 shows the distribution of subtypes in different countries. In the Dutch population, DRB1*1501 is the most frequent allele, accounting for over 95% of the DRB1*15 alleles. In our patient population, the majority of DRB1*15-positive individuals had DRB1*1501, which makes it unlikely that DRB1*1502 is the susceptibility allele for UC.

There is some evidence that genes in the HLA region may play a role in the severity of inflammatory bowel diseases and the development of certain complications (e.g. granulomas, erythema nodosum, and course of disease). It has been noted that the association of HLA-DR2 with UC appears to be stronger in patients with extensive disease[2]. Similarly, in the Japanese data, HLA-DR2 was found in 64% of patients with pancolitis, 35% of patients with subtotal colitis and 30% of controls[19].

Table 1 HLA-DRB1 genes in different populations of patients with ulcerative colitis and in ethnically matched control populations

HLA-DRB1*	Country (Reference)	UC patients		Controls		p	OR
		n	%	n	%		
DR2 (*15&*16)	Spain[21,30]	36	33.6	49	24.5	NS	1.6
*15		34	31.8	40	20.0	0.02	1.9
*16		2	1.9	11	5.5	NS	0.3
*15	Holland[27]	15	26.0		41.0	0.001	2.0
*16		2	1		0.5	NS	0.5
DRB1*1501	Spain[21,30]		29.9		17.5		2.1
DRB1*1501	Turkey[24,31]		16.9		13.9		
DRB1*1502	Spain[21,30]		5.6		3.0		
DRB1*1502	Turkey[24,31]		16.9		6.6		2.9
DRB1*1501	Israel[23]		27.7				
DRB1*1502			55.5				
DRB1*16			16.8				
DRB1*1501	Japan[22,32,33]		39.5				
DRB1*1502			57.0				
DRB1*16			3.5				
DRB1*0103	Holland[27]		12.0		0.2	0.0002	27.6
DRB1*03	Spain[21,30]	12	11.2	53	26.5	0.001	NS
DRB1*03	Holland[27]	25	21.0		22.0	0.8	NS

Several studies found that the frequency of the allele HLA-DRB1*0103, which is extremely rare in the general population, is increased in patients with UC[9,25–27]. Both the HLA-DRB1*15 and the HLA-DRB1+0103 are associated with extensive disease, as can be seen in Figures 1 and 2, respectively. Apart from the increased prevalence of DRB1*15 and DRB1*0103, in some studies, it was observed that the DRB1*04 allele frequency is decreased in UC patients, suggesting that this allele may provide protection[1,4,25,28,29].

These results suggest that genes in the HLA region may contribute to the severity of the disease and therefore play a role in the prognosis. In this regard, the study of Sugimura et al. is of particular interest[1]. These authors have suggested that the association in Japanese patients between UC and HLA-DR2 (*1502) is due to the presence of the Aw24-Bw52-DRB1*1502-DPw9 haplotype. The relative risk with different alleles suggests a stronger association with the HLA-B locus. The alleles, HLA-Bw52, HLA-B13, and HLA-B44, occurred more frequently in Japanese UC patients not carrying this haplotype. These alleles share unique amino acids, serine and aspartic acid at positions 67 and 77, respectively, thus suggesting that the HLA-B locus itself plays an important role[1]. However, in Caucasians, such as the Dutch population, the HLA-DR2 allele is associated with a different HLA-B allele. Therefore, further studies are necessary to define the biological basis of the association between HLA-DR2 and UC.

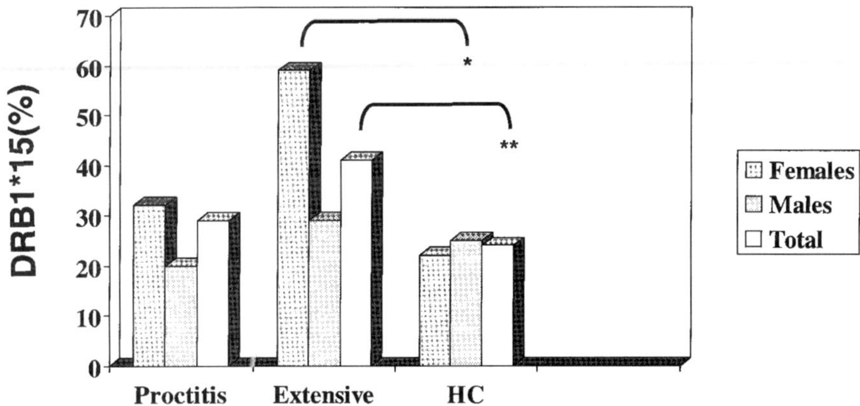

Figure 1   HLA-DRB1*15 frequency in relation to the extent of UC disease

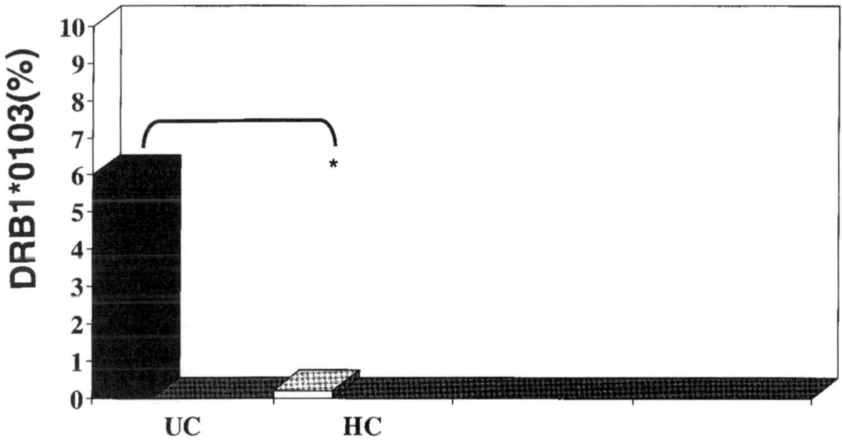

Figure 2   HLA-DRB*0103 frequency in UC patients and healthy controls (HC)

HLA AND CROHN'S DISEASE

The various forms in which Crohn's disease appears are so diverse that it has been hypothesized that CD might be a syndrome, with different pathogenic mechanisms leading to the various clinical phenotypes. This may offer a plausible explanation for the conflicting and inconclusive results with regard to HLA associations in these patients. In 95 CD patients in the United States, a positive association was found with the combination of DR1 and DQw5 alleles. The association was with the haplotype and not with either of the alleles individually.

The power of genetic-association studies may increase when disease heterogeneity is taken into account. It has been proposed that fistulizing CD occurs in a distinct subgroup of patients with CD. Our group in Amsterdam has recently studied the phenotype frequencies of the DRB1 alleles in 35 unrelated white Dutch CD patients with proven perianal fistulas. A strikingly lower incidence of the DRB1*03 allele was found in those patients with perianal fistulas when compared with 2400 healthy controls (HC) (3% vs. 25%; $p = 0.005$; OR $= 0.09$). The DRB1*03 allele is in strong linkage disequilibrium with a polymorphism at position -308 in the promoter region of the TNF-α gene (TNFA-308*2). We investigated whether the incidence of this allele was decreased as well. Surprisingly, the PF of TNFA-308*2 was 29%, not different from the PF of 98 HC (34%; $p = 0.7$; OR $= 0.8$)[12]. This is the first study showing a significant negative association between DRB1*03 and a particular subgroup of CD patients. Thus, patient selection may largely determine the outcome of genetic association studies in CD, as we observed no association with this allele in an unselected population of CD patients.

References

1. Sugimura K, Asakura H, Mizuki M, *et al.* Analysis of genes within the HLA region affecting susceptibility to ulcerative colitis. Hum Immunol. 1993;36:112–18.
2. Masuda H, Nakamura Y, Tanaka T, Hayakawa S. Distinct relationship between HLA-DR genes and intractability of ulcerative colitis. Am J Gastroenterol. 1994;89:1957–62.
3. Futami S, Aoyama N, Honsako Y, *et al.* HLA-DRB1 * 1502 allele, subtype of DR15, is associated with susceptibility to ulcerative colitis and its progression. Dig Dis Sci. 1995;40:814–18.
4. Toyoda H, Wang SJ, Yang HY, *et al.* Distinct associations of HLA class II genes with inflammatory bowel disease. Gastroenterology. 1993;104:741–8.
5. Caruso C, Palmeri P, Oliva L, Orlando A, Cottone M. HLA antigens in ulcerative colitis; a study in the Sicilian population. Tissue Antigens. 1985;25:47–9.
6. Bouma G, Oudkerk Pool M, Crusius JBA, *et al.* Evidence for genetic heterogeneity in inflammatory bowel disease (IBD); HLA genes in the predisposition to suffer from ulcerative colitis (UC) and Crohn's disease (CD). Clin Exp Immunol. 1997;109(1):175–9.
7. Satsangi J, Welsh KI, Bunce M, *et al.* Contribution of genes of the major histocompatibility complex to susceptibility and disease phenotype in inflammatory bowel disease. Lancet. 1996;347:1212–17.
8. Satsangi J, Parkes M, Jewell DP. Genetics of ulcerative colitis. Lancet. 1996;348:624–5.
9. Roussomoustakaki M, Satsangi J, Welsh K, *et al.* Genetic markers may predict disease behavior in patients with ulcerative colitis. Gastroenterology. 1997;112:1845–63.
10. Naom I, Lee J, Ford D, *et al.* Analysis of the contribution of HLA genes to genetic predisposition in inflammatory bowel disease. Am J Hum Genet. 1996;59:226–33.
11. Mathew CG, Easton DF, Lennard-Jones JE. HLA and inflammatory bowel disease. Lancet. 1996;348:68.
12. Bouma G, Poen AC, García-González MA, *et al.* HLA-DR3, but not the TNFalpha −308 promoter gene polymorphism confers protection against fistulising Crohn's disease. Immunogenetics. 1998;47:451–5.
13. Lennard-Jones JE. Classification of inflammatory bowel disease. Scand J Gastroenterol. 1989;24(Suppl. 170):2–6.
14. Sachar DB, Andrews HA, Farmer RG, *et al.* Proposed classification of patients subgroups in Crohn's disease. Working team report. Gastroenterol Int. 1992;5:141–54.
15. Winchester R. The molecular basis of susceptibility to rheumatoid arthritis. Adv Immunol. 1994;56:389.
16. She J-X. Susceptibility to type I diabetes: HLA-DQ and DR revisited. Immunol Today. 1996;17:323.
17. Kong YC, Lomo LC, Motte RW, *et al.* HLA-DRB1 polymorphism determines susceptibility to autoimmune thyroiditis in transgenic mice: definitive association to autoimmune thyroiditis in

transgenic mice: definitive association with HLA-DRB1*0301(DR3) gene. J Exp Med. 1996;184:1167.

18. Stretell MDJ, Donalson PT, Thomson LJ, *et al*. Allelic basis for HLA-encoded susceptibility to type 1 autoimmune hepatitis. Gastroenterology. 1997;112:2028.

19. Asakura H, Tsuchiya M, Aiso S, *et al*. Association of the human lymphocyte DR2 antigen with Japanese ulcerative colitis. Gastroenterology. 1982;82:413–18.

20. De la Concha EG, Fernandez-Arquero M, Santa-Cruz S, *et al*. Positive and negative associations of distinct HLA-DR2 subtypes with ulcerative colitis (UC). Clin Exp Immunol. 1997;108:392–5.

21. Fernández-Arquero M, López-Nava G, De la Concha EG, *et al*. HLA-DR2 gene and Spanish patients with ulcerative colitis [see comments]. Rev Esp Enf Digest. 1988;90:243–9.

22. Hashimoto M, Kinoshita T, Yamasaki M, *et al*. Gene frequencies and haplotypic associations within the HLA region in 916 unrelated Japanese individuals. Tissue Antigens. 1994;44(3):166–73.

23. Roitberg-Tambur A, Friedmann A, Korn S, *et al*. Serologic and molecular analysis of the HLA system in Israeli Jewish patients with oral erosive lichen planus. Tissue Antigens. 1994;43(4):219–23.

24. Uyar A, Imeryuz N, Direskereli-Saruhan G, *et al*. The distribution of HLA-DRB alleles in ulcerative colitis patients in Turkey [In Process Citation]. Eur J Immunogenet. 1998;25:293–6.

25. Satsangi J, Welsh KI, Bunce M, *et al*. Contribution of genes of the major histocompatibility complex to susceptibility and disease phenotype in inflammatory bowel disease. Lancet. 1996;347(9010):1212–17.

26. Duerr RH, Chensny LJ. Associations between HLA-DR alleles and subsets of ulcerative colitis defined by extent of colitis. Gastroenterology. 1997;112(4):A963.

27. Bouma G, Crusius JBA, García-González MA, *et al*. Genetic markers in clinically well defined patients with ulcerative colitis. Clin Exp Immunol. 1999;115:(in press).

28. Kobayashi K, Atoh M, Yagita A, *et al*. Crohn's disease in the Japanese is associated with the HLA-DRw53. Exp Clin Immunogenet. 1990;7:101–8.

29. Leidenius MH, Koskimies SA, Kellokumpu IH, Hockerstedt KA. HLA antigens in ulcerative colitis and primary sclerosing cholangitis. APMIS. 1995;103(7–8):519–24.

30. De la Concha EG, Arroyo R, Crusius JBA, *et al*. Combined effect of HLA-DRB1*1501 and interleukin-1 receptor antagonist gene allele 2 in susceptibility to relapsing/remitting multiple sclerosis. J Neuroimmunol. 1997:80:172–8.

31. Saruhan-Direskeneli G, Esin S, Baykan-Kurt B, Ornek I, Vaughan R, Eraksoy M. HLA-DR and -DQ associations with multiple sclerosis in Turkey. Hum Immunol. 1997;55(1):59–65.

32. Hiwatashi N, Kikuchi T, Masamune O, Ouchi E, Watanabe H, Goto Y. HLA antigens in inflammatory bowel disease. Tohoku J Exp Med. 1980;131(4):381–5.

33. Kobayashi K, Atoh M, Konoeda Y, Yagita A, Inoko H, Sekiguchi S. HLA-DR, DQ and T cell antigen receptor constant beta genes in Japanese patients with ulcerative colitis. Clin Exp Immunol. 1990;80:400–3.

4
Autoantibodies in IBD

F. SEIBOLD and M. SCHEURLEN

INTRODUCTION

The first autoantibodies in inflammatory bowel disease (IBD) were described by Broberger and Perlmann in 1959[1]. Since then a variety of antibodies in IBD have been found. The early autoantibody research in IBD was predominantly focused on a possible significance of autoantibodies in the pathogenesis of IBD, but since then no antibodies have been proven to be of pathogenetic relevance in these diseases. Recently, the question arose as to whether autoantibodies in IBD can be used as diagnostic tools to differentiate between ulcerative colitis (UC) and Crohn's disease (CD), or to define subgroups of these diseases. Some of the autoantibodies may be useful as genetic markers.

The most important autoantibodies are summarized in Table 1. In this chapter we focus on antineutrophil antibodies (pANCA), antibodies to *Saccharomyces cerevisiae cerevisiae* (ASCCA) and antibodies to pancreatic secretions (PAB).

Table 1 Autoantibodies in IBD: an overview

Antigen/antibodies	*Specificity*	*Ref.*
Lymphocytotoxic antibodies	CD	26
Epithelial cell-associated macromolecules	CD/UC	27
Pancreas (PAB)	CD	19
AEA 15	CD	31
ASCCA	CD	23, 24
Colon extract	UC	1, 14
Goblet cells	UC	18, 19
40 kDa protein	UC	22
Neutrophils (pANCA)	UC, PSC (subgroup CD?)	2, 3

ANTIBODIES TO NEUTROPHILS (pANCA)

Perinuclear antineutrophil cytoplasmic antibodies (pANCA) have been extensively studied because of their high prevalence in patients with UC[2,3]. The typical staining pattern of pANCA is characterized by a perinuclear fluorescence on cytospin slides of neutrophils. According to data from our group, the prevalence of pANCA in patients with UC is about 70% if titres higher than 1:10 are considered. This is in contrast to patients with CD, which are positive for pANCA in only 6% of cases. In primary sclerosing cholangitis (PSC), however, pANCA are found in high frequencies, whereas all healthy controls are pANCA-negative. In other studies the frequency of pANCA varied between 23% and 88% in UC, and between 0% and 43% in CD. This variability may be due to differences in the genetic background of the populations studied. Furthermore, methodological differences are of major importance and will continue to cause apparent variations in frequencies and titres unless the specific pANCA antigen is discovered. Many isolated neutrophil antigens have been tested for their reactivity with pANCA. Antigens such as myeloperoxidase, elastase, cathepsins C and G, glucosidase, galactosidase, lactoferrin, bactericidal permeability increasing protein (BPI), histone and others were tested, but none was proven to be the exclusive pANCA antigen[4,5].

Recently, pANCA were found in colitic mouse models such as IL-10–/– mice and T-cell receptor alpha (TCR-α)-deficient mice[6,7]. Absorption of either human or mouse pANCA-positive sera with enteric bacterial antigens greatly reduced or abolished the specific perinuclear staining of pANCA. Thus pANCA probably represent a cross-reactivity with enteric bacterial antigens[6].

The significance of antibodies is defined by the specificity and sensitivity of an antibody. Additionally it is of relevance whether an antibody defines a clinical subgroup of patients. We found no correlation of pANCA with disease activity, or extension; however, pANCA tends to occur more often in UC patients with a more severe course of disease. For example, we found four patients with severe colitis refractory to medical treatment, all of whom had high pANCA titres (> 1/100). All four patients later required colectomy[3].

Another study showed that pANCA occur more frequently in UC patients who later develop pouchitis after colectomy[8]. We have demonstrated that pANCA persist after colectomy or liver transplantation in primary sclerosing cholangitis (PSC) patients with constantly elevated titres for more than 3 years[3]. This is an important clue showing that pANCA are not only an epiphenomenon secondary to damage of the bowel or liver.

In CD, pANCA are less frequently found, but it seems that pANCA define a subgroup of patients with CD and left-sided colitis. All patients with CD who expressed pANCA had UC-like features[9].

To obtain further evidence of whether pANCA play a role as a genetic marker, family studies have been performed[10,11]. In our study, 43 patients with UC and their 142 first-degree relatives, 11 patients with PSC and their 40 relatives, 11 patients with CD and their 33 relatives and healthy controls were included. In 30% of the total relatives of patients with UC, pANCA were detectable. In a French and an English study, however, pANCA were not detected in sera of the relatives of patients with UC[12,13]. Technical or genetic differences could explain this difference. We found 35% of pANCA-positive relatives in the group of pANCA-positive patients in contrast to 20% of pANCA-positive relatives in the group of pANCA-negative patients. If only titres higher than 1:100 were considered, the difference between both groups became larger, but not statistically significant. However, another group found a statistically significant difference between relatives of pANCA-positive versus pANCA-negative patients[10]. Dividing our probands into two groups we have attempted to determine whether environmental factors play a role in the induction of pANCA. We stratified the families into persons living in the same household with the patients or living separately. No difference was found in the frequency of pANCA between the groups.

OTHER ANTIBODIES IN ULCERATIVE COLITIS

Besides pANCA, there are some other antibodies in patients with UC that are worth mentioning. In order to evaluate autoimmunity as a pathogenetic factor the first studies from the 1960s focused on autoantibodies to colonic mucosa. Antibodies to a fraction of crude colon mucosa were found to be specific for patients with UC[1,14]. A cross-reactivity of these antibodies with the *E. coli* bacterial antigen 0:14 has been described[15].

Anti-goblet cell antibodies have been described by many authors[16–18]. Some investigators refer to these antibodies as anticolon antibodies. In our study these antibodies were found to be very specific for UC with a prevalence of 26%[19]. In another group[20], a mucin-producing cell line was used as antigen. Antibodies to these goblet cells were found not only in patients with UC, but also in patients with CD. Recently, a family study showed a high prevalence of goblet cell antibodies (GAB) in healthy first-degree family members of patients with UC and CD. The prevalence of GAB in families with a GAB-positive patient was significantly higher than in families with a GAB-negative patient[21]. Our own results, however, showed only a very low prevalence of GAB in families of patients with UC, and in families of CD patients no GAB were detectable.

Antibodies to tropomyosin were first described as colonic tissue-bound IgG antibody to a 40 kDa protein. The detection of the antigen in skin and bile ducts may explain the phenomenon of extraintestinal manifestations[22].

ANTI-*SACCHAROMYCES* ANTIBODIES

Several groups have described antibodies to *Saccharomyces cerevisiae* in CD[23,24]. Generally, an ELISA system was used to detect these antibodies. Antibody titres to *Saccharomyces* in patients with CD were significantly higher than in UC patients or controls. We found antibodies to *Saccharomyces cerevisiae cerevisiae* (ASCCA) in 77% of patients with CD and in 8% of patients with UC using an ELISA with mannan as antigen or an indirect fluorescence technique. The test was more specific when only titres higher than 1:200 were respected. In this case ASCCA were detectable in 61% of CD patients, in only 2% of UC patients, and in none of the controls. We tested various substrains of *Saccharomyces* for their reactivity with ASCCA-positive sera and found that an optimal discrimination between CD and UC was obtained only with two sub-strains of *Saccharomyces cerevisiae cerevisiae*. ASCCA detect a mannose-rich carbohydrate antigen of the *Saccharomyces cerevisiae* cell wall.

In most studies ASCCA-positivity did not correlate with clinical features such as disease activity or bowel involvement. In another study, however, ASCCA together with the tumour necrosis factor (TNF) microsatellite A2B1C2D4E1 haplotype were found to define a subgroup of UC patients with medically resist-ant disease (to anti-TNF therapy)[25].

PANCREATIC ANTIBODIES

Pancreatic antibodies (PAB) are highly specific for CD and are found at a fre-quency of 31% in these patients[18,19]. PAB were not found in 300 controls with various autoimmune disorders, colon carcinoma, diverticulitis, coeliac disease or pancreatitis. Titres of PAB varied between 1:10 and 1:1280 in CD, whereas in UC titres did not exceed 1:20. No significant fluctuation of antibody titres was observed during long-term follow-up. PAB did not correlate with clinical activ-ity, disease pattern, or extraintestinal manifestations of CD. Patients with CD and concomitant pancreatic insufficiency, however, were significantly more fre-quently PAB-positive than patients without pancreatic insufficiency[26]. Thus, pancreatic insufficiency may be due to chronic pancreatic inflammation and PAB may play a role in this context. In patients with CD and acute pancreatitis, however, PAB occur no more frequently than in CD patients without acute pan-creatitis[27]. PAB are directed against an antigen with a molecular weight of greater than 1300 kDa that is localized in the pancreatic secretions.

In order to determine whether PAB are of significance as a genetic marker we studied 70 families of patients with CD and 26 families of patients with UC. Of the 233 first-degree realatives of patients with CD, only five had detectable PAB. Four of five relatives positive for PAB had frequent diarrhoea, and in one of these relatives CD was diagnosed. Only one PAB-positive relative was asympto-matic[28]. Thus, PAB are probably not useful as genetic markers, but their high specificity may help to detect patients with CD.

OTHER ANTIBODIES IN CROHN'S DISEASE

Lymphocytotoxic antibodies were found in 40% of the patients with IBD. In a study of 17 families of patients with CD and five families of patients with UC these antibodies were found in 30% of the relatives. There is evidence, however, that the occurrence of this antibody is influenced by environmental factors[29].

In another study, autoantibodies to epithelial cell-associated components were detected in 69% of IBD patients (12 UC, 31 CD) and 55% of their relatives, but at a lower frequency also in other gastrointestinal diseases (27%) and systemic autoimmune diseases (10%)[30].

Furthermore, anti-erythrocyte antibodies have been described[31]. They occur at a high frequency in patients with CD (90%) and *Campylobacter jejuni* (100%), but only at a low frequency in patients with UC (30%) and in healthy controls[31].

This antibody, therefore, might be of relevance because of its high prevalence in patients with CD.

SUMMARY

During the past 40 years a variety of antibodies have been described in IBD. Antibodies to neutrophils (pANCA) are found at a high frequency in patients with UC, antibodies to *Saccharomyces cerevisiae cerevisiae* (ASCCA) are found at a high frequency in patients with CD. Together with pancreatic antibodies (PAB), which are very specific for CD, these antibodies may become useful as diagnostic tools. Further studies are necessary to show the possible role of some antibodies in the definition of a clinical subgroup of patients, e.g. non-responders to immunosuppressive therapy. None of the antibodies is of pathogenetic relevance, but may be the consequence of a disturbed regulation of the immune system. pANCA probably represent a cross-reactivity with enteric bacterial antigens.

References

1. Broberger O, Perlmann P. Autoantibodies in human ulcerative colitis. J Exp Med. 1959;110: 657–74.
2. Saxon A, Shanahan F, Landers C, Ganz T, Targan S. A subset of antineutrophil anticytoplasmic antibodies is associated with inflammatory bowel disease. J Allergy Clin Immunol. 1990;86:202–10.
3. Seibold F, Weber P, Klein R, Berg PA, Wiedmann KH. Clinical significance of antibodies against neutrophils in patients with inflammatory bowel disease and primary sclerosing cholangitis. Gut. 1992;33:657–62.
4. Seibold F, Weber P, Schöning A, Mörk H, Goppel S, Scheurlen M. Neutrophil antibodies in chronic liver disease and inflammatory bowel disease: do they react with different antigens? Eur J Gastroenterol Hepatol. 1996;8:1095–100.
5. Walsmley RS, Zhao MH, Hamilton MI *et al*. Antineutrophil cytoplasmic autoantibodies against bactericidal/permeability increasing protein in inflammatory bowel disease. Gut. 1997;40:105–9.
6. Seibold F, Brandwein S, Simpson S, Terhorst S, Elson CO. pANCA represents a cross-reactivity to enteric bacterial antigens. J Clin Immunol. 1998;18:153–60.
7. Mizoguchi E, Mizoguchi A, Chiba C, Niles JL, Bhan AK. Antineutrophil cytoplasmic antibodies in T-cell receptor α-deficient mice with chronic colitis. Gastroenterology. 1997;113:1828–36.
8. Sandborn WJ, Landers CJ, Tremaine WJ, Targan SR. The presence of antineutrophil cytoplasmic antibodies correlates with pouchitis after ileal pouch–anal anastomosis for ulcerative colitis. Gastroenterology. 1993; 104:A774.
9. Vasiliauskas EA, Plevy SE, Landers CJ *et al*. Perinuclear antineutrophil cytoplasmic antibodies in patients with Crohn's disease define a clinical subgroup. Gastroenterology. 1996;110:1810–19.
10. Shanahan F, Duerr R, Rotter JI *et al*. Neutrophil autoantibodies in ulcerative colitis: Familial aggregation and genetic heterogeneity. Gastroenterology. 1992;103:456–61.
11. Seibold F, Slametschka D, Gregor M, Weber P. Neutrophil autoantibodies: genetic marker in primary sclerosing cholangitis and ulcerative colitis. Gastroenterology. 1994;107:532–6.
12. Reumaux D, Colombel JF, Delecourt L, Noel LH, Cortot A, Duthilleul P. Antineutrophil cytoplasmic autoantibodies in relatives of patients with ulcerative colitis. Gastroenterology. 1992;103:1706.
13. Lee CW, Lennard-Jones JE, Cambridge G. Antineutrophil antibodies in familial inflammatory bowel disease. Gastroenterology. 1995;108:428–33.
14. Broberger O, Perlmann P. Demonstration of an epithelial antigen in colon by means of fluorescent antibodies from children with ulcerative colitis. J Exp Med. 1962;115:13–26.
15. Lagercrantz R, Perlmann P, Hammarström S. Immunological studies in ulcerative colitis. V. Family studies. Gastroenterology. 1971;60:381–8.

16. Koffler D, Minkowitz S, Rothman W, Garloch J. Immunocytochemical studies in ulcerative colitis and regional ileitis. Am J Pathol. 1962;41:733–42.
17. Harrison WJ. Autoantibodies against intestinal and gastric mucous cells in ulcerative colitis. Lancet. 1965;1:1346–50.
18. Stöcker W, Otte M, Ulrich S *et al.* Autoimmunity: pancreatic juice in Crohn's disease. Scand J Gastroenterol. 1987;22:41–52.
19. Seibold F, Weber P, Jenss H, Wiedmann KH. Antibodies to a trypsin sensitive pancreatic antigen in chronic inflammatory bowel disease: specific markers for a subgroup of patients with Crohn's disease. Gut. 1991;32:1192–7.
20. Hibi T, Kobayashi K, Brown WR *et al.* Enzyme linked immunosorbent assay and immuno-precipitation studies on anti-goblet cell antibody using a mucin producing cell line in patients with inflammatory bowel disease. Gut. 1994;35:224–30.
21. Folwaczny C, Noehl N, Tschöp K *et al.* Goblet cell antibodies in patients with inflammatory bowel disease and their first-degree relatives. Gastroenterology. 1997;113:101–6.
22. Das KM, Vecchi M, Sakamaki S. A shared and unique epitope on human colon, skin, and biliary epithelium detected by a monoclonal antibody. Gastroenterology. 1990;98:464–8.
23. Giaffer MH, Clark A, Holdsworth CD. Antibodies to *Saccharomyces cerevisiae* in patients with Crohn's disease and their possible pathogenic importance. Gut. 1992;33:1071–5.
24. Sendid B, Colombel JF, Jacquinot PM *et al.* Specific antibody response to oligomannosidic epitopes in Crohn's disease. Clin Diagn Lab Immunol. 1996;3:219–26.
25. Plevy SE, Vasiliauskas EA, Taylor K *et al.* The Crohn's disease associated tumor necrosis factor microsatellite A2B1C2D4E1 haplotype and anti-*Saccharomyces cerevisiae* antibody define medically resistant forms of ulcerative colitis. Gastroenterology. 1997;112:1112.
26. Seibold F, Scheurlen M, Müller A, Jenss H, Weber P. Impaired pancreatic function in patients with Crohn's disease with and without pancreatic antibodies. J Clin Gastroenterol. 1996;22:202–6.
27. Weber P, Seibold F, Jenss H. Acute pancreatitis in Crohn's disease. J Clin Gastroenterol. 1993;17:286–91.
28. Seibold F, Mörk H, Tanza S *et al.* Pancreatic autoantibodies in Crohn's disease: a family study. Gut. 1997;40:481–4.
29. Korsmeyer SJ, Williams RC, Wilson D, Strickland RG. Lymphocytotoxic antibody in inflammatory bowel disease. N Engl J Med. 1975;22:1117–20.
30. Fiocchi C, Roche JK, Michener WM. High prevalence of antibodies to intestinal epithelial antigens in patients with inflammatory bowel disease and their relatives. Ann Intern Med. 1989;110:786–94.
31. Berberian LS, Valles-Ayoub Y, Gordon LK, Targan SR, Braun J. Expression of a novel auto-antibody defined by the Vh3-15 gene in inflammatory bowel disease and *Campylobacter jejuni* enterocolitis. J Immunol. 1994;153:3756–63.

Section II
Experimental Models of IBD

5
Experimental models of IBD: old hypotheses confirmed and new paradigms generated

C. O. ELSON, Y. CONG, S. BRANDWEIN, C. T. WEAVER,
M. MÄHLER and J. SUNDBERG

The inflammatory bowel diseases are complex disorders in humans whose aetiology and pathogenesis have been elusive. Patients present to clinic after their disease has become fairly advanced and symptomatic and this has made understanding of the early events leading to disease, which may have occurred decades before presentation, very difficult. Experimental models have some advantages over study of the human disease in this regard in that the onset of disease can be precisely controlled and hypotheses about the early events in the process tested.

NEWER MODELS OF INTESTINAL INFLAMMATION

The inflammatory bowel diseases appear to involve interactions among immune, environmental and genetic factors and it is the combination of these factors that results in induction of inflammation, subsequent tissue damage, and then processes of restitution and repair. Experimental models have been developed that can examine each phase of this cascade of events, including those early events that seem to be crucial to disease induction[1]. Some of these models involve environmental stressors, such as the feeding of dextran sulphate sodium, a highly sulphated polysaccharide that reproducibly induces colitis when added to the drinking water of rodents, possibly due to damage to colonic enterocytes[2,3]. Repeated administration of this agent in cycles can induce chronic colitis. Another environmental stressor is the administration by enema of trinitrobenzenesulphonic acid (TNBS) in ethanol. The ethanol breaks the mucosal barrier and allows this contact sensitizing agent to reach the deeper tissues of the colon. There is acute damage followed by a contact hypersensitivity reaction which can result in chronic inflammation[4].

A number of other models have arisen from new technologies that allow the insertion or deletion of a gene into or from an animal. Animals resulting from such manipulations have been termed collectively 'induced mutants' to distinguish them from mutants that arise spontaneously. In the case of gene deletions, a new strain deficient in a given gene and its product is created. The major purpose of these sorts of experiments in immunology has been to determine whether deficiency of a given molecule results in a functional disturbance in the immune system. One of the major surprises coming from such experiments is how often the immune system is able to carry on its functions with no identifiable effect of a gene deletion, due to the great redundancy of function among the molecules of immunity. A small subset of immune-gene-deleted mutant mice have developed inflammatory bowel disease in the absence of any further manipulation. This subset represents a small fraction of the total number of immunological genes that have been deleted, which argues that they represent critical non-redundant mechanisms of mucosal homeostasis. Most of these mutations affect T-cell function in some way; others may have a predominant effect on the epithelium.

One of the first reports of induced mutants developing colitis was the interleukin-2-deficient mouse. In the original report these mice developed pancolitis starting at about 10 weeks of age[5]. There were increased numbers of B cells and T cells infiltrating the colon lamina propria, increased serum immunoglobulins such as IgG_1 and IgE, and anticolon antibodies. Subsequent work has found that the major cytokine expressed in the colon is interferon-γ (IFN-γ), not IL-4 as was originally suspected[6]. In fact, mice with a deficiency of both IL-2 and IL-4 still get colitis, indicating that IL-4 is not required for this disease to develop. Mice deficient in both B cells and IL-2[7] and those deficient in both CD8+ T cells and IL-2 still develop disease[8], indicating that the CD4+ T cell is the critical effector cell. As will be discussed below, when these mice are rendered germ free, they no longer develop colitis[5]. In addition, when the IL-2 null mutation is bred onto other inbred strains, disease expression is markedly altered, indicating a strong influence of background modifier genes on this mutation[9].

THE ROLE OF MUCOSAL CD4+ T CELLS

These results in IL-2-deficient mice have been mirrored in many other models. The CD4+ T cell expressing a T$\alpha\beta$ receptor has been found to be the critical effector cell in most models where the effector has been identified. In addition, in most of these models, overproduction of IFN-γ in the colon seems to be a major pathogenetic event. IFN-γ production by CD4+ T cells is stimulated by the cytokine interleukin-12 (IL-12)[10]. In turn, IFN-γ stimulates macrophages to produce more IL-12, setting up a self-reinforcing feedback loop that can maintain chronic intestinal inflammation. Monoclonal antibodies to IL-12 can both prevent induction of colitis as well as treat active colitis in a number of animal models[6,10]. There are data from human studies that IFN-γ is overexpressed in the lesions of Crohn's disease, as is IL-12[11]. Thus, antibodies to IL-12 are an attractive candidate for therapy of patients with Crohn's disease and clinical trials with such an agent are planned.

THE Th-1/Th-2 PARADIGM AND EXPERIMENTAL IBD

CD4+ T cells can be subdivided into several important functional subsets based on the types of cytokines that they produce. Th-1 cells produce IL-2, IFN-γ and TNF-β, cytokines that are important in cellular immunity and delayed hypersensitivity. Th-2 cells do not produce these cytokines, but rather produce IL-4, IL-5, IL-6, IL-10 and IL-13, cytokines important in providing help for antibody responses and thus humoral immunity. The type of CD4+ T cell response to a given pathogen can be a life or death matter in that inbred mouse strains that respond to a microbial pathogen such as *Leishmania major* with a Th-2 response succumb to the infection and die, whereas inbred strains that respond to the same agent with a predominantly Th-1 response clear the infection and are resistant to reinfection[12]. The predominance of IFN-γ production in the colon of most of the models tested to date has led to the concept that Th-1 responses are deleterious and Th-2 responses are beneficial. However, results from one of the other models contradict this assumption. The T-cell receptor α chain-deficient mouse develops a pancolitis with a striking crypt hyperplasia beginning at 3 months of age[13]. These mice lack CD4+ TCR$\alpha\beta$+ T cells but do have TCR $\gamma\delta$ cells, as well as a small subset of CD4+ TCRα–β+ cells. They have increased serum IgG$_1$, IgG$_2$ and IgA during colitis, as well as antibodies to tropomyosin, an antibody present in the majority of patients with ulcerative colitis. Cells in the mesenteric lymph nodes draining the inflamed gut demonstrated decreased IL-2 and increased IL-4 production by T cells, and some IFN-γ production by non-T cells in the colitic mice[14]. One of the interesting features of this model is that resection of the proximal caecum containing a prominent lymphoid follicle between 3 and 5 weeks of age reduces the frequency of colitis as the mice age, from 80% in controls down to 3% in operated mice[15]. This follicle may be the equivalent of an appendix in humans and thus is somewhat analogous to the observation that appendectomy is protective against development of ulcerative colitis. Colitis in this model is a Th-2-type of response in that the CD4+ TCRβ+ cells produce only IL-4 and their deletion (or neutralization of IL-4 with monoclonal antibodies) completely suppresses the development of colitis[16]. These results do not support the concept that Th-2 responses are always beneficial. Instead, it appears that strong polarization of mucosal T-cell responses along either pathway can result in inflammatory bowel disease. Interestingly, the tissue pathology seen in the IL-2-deficient mouse and the TCRα-deficient mouse is not all that different, indicating that the pathology itself gives few clues as to the underlying pathogenetic process.

MUCOSAL IMMUNE REGULATION

The mucosal immune system encounters an enormous antigenic load in the form of food or commensal bacterial antigens, much of which is innocuous. Although immune cells are present in the intestine and primed, inflammation is normally limited by processes of mucosal immune regulation. Much of this regulation is exerted by T cells. Given the enormous quantity of antigens within and transiting the gut, abnormalities of mucosal regulatory processes could easily result in intestinal inflammation. This has been a hypothesis for human disease for some years and now evidence is arising in the animal models confirming this hypothesis. One of the features of the immune system is that effector cells are counterbalanced by regulatory cells. One example is the balance between Th-1 and Th-2 subsets, which reciprocally regulate one another via IFN-γ inhibition of Th-2 responses and IL-10 inhibition of Th-1 responses. However, other T-cell subsets have been identified that have regulatory functions distinct from Th-1 and Th-2 cells. One of these, denoted 'Tr-1', produces predominantly interleukin-10[17]. Another, denoted 'Th-3', produces transforming growth factor β_1 (TGF-β)[18]. The evidence supporting the existence of Tr-1 is given in Table 1. Both subsets may also be involved in the phenomenon known as oral tolerance in which the feeding of an antigen reduces the subsequent immune response to it following parenteral immunization. Recent studies in TCR transgenic mice indicate that there are two major cytokine-producing CD4+ T cells in the intestinal lamina propria of mice, one that produces IFN-γ and another that produces IL-10, suggesting that the Tr-1 subset may be represented predominantly in the intestinal mucosa[19]. Indeed, functional Tr-1 activity has been demonstrated in the intestine *in vivo*. This comes from an experiment in which Tr-1 cells producing high levels of IL-10 in response to ovalbumin were generated by culturing these cells *in vitro* with ovalbumin in the presence of IL-10. Prolonged culture under these conditions generates a subset of cells that produces large amounts of IL-10, as well as significant amounts of IL-4 and IFN. These Tr-1, OVA-specific T cells were administered to SCID mice along with disease-inducing CD4+, CD45RB[hi] cells from normal histocompatible donors[17]. The latter cells induced colitis in the recipients when transferred alone or with Tr-1 cells in the absence of OVA. However, colitis was prevented if the mice were fed ovalbumin in order to trigger the Tr-1 regulatory subset. This is an example of what has been termed 'bystander suppression' and represents a possible new approach to future therapy for patients with inflammatory bowel disease. Somewhat similar results were obtained with T cells from a mouse transgenic for IL-10 under the regulation of the IL-2 promoter[20]. Because this promoter is restricted to the T-cell lineage, IL-10 is overproduced only when such T cells are activated. CD4+, CD45RB[hi] T cells from these IL-10 transgenic mice did not induce disease in SCID recipients and, moreover, they prevented colitis when cotransferred with control non-transgenic CD4+, CD45RB[hi] T cells. Thus, high local production of

Table 1 Mucosal immune regulation: evidence for a T-regulatory-1 (Tr-1) subset producing IL-10

IL-10-deficient mice develop enterocolitis[31]

There are two major cytokine-producing CD4+ cells in lamina propria of TCR Tg mice: one producing IFN-γ and the other producing IL-10[19]

'Protective' CD4+, CD45RB[lo] T cells from IL-10-deficient mice cause colitis in RAG-2 –/– recipients[32]

Tr-1 regulatory T cells producing high levels of IL-10 prevent colitis in the CD4+, CD45RB[hi] transfer model[17]

CD4+, CD45RB[hi] T cells from mice transgenic for IL-10 (under the IL-2 promotor) do not cause colitis in SCID mice and prevent colitis due to transfer of pathogenic CD4+ CD45RB[hi] T cells[20]

---

interleukin-10 either by the Tr-1 subset or by a transgenic IL-10 producing T-cell subset can prevent the induction of colitis in the CD45Rb[hi] transfer model. Whether the same will be true in other models and whether this subset can treat established active disease remains to be tested.

The other regulatory subset is one that produces TGF-β_1. These cells have been given the designation 'Th-3' to distinguish them from the Th-1 and Th-2 subsets. They have been identified in experiments examining mechanisms of oral tolerance induced by autoantigen feeding in mice[21,22] and in patients with multiple sclerosis[18]. These cells produce large amounts of TGF-β_1 when stimulated with antigen. Cells producing TGF-β mediate protective oral tolerance in the TNBS-induced colitis model after feeding TNP-colon proteins[23]. Neutralization of TGF-β_1 abolishes the protective effect of CD+, CD45RB[lo] cells in the CD+ CD45RB-induced transfer model of colitis[24]. Lastly, TGF-β_1 appears to regulate the development of TNP-KLH-induced colitis in IL-2-deficient mice[25].

INFLUENCE OF THE MICROBIAL ENVIRONMENT

There are clear environmental effects which influence the development of inflammatory bowel disease in humans. The same is true in the experimental models. However, in these models, the major environmental factor is the enteric bacterial flora in that germ-free animals do not develop colitis. These include IL-2-deficient mice, IL-10-deficient mice, TCRα-deficient mice, and HLAB27/β_2M transgenic rats. In addition, disease is reduced by maintaining a restricted bacterial colonization or by administration of antibiotics. The bacterial flora contains a complex mixture of materials that could interact with the immune system, including mitogens, superantigens and nominal protein antigens. Some insights into what might be stimulating disease in these models come from studies done in the C3H/HeJBir mouse. This mouse was originally generated by selective breeding for a phenotype of spontaneous colitis[26]. These mice developed focal to locally extensive inflammation in the caecum early in life, from which they recovered. The peak incidence was at 3–7 weeks of age and, in virtually all of the animals, the inflammation had resolved by 3 months of age. A search for reactivity to food antigens or epithelial cell antigens was negative. However, these mice do show strong serum reactivity to a small highly selected subset of bacterial antigens using Western immunoblotting[27]. These antibodies do not appear to be involved in the pathogenesis in that they reach maximal expression after three months of age, a time when the colitis has resolved. However, they do indicate that the immune system responds to only a highly select subset of the total bacterial protein antigens present in the intestinal lumen. CD4+ T cells from such mice respond strongly to freshly obtained caecal bacterial antigen preparations[28]. The stimulatory material is protein in origin and is presented to T cells via MHC Class II molecules. Superantigens do not appear to be involved. The C3H/HeJBir T cells overproduce IFN-γ and IL-2 when stimulated with these bacterial antigens in vitro and are able to mediate colitis in histocompatible immunodeficient recipient mice when activated by bacterial antigens and transferred. Interestingly, the lesions in the recipient mice are focal as they are in the donor strain. A number of cell lines reactive to enteric bacterial antigens have now been generated, some of which uniformly induce colitis in the recipients and overproduction of IFN-γ and IL-12 in the lesions. Only a restricted set of T-cell receptors are being utilized to recognize these antigens, which is compatible with the concept that only a select subset of enteric bacterial antigens are triggering the pathogenic response.

SUSCEPTIBILITY TO COLITIS IS A GENETIC TRAIT

It has been recognized for some time that there is a genetic component to inflammatory bowel disease. Because this genetic aspect is not inherited in a simple Mendelian fashion, it has been postulated that multiple genes are interacting to cause susceptibility. The newer experimental models have provided strong evidence in support of this concept. Different inbred strains show reproducible susceptibility or resistance to colitis, independent of the stimulus used to induce that colitis. We have used the feeding of dextran sulphate sodium (DSS) as an environmental stressor to quantitatively define the severity and frequency of lesions in the caecum and colon of many different inbred strains. These data indicate that there are quantifiable differences that are reproducible from strain to strain, with some strains significantly more susceptible than others[29]. Interestingly, C3H/HeJBir and C3H/HeJ mice are among the most susceptible. The 129/SvJ strain was found to be highly susceptible in the colon but highly resistant in the caecum, indicating that the genetic control of susceptibility in these two regions may well be different. This work has now been extended by breeding a highly susceptible substrain, C3H/HeJ, to a moderately resistant strain, C57BL/6. The F1 animals resulting from this cross were intercrossed with one another, as well as backcrossed with each parental strain. DSS was then fed to the resulting progeny and the severity of the inflammation in colon and caecum correlated with the inheritance pattern of multiple microsatellite markers in a genome scan. This analysis has identified loci on five different chromosomes, two of which have a very high level of statistical probability and have been assigned the designations Dssc1 and Dssc2 for dextran sulphate sodium colitis-gene 1 and -gene 2[30]. Interestingly, both parental strains contributed susceptibility genes to the progeny. These results confirm the hypothesis that susceptibility to colitis is a multigenic trait and provides some new candidate regions for testing in humans. Studies utilizing a similar approach using IL-10 deficiency as the inducing stimulus for colitis are now underway.

In conclusion, there has been a virtual explosion of information coming from experimental models in recent years. Some of these results have provided support and confirmation for long-standing hypotheses concerning human IBD, particularly the importance of T cells, specifically CD4+ T cells, in mediating disease. These studies have emphasized the role of antigens of the enteric bacteria in driving such pathogenic T cells, a finding that now needs to be tested in patients. Some of these data point to new strategies for therapeutic invention, such as inhibitors of IL-12 and selective stimulation of critical regulatory cells. Genetic analysis has confirmed the multigenic nature of susceptibility and has offered new approaches to identification of the genes and genetic pathways involved in such susceptibility. Studies in experimental animals are complementary to those in humans but do have great value in clarifying concepts and generating new hypotheses and paradigms to be tested in our patients.

References

1. Elson CO, Sartor RB, Tennyson GS, Riddell RH. Experimental models of inflammatory bowel disease. Gastroenterology. 1995;109(4):1344–67.
2. Okayasu I, Hatakeyama S, Yamada M, Ohkusa T, Inagaki Y, Nakaya R, A novel method in the induction of reliable experimental acute and chronic ulcerative colitis in mice. Gastroenterology 1990;98:694–702.
3. Dieleman LA, Ridwan BU, Tennyson GS, Beagley KW, Bucy RP, Elson CO. Dextran sulfate sodium-induced colitis occurs in severe combined immunodeficient mice. Gastroenterology. 1994;107(6):1643–52.
4. Elson CO, Beagley KW, Sharmanov AT *et al*. Hapten-induced model of murine inflammatory bowel disease – mucosal immune responses and protection by tolerance. J Immunol. 1996;157(5):2174–83.
5. Sadlack B, Merz H, Schorle H, Schimpl A, Feller AC, Horak I. Ulcerative colitis-like disease in mice with a disrupted interleukin-2 gene. Cell. 1993;75(2):253–61.
6. Ehrhardt RO, Ludviksson BR, Gray B, Neurath M, Strober W. Induction and prevention of colonic inflammation in IL-2-deficient mice. J Immunol. 1997;158(2):566–73.
7. Ma A, Datta M, Margosian E, Chen J, Horak I. T cells, but not B cells, are required for bowel inflammation in interleukin 2-deficient mice. J Exp Med. 1995;182(5):1567–72.
8. Simpson SJ, Mizoguchi E, Allen D, Bhan AK, Terhorst C. Evidence that CD4+, but not CD8+ T cells are responsible for murine interleukin-2-deficient colitis. Eur J Immunol. 1995;25(9):2618–25.
9. Mähler M, Serreze D, Evans R, Linder CD, Leiter EH, Sundberg JP. IL-2[tm1Hor], an interleukin-2 gene targeted mutation: In: Bar Harbor, ME: The Jackson Laboratory 1996.
10. Neurath MF, Fuss I, Kelsall BL, Stuber E, Strober W. Antibodies to interleukin 12 abrogate established experimental colitis in mice. J Exp Med. 1995;182(5):1281–90.
11. Parronchi P, Romagnani P, Annunziato F *et al*. Type 1 T-helper cell predominance and interleukin-12 expression in the gut of patients with Crohn's disease. Am J Pathol. 1997;150(3):823–32.
12. Mosmann TR, Sad S. The expanding universe of T cell subsets: Th1, Th2 and more. Immunol Today. 1996;17:138–46.
13. Mombaerts P, Mizoguchi E, Grusby MJ, Glimcher LH, Bhan AK, Tonegawa S. Spontaneous development of inflammatory bowel disease in T cell receptor mutant mice. Cell. 1993;75(2):1–20.
14. Mizoguchi A, Mizoguchi E, Chiba C *et al*. Cytokine imbalance and autoantibody production in T cell receptor-alpha mutant mice with inflammatory bowel disease. J Exp Med. 1996;183(3):847–56.
15. Mizoguchi A, Mizoguchi E, Chiba C, Bhan AK. Role of appendix in the development of inflammatory bowel disease in TCR-alpha mutant mice. J Exp Med. 1996;184(2):707–15.
16. Takahashi I, Kiyono H, Hamada S. A CD4+ T-cell population mediates development of inflammatory bowel disease in T-cell receptor alpha-deficient mice. Gastroenterology. 1997;112:1876–82.
17. Groux H, O'Garra A, Bigler M *et al*. A CD4+ T cell subset inhibits antigen-specific T-cell responses and prevents colitis. Nature. 1997;389:737–42.
18. Fukaura H, Kent SC, Pietrusewicz MJ, Khoury SJ, Weiner HL, Hafler DA. Induction of circulating myelin basic protein and proteolipid protein-specific transforming growth factor-beta 1-secreting Th3 T cells by oral administration of myelin in multiple sclerosis patients. J Clin Invest. 1996;98(1):70–7.
19. Saparov A, Elson CO, Devore-Carter D, Bucy RP, Weaver CT. Single-cell analyses of CD4+ T cells from alpha beta T cell receptor-transgenic mice: a distinct mucosal cytokine phenotype in the absence of transgene-specific antigen. Eur J Immunol. 1997;27(7):1774–81.
20. Hagenbaugh A, Sharma S, Dubinett SM *et al*. Altered immune responses in interleukin 10 transgenic mice. J Exp Med. 1997;185(12):2101–10.
21. Santos LM, al-Sabbagh A, Londono A, Weiner HL. Oral tolerance to myelin basic protein induces regulatory TGF-beta-secreting T cells in Peyer's patches of SJL mice. Cell Immunol. 1994;157(2):439–47.

22. Chen Y, Kuchroo VK, Inobe J, Hafler DA, Weiner HL. Regulatory T cell clones induced by oral tolerance: suppression of autoimmune encephalomyelitis. Science. 1994;265(5176):1237–40.
23. Neurath MF, Fuss I, Kelsall BL, Presky DH, Waegell W, Strober W. Experimental granulomatous colitis in mice is abrogated by induction of TGF-beta-mediated oral tolerance. J Exp Med. 1996;183(6):2605–16.
24. Powrie F, Carlino J, Leach MW, Mauze S, Coffman RL. A critical role for transforming growth factor-beta but not interleukin 4 in the suppression of T helper type 1-mediated colitis by CD45RB(low) CD4+ T cells. J Exp Med. 1996;183(6):2669–74.
25. Ludviksson BR, Ehrhardt RO, Strober W. TGF-beta production regulates the development of the 2,4,6-trinitrophenol-conjugated keyhole limpet hemocyanin-induced colonic inflammation in IL-2-deficient mice. J Immunol. 1997;159(7):3622–8.
26. Sundberg JP, Elson CO, Bedigian H, Birkenmeier EH. Spontaneous, heritable colitis in a new substrain of C3H/HeJ mice. Gastroenterology. 1994;107(6):1726–35.
27. Brandwein SL, McCabe RP, Cong Y *et al.* Spontaneously colitic C3H/HeJBir mice demonstrate selective antibody reactivity to antigens of the enteric bacterial flora. J Immunol. 1997;159(1):44–52.
28. Cong Y, Brandwein SL, McCabe RP *et al.* CD4+ T cells reactive to enteric bacterial antigens in spontaneously colitic C3H/HeJBir mice. Increased Th1 response and ability to transfer disease. J Exp Med. 1998;187(6):855–64.
29. Mähler M, Briostol IJ, Leiter EH, Birkenmeier EH, Elson CO, Sundberg JP. Differential susceptibility of inbred mouse strains to dextran sulfate sodium-induced colitis. Am J Physiol. 1998;274:G544–51.
30. Mähler M, Sundberg J, Birkenmeier EH, Bristol IJ, Elson CO, Leiter EH. Chromosomal location of genes determining susceptibility of mice to dextran sulfate sodium (DSS)-induced colitis. Gastroenterology. 1997;112(4):A1031.
31. Kuhn R, Lohler J, Rennick D, Rajewsky K, Muller W. Interleukin-10-deficient mice develop chronic enterocolitis. Cell. 1993;75(2):263–74.
32. Rennick DM, Fort MM, Davidson NJ. Studies with IL-10-/- mice: an overview. J Leukocyte Biol. 1997;61(4):389–96.
33. Miller A, Lider O, Roberts AB, Sporn MB, Weiner HL. Suppressor T cells generated by oral tolerization to myelin basic protein suppress both *in vitro* and *in vivo* immune responses by the release of transforming growth factor beta after antigen-specific triggering. Proc Natl Acad Sci USA. 1992;89(1):421–5.

6
Neuroimmune interactions in IBD

M. REINSHAGEN, H. ROHM, J. LAKSHMANAN and
V. E. EYSSELEIN

INTRODUCTION

The sensory nervous system of the gut has a variety of efferent functions besides its well-known afferent action in the gastrointestinal tract[1]. Transmission of sensory information about site and kind of injury to the central nervous system is pivotal for maintaining the integrity of the body in response to injury.

Enhancement of the inflammatory tissue response after injury ('neurogenic inflammation') and consequent promotion of tissue healing are examples of this afferent function. Examples for this 'neurogenic inflammation' have been demonstrated in various tissues such as the eye[2], skin[3] and joints[4]. In the gastrointestinal system these mechanisms are still incompletely understood. The phenomenon of neurogenic inflammation induced by sensory neurones by release of sensory neuropeptides seems to be contradictory to a subsequent wound healing promoting action. However, it is conceivable that the nervous system is needed to defend injury by modulating the inflammatory response which is needed for the subsequent healing process.

Especially the interaction of the sensory nervous system in the gut with different cells of the immune system during the inflammatory response, and how this interaction is mediated, has not yet been clearly defined. An imbalance of this system may lead to chronic inflammation, and might be involved in the pathophysiology of inflammatory bowel disease (IBD).

STUDIES IN EXPERIMENTAL MODELS OF COLITIS AND IBD

Chronic treatment with the neurotoxin *capsaicin* in adult rats damages small sensory nerve fibres in the gut[5]. In an acute model of colitis (immune-complex colitis of the rabbit) capsaicin-pretreated animals showed a significantly enhanced severity of the experimental colitis[6,7]. This effect could be reproduced in a chronic model of colitis (TNB colitis of the rat)[8], suggesting that these capsaicin-sensitive sensory fibres have an overall protective function in these experimental colitis models. Using a CGRP (calcitonin gene-related peptide) antagonist or an immunoneutralizing CGRP antibody this effect could again be reproduced, while a substance P (SP) antagonist had no significant effect on the severity of the TNB colitis[9]. These data suggest that CGRP but not SP mediates this protective sensory function in this model. Other groups have confirmed this observation that SP might serve in the early phase of inflammation as a proinflammatory neuropeptide, while CGRP subsequently promotes tissue protection by its potent vasodilatory properties[10,11].

Recent studies in patients with Crohn's disease' by Mantyh *et al.*, have shown an up-regulation of SP-receptor density not only in inflamed tissue but also in non-inflamed gut tissue of these patients, suggesting an increased tissue suscept-ibility to SP in the gut of patients with Crohn's disease[12].

Nerve growth factor (NGF) is a multipotent growth factor supporting growth and differentiation of sympathetic and sensory neurones in the peripheral nervous system[13,14]. Furthermore NGF controls synthesis and release of sensory neuropeptides in the enteric nervous system[15].

Immunoneutralization of NGF in adult rats decreased the amount of mucosal CGRP by about 50%, while SP contents were not significantly reduced[16].

Immunoneutralization of NGF or neurotrophin-3 (NT-3), another member of the neurotrophin family of growth factors, again significantly increased the severity of experimental colitis in the TNB model of colitis[16]. Whether this effect was due only to the reduced CGRP content in the mucosa was not clear from this study.

Since NGF might be an important regulator and mediator during the inflammatory response we looked for the expression of NGF during the time-course of different experimental models of colitis and in patients with IBD. We could show that NGF, BDNF (brain-derived neurotrophic factor) and NT-3, as well as their tyrosine kinase receptors Trk A, Trk B and Trk C, are differentially regulated during the inflammatory response in experimental colitis, as well as in patients with Crohn's disease and ulcerative colitis[17].

IL-2 knockout mice develop ulcerative colitis resembling human Crohn's disease about 12 weeks after birth when they are housed under conventional conditions. This inflammation is driven by a CD4+ Th1-type lymphocyte popu-lation[18,19]. In the first 4 weeks after birth there are no signs of inflammation in the colon and there is a low expression of neurotrophins in the gut. Between 4 and 8 weeks of life there is still no histological evidence of inflammation, but we could show that there is already a significant increase of NGF expression in the colon. From 8 to 12 weeks ulcerative colitis develops and there is a highly significant increase of NGF, whereas BDNF and its receptor Trk B are sharply down-regulated[20]. This up-regulation of NGF and down-regulation of BDNF implies a regulatory role of neurotrophins in this clearly immunological defined model of colitis.

When SCID mice, which lack B and T cells, are repopulated with congenic CD4+ cells, the CD4+ cells proliferate in the colon and induce ulcerative colitis resembling human Crohn's disease[21,22]. These CD4+ cells have a clearly defined Th1 phenotype. As in the IL-2 knockout mouse during the first 4 weeks after CD4+ repopulation there are no signs of histological inflammation, and there is only a marginal expression of NGF in the colon or in proliferating CD4+ cells extracted from the colon. After 6–8 weeks there is a significant up-regulation of

NGF in the CD4+ cells extracted from the colon, while no significant histological signs of inflammation can be observed. After 8–10 weeks there is a highly significant up-regulation of NGF in the inflamed colon and in the CD4+ cells extracted from the colon[23].

NGF is able to regulate a wide range of immune cells, such as T cells[24–26], B cells[27] and mast cells[28]. The fact that these cells not only express Trk A but also release active NGF[29] indicates that NGF is an autocrine and/or paracrine mediator in the regulation of immune responses, and that it therefore serves as an important link between the nervous and immune systems[14].

CONCLUSION

The sensory enteric nervous system is involved in the regulation of inflammation by releasing proinflammatory and anti-inflammatory sensory neuropeptides in response to the inflammatory stimulus. Our data suggest that this system is under control of neurotrophic mediators such as nerve growth factor (NGF), which might serve as the prototypic mediator of neuroimmune interactions in the gut, since it is expressed and up-regulated in the nervous system as well as in a variety of immune cells which initiate the damage during intestinal inflammation.

References

1. Maggi CA, Meli A. The sensory-efferent function of capsaicin-sensitive sensory neurons. Gen Pharmacol. 1988;19:1–43.
2. Bill A, Stiernschantz J, Mandahl A, Brodin E, Nilsson G. Substance P release on trigeminal nerve stimulation, effects in the eye. Acta Physiol Scand. 1979;106:371–3.
3. Haegermark O, Hoekfelt T, Pernow P. Flare and itch produced by substance P in human skin. J Invest Dermatol. 1978;71:233–6.
4. Levine JD, Clark R, Devor M, Helms C, Moskowitz MA, Basbaum AI. Intraneuronal substance P contributes to the severity of experimental arthritis. Science. 1984;226:547–9.
5. Holzer P. Capsaicin: cellular targets, mechanisms of action, and selectivity for thin sensory neurons. Pharmacol Rev. 1991;43:143–204.
6. Eysselein VE, Reinshagen M, Cominelli F et al. Calcitonin gene-related peptide and substance P decrease in the rabbit colon during colitis. A time study. Gastroenterology. 1991;101:1211–19.
7. Reinshagen M, Patel A, Sottili M et al. Protective function of extrinsic sensory neurons in acute rabbit experimental colitis. Gastroenterology. 1994;106:1208–14.
8. Reinshagen M, Patel A, Sottili M, French S, Sternini C, Eysselein VE. Action of sensory neurons in an experimental rat colitis model of injury and repair. Am J Physiol. 1996;270:G79–86.
9. Reinshagen M, Flämig G, Ernst S et al. Calcitonin gene-related peptide mediates the protective effect of sensory nerves in TNB rat colitis. J Pharmacol Exp Ther. 1998;286:657–61.
10. McCafferty DM, Sharkey KA, Wallace JL. Beneficial effects of local or systemic lidocaine in experimental colitis. Am J Physiol. 1994;266:G560–7.
11. Wallace JL, McCafferty DM, Sharkey KA. Lack of beneficial effect of a tachykinin receptor antagonist in experimental colitis. Regul Pept. 1998;73:95–101.
12. Mantyh CR, Vigna SR, Bollinger RR, Mantyh PW, Maggio JE, Pappas TN. Differential expression of substance P receptors in patients with Crohn's disease and ulcerative colitis. Gastroenterology. 1995;109:850–60.
13. Levi Montalcini R, Dal Toso R, della Valle F, Skaper SD, Leon A. Update of the NGF saga. J Neurol Sci. 1995;130:119–27.
14. Levi Montalcini R, Skaper SD, Dal Toso R, Petrelli L, Leon A. Nerve growth factor: from neurotrophin to neurokine. Trends Neurosci. 1996;19:514–20.
15. Lindsay RM, Harmar AJ. Nerve growth factor regulates expression of neuropeptides genes in adult sensory neurons. Nature. 1989;337:362–4.

16. Reinshagen M, Rohm H, Geerling I, Eysselein VE, Adler G. Role of neurotrophin-3 and nerve growth factor in chronic experimental colitis in the rat. Gastroenterology. 1996;110:A1111.
17. Reinshagen M, Rohm H, Geerling I *et al*. Expression of nerve growth factor prohormones in experimental colitis and inflammatory bowel disease. Gastroenterology. 1996;110:A1111.
18. Sadlack B, Merz H, Schorle H, Schimpl A, Feller AC, Horak I. Ulcerative colitis-like disease in mice with a disrupted interleukin-2 gene. Cell. 1993;75:253–61.
19. Ehrhardt RO, Ludviksson BR, Gray B, Neurath M, Strober W. Induction and prevention of colonic inflammation in IL-2-deficient mice. J Immunol. 1997;158:566–73.
20. Rohm H, Lakshmanan J, Adler G, Reinshagen M. Differential expression of neurotrophins and their Trk tyrosine kinase receptors in the inflamed colon of IL-2 knockout mice. Gastroenterology. 1998;114:A1071.
21. Leach MW, Bean AG, Mauze S, Coffman RL, Powrie F. Inflammatory bowel disease in C.B-17 scid mice reconstituted with the CD45RBhigh subset of CD4+ T cells. Am J Pathol. 1996;148:1503–15.
22. Rudolphi A, Boll G, Poulsen SS, Claesson MH, Reimann J. Gut homing CD4+ T cell receptor ab+ T cells in the pathogenesis of murine inflammatory bowel disease. Eur J Immunol. 1994;24:2803–12.
23. Reinshagen M, Rohm H, Bonhagen K *et al*. Expression of NGF prohormone in the lamina propria CD4+ lymphocytes repopulating SCID mice. Gastroenterology. 1996;112:A1070.
24. Lambiase A, Bracci Laudiero L, Bonini S *et al*. Human CD4+ T cell clones produce and release nerve growth factor and express high-affinity nerve growth factor receptors. J Allergy Clin Immunol. 1997;100:408–14.
25. Ehrhard PB, Erb P, Graumann U, Schmutz B, Otten U. Expression of functional trk tyrosine kinase receptors after T cell activation. J Immunol. 1994;152:2705–9.
26. Ehrhard PB, Erb P, Graumann U, Otten U. Expression of nerve growth factor and nerve growth factor receptor tyrosine kinase Trk in activated CD4-positive T-cell clones. Proc Natl Acad Sci USA. 1993;90:10984–8.
27. Otten U, Scully C, Ehrhard P, Gadient RA. Neurotrophins: signals between the nervous and the immune systems. Progr Brain Res. 1994;103:293–305.
28. Aloe L, Tuveri MA, Levi Montalcini R. Studies on carrageenan-induced arthritis in adult rats: presence of nerve growth factor and role of sympathetic innervation. Rheumatol Int. 1992;12:213–16.
29. Santambrogio L, Benedetti M, Chao MV *et al*. Nerve growth factor production by lymphocytes. J Immunol. 1994;153:4488–95.

7
Interleukin-12 and anti-interleukin-12

M. F. NEURATH

Inflammatory bowel disease (IBD) encompasses Crohn's disease (CD) and ulcerative colitis, the major chronic inflammatory diseases of the gastrointestinal tract in humans[1,2]. Recently, various animal models of chronic intestinal inflammation have been established which will probably provide new insights into the pathogenesis of IBD (reviewed in ref. 3). These include rats carrying transgenes for HLA-B27 and β_2-microglobulin[4], T cell reconstituted Tgε26 mice transgenic for the human CD3ε gene[5], and mice in which the genes for IL-2[6], IL-10[7], Gα_{i2}[8] and the alpha or beta chain of the T cell receptor[9] have been inactivated by homologous recombination. In addition, a Th1-mediated granulomatous colitis model has been established by the adoptive transfer of normal CD45RB^{hi} T cells from BALB/c mice to C.B.-17 *scid* mice[10]. Importantly, in this model, the CD45RB^{lo} CD4+ T cell population did not cause disease and, if injected together with the CD45RB^{hi} population, prevented disease induction[11]; in addition, this prevention could be reversed by adding antibodies to transforming growth factor beta (TGF-β), suggesting a key negative role for this cytokine in disease induction.

Interestingly, it was shown that in most animal models of IBD production of Th1-type cytokines such as interferon-γ (IFN-γ) by CD4+ T cells is a major feature of the inflammation. This overproduction of IFN-γ leads to a dysbalance between protective Th2 and Th3 cytokines and pathogenic Th1 cytokines in the mucosal immune system (Figure 1). Furthermore, it has been shown that the Th1 cytokine production in these models is triggered by increased production of IL-12 heterodimer, a cytokine that plays a major role in driving Th1 cell differentiation[12,13]. IL-12 is a recently characterized cytokine with unique structure and pleiotropic effects[14–17]. It consists of two disulphide-linked subunits, p40 and p35, that form functionally active p40/p35 heterodimers or inhibitory p40 homodimers. IL-12 is produced mainly by macrophages/monocytes and to a lesser extent by activated B cells and follicular dendritic cells. It can be efficiently induced by intracellular parasites, bacteria and bacterial products. Functional studies showed that IL-12 enhances cytolytic activity of NK cells and macrophages and induces, in synergism with the B7/CD28 interaction, cytokine production and proliferation of activated NK cells and T cells[18,19].

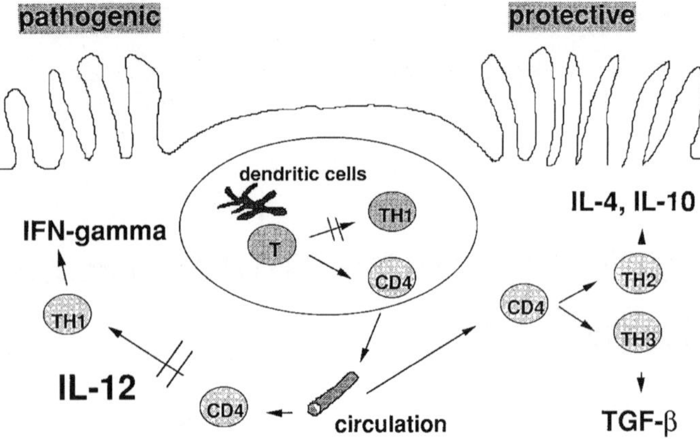

Figure 1 Protective and pathogenic roles of cytokines in the mucosal immune system in Th1-colitis models

Furthermore, IL-12 plays a pivotal role in Th1 T cell differentiation and induces naive T cells to produce IFN-γ via binding to a specific receptor and activation of a specific signalling protein (STAT-4; Figure 2). As a result of this ability to drive T cell responses to the Th1 phenotype, IL-12 has been shown to be an effective treatment of established parasitic infections in mice[20–22], which elicit a Th2 T cell response. In addition, antibodies to IL-12 have been shown to prevent experimental autoimmune encephalitis, a disease mediated by Th1 T cells[23].

With regard to experimental colitis, we have previously shown that the murine TNBS model is mediated by IL-12-driven Th1 CD4+ T cells and can be treated with anti-IL-12[12]. Furthermore, it was shown that TNBS-induced colitis can be

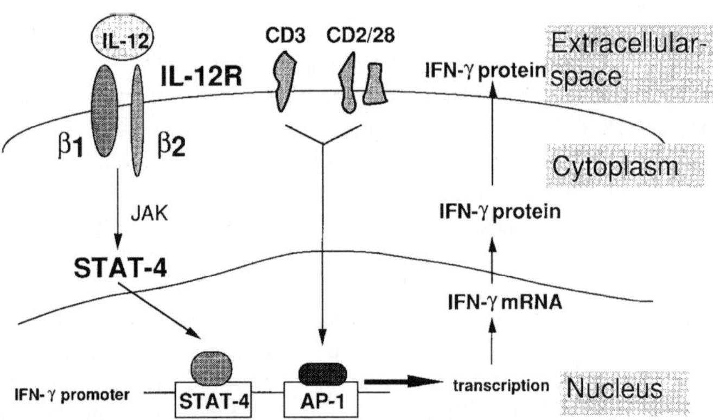

Figure 2 Function of IL-12. Upon binding to its receptor IL-12 activates the STAT-4 protein. Simultaneous activation of AP-1 then leads to enhanced IFN gene transcription in T lymphocytes (from Jacobsen *et al.*, JEM. 1995; Barbulescu and Neurath, J Immunol. 1998)

actively suppressed via oral tolerance by feeding of haptenized colonic proteins (HCP), and that such tolerance is critically dependent on TGF-β production by intestinal cells. TGF-β has been shown to be a potent inhibitor of IL-12-induced Th1 development[13] and TGF-β-producing cells generated upon feeding may prevent IL-12-dependent Th1 cell development upon which TNBS-induced colitis is critically dependent.

The relevance of these findings on IL-12 to Crohn's disease in humans is underlined by recent studies showing that this disease is also associated with an excessive Th1 T cell response (Figure 3) driven by IL-12-sensitive lamina propria T cells that exhibit large amounts of nuclear STAT-4 (Neurath *et al.*, unpublished data; Figures 4 and 5). These studies suggest that activation of IL-12 is a key element in the pathogenesis of Crohn's disease, and therapeutic blockade of IL-12 may be a promising way to treat patients with this disease.

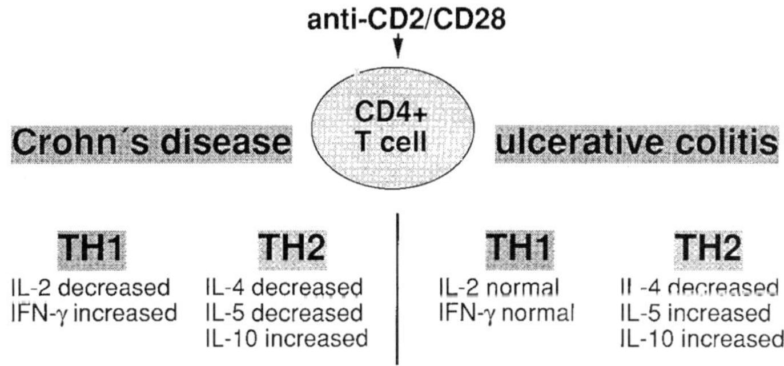

Figure 3 Cytokine profiles by activated CD4+ T cells in IBD (from Fuss *et al.* 1997)

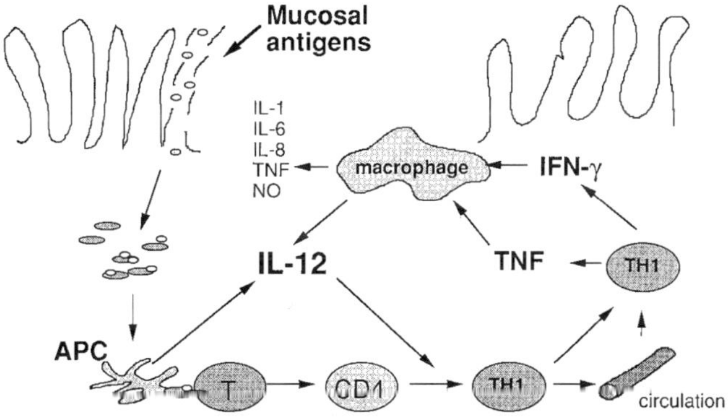

Figure 4 Central role of IL-12 in the pathogenesis of Crohn's disease

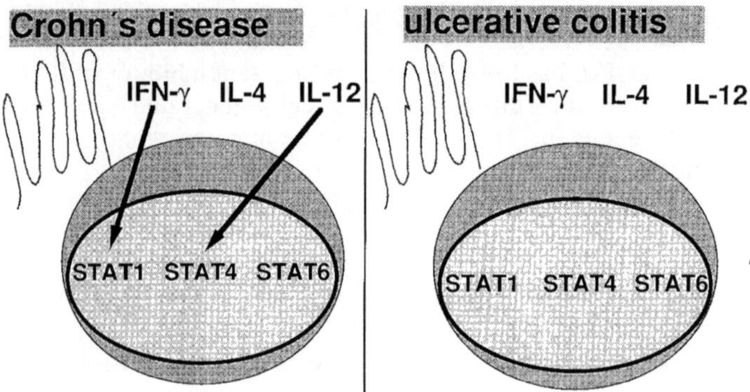

Figure 5 Cytokine signalling in IBD. Activation of IL-12 in Crohn's disease causes activation of STAT-4 but not STAT-6

References

1. Podolsky DK. Inflammatory bowel disease. N Engl J Med. 1991;325:928–35.
2. Strober W, Neurath MF. Immunological diseases of the gastrointestinal tract. In: Rich RR, editor. Clinical Immunology. St Louis: Mosby; 1995;1401–28.
3. Strober W, Ehrhardt RO. Chronic intestinal inflammation: an unexpected outcome on cytokine or T cell receptor mutant mice. Cell. 1993;75:203–5.
4. Hammer RE, Maika SD, Richardson JA, Tang YP, Taurog JD. Spontaneous inflammatory disease in transgenic rats expressing HLA-B27 and human β2m: an animal model of HLAB-27-associated human disorders. Cell. 1990;63:1099–112.
5. Holländer GA, Simpson SJ, Mizoguchi E *et al.* Severe colitis in mice with aberrant thymic selection. Immunity. 1995;3:27–38.
6. Sadlack B, Merz H, Schorle H, Schimpl A, Feller AC, Horvak I. Ulcerative colitis-like disease in mice with a disrupted interleukin-2 gene. Cell. 1993;75:253–61.
7. Kühn R, Löhler J, Rennick D, Rajewsky K, Müller W. Interleukin-10-deficient mice develop chronic enterocolitis. Cell. 1993;75:263–74.
8. Rudolph U, Finegold MJ, Rich SS *et al.* Ulcerative colitis and adenocarcinoma of the colon in $G\alpha_{i2}$-deficient mice. Nature Genet. 1995;10:143–6.
9. Mombaerts P, Mizoguchi E, Grusby MJ, Glimcher LH, Bahn AK, Tonegawa S. Spontaneous development of inflammatory bowel disease in T cell receptor mutant mice. Cell. 1993;75:275–82.
10. Powrie F, Leach MW, Mauze S, Menon S, Caddle LB, Coffman RL. Inhibition of Th1 responses prevents inflammatory bowel disease in scid mice reconstituted with CD45RBhi CD4+ T cells. Immunity. 1994;1:553–62.
11. Powrie F, Correa-Oliveira R, Mauze S, Coffman RL. Regulatory interactions between CD45RBhi and CD45RBlo CD4+ T cells are important for the balance between protective and pathogenic cell-mediated immunity. J Exp Med. 1994;179:589–600.
12. Neurath MF, Fuss I, Kelsall BL, Stüber E, Strober W. Antibodies to IL-12 abrogate established experimental colitis in mice. J Exp Med. 1995;182:1281–90.
13. Schmitt E, Hoehn P, Huels C, *et al.* T helper type 1 development of naive CD4+ T cells requires the coordinate action of interleukin-12 and interferon-γ and is inhibited by transforming growth factor-β. Eur J Immunol. 1994;24:793–8.
14. Kobayashi M, Fitz L, Ryan M *et al.* Identification and purification of natural killer cell stimulatory factor (NKSF), a cytokine with multiple biological effects on human lymphocytes. J Exp Med. 1989;170:827.
15. Seder RA, Gazzinelli R, Sher A, Paul WE. IL-12 acts directly on CD4+ T cells to enhance priming for IFN-γ production and diminishes IL-4 inhibition of such priming. Proc Natl Acad Sci USA. 1993;90:10188.

16. Ling P, Gately MK, Gubler U *et al.* Human IL-12 p40 homodimer binds to the IL-12 receptor but does not mediate biologic activity. J Immunol. 1995;154:116.
17. Podlaski FJ, Nanduri VB, Hulmes JD *et al.* Molecular characterization of interleukin 12. Arch Biochem Biophys. 1992;294:230.
18. Chua AO, Chizzonite R, Desai BB *et al.* Expression cloning of a human IL-12 receptor component. A new member of the cytokine receptor superfamily with strong homology to gp130. J Immunol. 1994;153:128.
19. Kubin M, Kamoun M, Trinchieri G. Interleukin 12 synergizes with B7/CD28 interaction in inducing efficient proliferation and cytokine production of human T cells. J Exp Med. 1994;180:211.
20. Alzona M, Jäck H-M, Fisher RI, Ellis TM. IL-12 activates IFN-γ production through the preferential activation of CD30+ T cells. J Immunol. 1995;154:9.
21. Wynn TA, Eltoum I, Oswald IP, Cheever AW, Sher A. Endogenous interleukin 12 (IL-12) regulates granuloma formation induced by eggs of *Schistosoma mansoni* and exogenous IL-12 both inhibits and prophylactically immunizes against egg pathology. J Exp Med. 1994;179:1551.
22. Murray HW, Hariprashad J. Interleukin 12 is effective treatment for an established systemic intracellular infection: experimental visceral leishmaniasis. J Exp Med. 1995;181:387.
23. Leonard JP, Waldburger KE, Goldman SJ. Prevention of experimental autoimmune encephalomyelitis by antibodies against interleukin 12. J Exp Med. 1995;181:381.

8
Spontaneous colitis and gastritis in HLA-B27/β_2-microglobulin transgenic rats and its association with normal luminal bacteria

H. C. RATH

THE MHC CLASS I MOLECULE HLA-B27/β_2 MICROGLOBULIN AND HUMAN DISEASES

The major histocompatibility complex (MHC) is a region of genetic loci which plays an important role in immunoregulation. Its highly polymorphic cell surface structures in humans are called human leukocyte antigens (HLA). HLA class I molecules, dimers with a variable α- (heavy-)chain and the invariant β_2-microglobulin, are expressed on all nucleated cells and platelets and present intracellular antigens to CD8 T lymphocytes[1]. HLA-B27 is the MHC class I molecule with the strongest association to human diseases[2]. More than 90% of patients with ankylosing spondylitis carry the HLA-B27 antigen and they suffer from a prolonged and more aggressive course of disease than those who are B27 negative[3]. It is also present in patients with reactive arthritis, psoriatic arthritis, juvenile spondyloarthropathy and arthritis occurring in inflammatory bowel disease (IBD). Some observations associate intestinal inflammation with HLA-B27 positive disorders: a high prevalence of spondyloarthropathy is found in patients with IBD; certain enteropathogenic bacteria predictably trigger B27-associated reactive arthritis; moreover, at least subclinical ileocolitis has been found in two-thirds of patients with HLA-B27 positive spondyloarthropathies examined by ileocolonoscopy[4].

HLA-B27/β_2 MICROGLOBULIN TRANSGENIC RATS

To investigate the influence of HLA-B27 on disorders stated above, HLA-B27 and human β_2-microglobulin genes were introduced by microinjection into fertilized one-cell eggs of rats on Lewis or Fischer background[5]. These rats spontaneously develop gastrointestinal inflammation, predominantly in the caecum and antrum, arthritis, dermatitis, orchitis and epididymitis, carditis, nail changes and neurological disorders. The influence of the genetic background is demonstrated by an earlier onset and more aggressive arthritis and the presence of seizures and nail changes in transgenic rats on Lewis background, but an earlier onset of colitis and the restriction of colonic ulcers, polyps, and adenocarcinomas to transgenic Fischer rats[6,7]. Disease susceptibility correlates with gene copy number and the quantity of B27 in the lymphoid cells[7]. Animals with high copy numbers of the transgene develop disease even in the hemizygous state, whereas disease in transgenic rats with moderate copy numbers is restricted to the homozygous state and animals with low level of gene expression fail to develop disease even in the homozygous state[7]. For investigations of gastrointestinal disorders, transgenic rats on Fischer background with high-level expression of the HLA-B27 gene were used. Gastrointestinal inflammation is the earliest sign of the multiorgan disease in transgenic Fischer rats beginning at approximately 2 months of age with an incidence of 100% at 3 months of age[7]. The colon is thickened with no grossly detectable signs of adhesions or ulcerations. Histological signs in the colon and a caecum are: infiltration of inflammatory cells, predominantly mononuclear cells, mostly limited to the mucosa; reduction of goblet cells; crypt hyperplasia; occasionally crypt abscesses and early ulcers. Histological inflammation is also detected in the stomach, more in the antrum, less in the proximal glandular stomach and not in the squamous portion[8]. Increased colonic levels of interferon-γ (INF-γ) and interleukin-1 (IL-1) and attenuation of inflammation with IL-11 therapy implicate activated T lymphocytes and macrophages in disease pathogenesis[8,9]. The chronic colitis seems to be associated with enhanced nitric oxide metabolism[10].

The pathomechanism of this model is not completely understood. Cell transfer experiments have investigated the cellular mechanisms of this model[11]. Bone marrow and fetal liver cells from transgenic rats could transfer disease to non-transgenic littermates but mature lymphocytes and spleen cells mostly failed to induce disease. Active disease in the donors was not necessary for disease induction. Engraftment of non-transgenic bone marrow led to remission of spontaneous disease in irradiated transgenic rats[11]. These results emphasize the essential role of HLA-B27 expression in bone marrow-derived cells and suggest that HLA-B27/β_2-microglobulin expression by epithelial, endothelial, and other non-immune cells is not necessary for disease induction. Recently it has been shown that low affinity of B27 to human β_2-microglobulin may result in free heavy chains which modify T-cell selection in the thymus and function in a similar way to MHC class II molecules by presenting exogenous bacterial antigen to CD4+ T cells[12]. HLA-B27 transgenic mice, where endogenous β_2-microglobulin gene was replaced with transgenic human β_2m gene, showed cell surface expression of HLA-B27 similar to that of human peripheral blood mononuclear cells. In addition, free heavy chains of HLA-B27 were also expressed on thymic epithelium and on a subpopulation of B27-expressing peripheral blood lymphocytes. These mice developed spontaneous arthritis and nail changes in the rear paws. Transgenic mice expressing HLA-B27 with mouse β_2-microglobulin have undetectable levels of free heavy chains on the cell surface and do not develop arthritis. *In-vivo* treatment with anti-heavy chain-specific antibody delayed the onset of disease[12].

HLA-B27 TRANSGENIC RATS AND THEIR ASSOCIATION WITH NORMAL LUMINAL BACTERIA

Both genetic and environmental factors have been documented in the pathogenesis of the idiopathic IBD, ulcerative colitis and Crohn's disease[13]. Substantial data from clinical observations and animal models incriminate commensal luminal bacteria or bacterial products in the initiation and perpetuation of chronic enterocolitis and associated systemic inflammation[14], although the critical bacterial components or antigen(s) are not yet known.

A bacterial influence on intestinal and joint inflammation was demonstrated by the lack of colitis and arthritis in B27 transgenic rats raised under germ-free conditions[15]. The aims of our studies were to examine systematically the effects of commensal luminal bacteria on the initiation and perpetuation of spontaneous gastrointestinal and systemic inflammation in HLA-B27 transgenic rats.

Evidence for commensal luminal bacteria in the pathogenesis of colitis, gastritis and arthritis

Transgenic and non-transgenic littermates raised in a germ-free environment were divided into two groups at 6–8 weeks of age[8]. One group remained in sterile isolators until necropsy at 3–9 months of age. The second group was conventionalized with specific pathogen-free rat bacterial flora. All rats were monitored weekly for clinical evidence of diarrhoea and arthritis, then were killed by CO_2 asphyxiation within 3 hours of removal from gnotobiotic isolators.

Transgenic conventionalized rats were the only group to show diarrhoea or clinical signs of arthritis. The onset of the non-bloody diarrhoea and arthritis was variable in the conventionalized transgenic rats, but peaked by 3 months of age. Arthritis followed an undulating pattern with spontaneous remission, and was relatively mild. There were no differences in weight gain, dermatitis, orchitis and epididymitis, or incidence of hair loss in transgenic conventionalized rats compared with transgenic germ-free littermates.

At necropsy transgenic conventionalized rats had overall more thickening of the caecal and colonic walls than transgenic germ-free and non-transgenic conventionalized littermates ($p < 0.001$); the latter two groups had no detectable lesions.

Similar to the gross observations, transgenic conventionalized rats had significantly more histological caecal inflammation ($p < 0.0001$) than germ-free and conventionalized non-transgenic littermates. These lesions were similar to those previously described in conventionally housed B27 transgenic rats[5,7,15]. Histological inflammatory scores were not significantly different between germ-free transgenic and non-transgenic conventionalized rats.

Colonic myeloperoxidase (MPO) activity was increased in transgenic conventionalized rats ($p < 0.005$) compared with transgenic germ-free and non-transgenic rats; no differences were seen between the transgenic germ-free and non-transgenic groups.

Tissue IL-1α protein concentrations in the transverse colon were increased in transgenic conventionalized rats compared with undetectable levels in transgenic germ-free and non-transgenic conventionalized rats ($p < 0.0001$). Elevated mRNA levels of the monokines IL-1α, IL-1β and tumour necrosis factor α (TNF-α) were demonstrated in the inflamed colonic tissues of the transgenic conventionalized rats but were undetectable in transgenic germ-free rats. In addition, we observed an increase in IL-6 mRNA expression in some of the transgenic conventionalized animals. All colons had detectable IL-1ra expression, which increased following bacterial exposure. IFN-γ mRNA was strongly elevated in rats with intestinal inflammation compared with the non-inflamed tissues of transgenic germ-free and non-transgenic conventionalized rats.

The stomach of transgenic conventionalized rats was inflamed predominantly in the antrum and less extensively in the proximal glandular portion. As in the caecum, the blinded histological scores of inflammation in these areas of the stomach were significantly increased in transgenic conventionalized rats ($p < 0.0001$) compared with germ-free littermates. Germ-free transgenic and conventionalized non-transgenic rats had similar histological scores. No inflammation was detectable in the squamous portion of the stomach in any group.

Duodenal inflammation in germ-free transgenic rats was less than in conventionalized littermates ($p < 0.005$) and was not different from conventionalized non-transgenic rats. No consistent inflammatory changes were seen in the jejunum and ileum of conventionalized transgenic rats and, when present, were less extensive than in the duodenum and colon. There were no significant differences in ileitis in germ-free and conventionalized transgenic rats.

Transgenic conventionalized rats had the highest degree of leukocytosis ($p < 0.001$), but germ-free transgenic rats also had elevated white blood cell (WBC) concentrations relative to non-transgenic controls ($p < 0.05$).

Time-course of inflammation after bacterial exposure

To determine the kinetics of the onset of inflammation following bacterial colonization, transgenic rats were observed for 1–4 weeks following exposure to SPF bacteria[8]. Colonic MPO levels progressively increased and were significantly elevated at 4 weeks ($p < 0.05$). Gross and histological assessment of colonic inflammation followed the same time-course. Arthritis was not seen during this brief period of bacterial exposure.

The role of anaerobic bacteria in the pathogenesis of colitis and gastritis

To address the question whether all bacteria are equally capable of inducing gastrointestinal inflammation transgenic rats raised in a SPF environment were divided into three groups at 2 months of age, when colitis is first becoming evident[16]. In one group a caecal self-filling blind loop (SFBL) was created, in the second the caecum was excluded from the faecal stream (EX), and the third group was sham operated (SHAM). Non-transgenic littermates were SHAM or SFBL operated and served as negative controls. All rats were monitored weekly for clinical evidence of diarrhoea and arthritis. One month after surgery, at the age of 3 months, all rats were killed by CO_2 asphyxiation.

All transgenic SFBL rats had diarrhoea 3–4 weeks after surgery compared with none of the SHAM and EX ($p < 0.0005$). One transgenic rat with SFBL developed active arthritis but no arthritis was seen in the SHAM and EX groups. Non-transgenic rats had no evidence of diarrhoea or arthritis.

The blinded gross gut score of the caecum was significantly increased in the transgenic SFBL compared with transgenic SHAM rats ($p < 0.0001$). There were no macroscopic signs of inflammation in the transgenic EX and non-transgenic SHAM groups ($p < 0.001$ vs. transgenic SHAM).

Mucosal inflammation increased in transgenic SFBL rats and extended to the submucosa compared to transgenic SHAM controls. The majority of transgenic SFBL rats (75%) had submucosal inflammation vs. 0% of transgenic SHAM rats ($p < 0.01$). More aggressive caecal inflammation in SFBL transgenic rats was confirmed by blinded histological inflammatory scores ($p < 0.005$). There was almost no evidence of caecal inflammation in transgenic EX rats, as confirmed by the lack of difference in histological scores of transgenic EX and non-transgenic SHAM rats (both $p < 0.0001$ vs. transgenic SHAM).

IL-1β protein concentrations in the caecal tissue of transgenic EX were significantly reduced compared with transgenic SHAM ($p < 0.01$). However, there were no differences evident between transgenic SHAM and SFBL or between transgenic EX and non-transgenic SHAM groups.

Non-transgenic SFBL rats had grossly detectable caecal thickening but had only very mild inflammation by histological criteria.

Antral gastritis, with mucosal thickening and mononuclear cell infiltration predominantly in the basal two-thirds of the crypts, was a consistent histological feature in transgenic SHAM and SFBL rats. Surprisingly, gastritis was significantly decreased in the transgenic EX group ($p < 0.0005$) and totally absent in some of these animals. There was no gastritis in non-transgenic SFBL animals.

In SHAM-operated rats the total, microscopically visible number of bacteria/ml luminal contents in the stomach, jejunum, and ileum was one log less than in the caecum and colon. Anaerobically and aerobically cultivatable bacterial concentrations were lowest in the jejunum and highest in the caecum and colon. Our results demonstrate a luxurious growth of bacteria in the rat stomach. Bacteria in the stomach and jejunum were predominantly Gram-positive rods and coccobacilli, and spores were present in the ileum. The microscopic picture of the caecal bacteria was quite complex, yet similar to the colon, dominated by Gram-positive bacilli and spores with less frequent Gram-negative bacilli. Using selective culture media, concentrations of presumed *Bacteroides* spp. were 3–6 logs higher in the caecum and colon compared with the small intestine. One out of three rats had no detectable *Bacteroides* spp. in the stomach. The concentrations of total visible bacteria in the caecal contents were equal between the SFBL and SHAM groups. However, the ratio of all anaerobic bacteria to only facultative anaerobic bacteria in the SFBL group and the concentrations of caecal *Bacteroides* spp. were up to 1000- and 10 000-fold, respectively, that of the SHAM group. Rats from the transgenic EX group had decreased total and viable caecal bacterial concentrations in the caecum than SHAM. Although bacterial concentrations/ml caecal contents were similar between the SFBL and SHAM groups, the enlarged caeca of SFBL rats were considerably heavier, due to increased luminal contents and the thickened caecal walls, leading to much higher bacterial loads in the SFBL caeca. The total concentrations of bacteria in the stomach and colon were not different between the groups.

This study emphasizes the direct influence of the caecal anaerobic bacterial load, especially *Bacteroides* spp., on local inflammation in the caecum, since the degree of inflammation correlates with levels of isolates on *Bacteroides*-selective medium. Moreover, it demonstrates that the caecal bacterial load influences remote inflammation in the distal colon and stomach through as-yet-undefined mechanisms.

The role of *Bacteroides vulgatus* in colitis and gastritis

At 2 months of age, germ-free transgenic rats were transferred into separate isolators and colonized with one of three different specific bacterial cocktails: Charles River Altered Schaedler (CRAS), DESEP (*Streptococcus faecium, Escherichia coli, Streptococcus avium, Eubacterium contortum, Peptostreptococcus productus*), and DESEP-B (DESEP and *Bacteroides vulgatus*). Transgenic control rats were either kept germ-free or conventionalized with SPF bacteria. Each group of colonized rats were maintained under gnotobiotic conditions. Successful bacterial colonization was confirmed by culturing and Gram staining faecal pellets 1 week after inoculation, and of the caecal content at necropsy.

Neither diarrhoea nor arthritis was observed in the gnotobiotic groups and germ-free or conventionalized controls over the 1 month of bacterial exposure[8]. Caecal inflammation occurred in CRAS and DESEP-B colonized transgenic animals, but not in DESEP and germ-free rats, as shown by gross and histological observations as well as tissue MPO and IL-1β protein concentration. Colitis was consistently highest in the DESEP-B group of gnotobiotic rats by all observed parameters. Gastritis was significantly higher than germ-free rats only in DESEP-B animals; however, gastritis and caecal inflammation in the DESEP-B group did not reach the degree of inflammation observed in transgenic conventionalized rats.

In the second experiment HLA-B27 transgenic rats raised under germ-free (sterile) conditions were divided in four groups at the age of 2 months[17]. One group remained germ-free and served as negative control, the other groups were transferred into separate isolators and colonized with different bacteria or bacterial cocktails. One group was colonized with *B. vulgatus*, another group with *E. coli*, and a third group with DESEP-B, which served as positive controls. Persistent selective bacterial colonization was documented by faecal Gram stain and culture. All rats were clinically observed for evidence of diarrhoea and arthritis and were killed at 3 months of age (1 month after colonization) by CO_2 asphyxiation within 3 hours of removal from the gnotobiotic isolators.

There was no evidence of grossly detectable inflammation in any group. By blinded microscopic scores rats monoassociated with *B. vulgatus* had almost as much caecal inflammation as the positive controls colonized with the six commensals, including *B. vulgatus* ($p = 0.06$). Rats monoassociated with *E. coli* had almost no caecal inflammation and were nearly identical to germ-free animals ($p = 0.06$). Transgenic rats monoassociated with *B. vulgatus* had more severe caecal inflammation than those monoassociated with *E. coli* ($p = 0.001$). Caecal MPO activity confirmed the lack of difference between DESEP-B and *B. vulgatus* colonized rats and significantly increased inflammation in both of these groups compared with *E. coli* monoassociated ($p < 0.03$) and germ-free rats ($p < 0.0001$). However, in contrast to the lack of histological inflammation in *E. coli* mono-associated rats, colonic MPO levels were significantly increased in the *E. coli* group compared with germ-free controls ($p < 0.0001$). IL-1β protein concentrations in the caecal tissue were not significantly different between the gnotobiotic groups, all of which were significantly elevated compared to germ-free rats ($p > 0.0005$ vs. germ-free; *B. vulgatus* vs. *E. coli* $p = 0.06$). Total luminal bacterial concentrations in the caecum were not different between the groups (1.0–4.4×10^{11} bacteria/ml caecal contents). By Gram staining *E. coli* outnumbered *B. vulgatus* by approximately 5:1 in DESEP-B rats.

Transgenic rats colonized with DESEP-B had active antral mucosal inflammation ($p < 0.05$ vs. germ-free). However, transgenic rats monoassociated with either *B. vulgatus* or *E. coli* had significantly less gastritis ($p < 0.04$ vs. DESEP-B) and were not different from germ-free rats.

These results indicate that the bacterial concentration and composition of the caecum is important, not only in inducing local colitis, but also in stimulating remote inflammation, including the stomach. Different bacteria have different roles in the inflammatory process: *B. vulgatus* has a key role in initiating colitis in B27 transgenic rats, and other strains, although they cannot initiate colitis, have an important role in mediating inflammation in remote organs such as the stomach. To prove this hypothesis we have performed the experiments described below.

The effect of antibiotic treatment on colitis

To address the hypothesis that a small subset of commensal luminal bacteria, although important in initiating colitis, is only one of a variety of bacteria capable of perpetuating disease, we administered several antibiotics to HLA-B27 transgenic rats[18].

Transgenic rats and non-transgenic littermates were treated with either antibiotics (ciprofloxacin 50 mg/kg, metronidazole 40 mg/kg, or vancomycin/imipenem 50/50 mg/kg) in drinking water or water alone as control. Prevention started soon after weaning (4 weeks); treatment was begun at 3 months of age. All rats were killed at 4 months of age.

Although preventive metronidazole significantly attenuated colitis ($p < 0.005$ vs. transgenic water controls) there was no benefit in treating with metronidazole once colitis was established. These results were confirmed by tissue-IL-1β. Antibiotic therapy with vancomycin/imipenem, a broad-spectrum combination, was effective in both treatment ($p < 0.0001$ vs. transgenic water control) and in prevention ($p < 0.0001$ vs. transgenic water control). However, even vancomycin/imipenem did not completely abrogate inflammation ($p < 0.005$ vs. non-transgenic water controls). Ciprofloxacin, which inhibits a variety of intestinal Gram-negative bacteria, had similar histological effects to metronidazole ($p < 0.05$ vs. transgenic water control in prevention and n.s. in treatment) but did not reduce tissue IL-1β.

These results suggest that defined bacterial subsets initiate colitis, but that a much broader range of commensal bacteria can provide the constant antigenic drive for chronic inflammation once mucosal permeability is altered.

SUMMARY

These results indicate that: (1) resident luminal bacteria are important in the initiation and perpetuation of chronic colitis and gastritis in HLA-B27 transgenic rats; (2) not all bacterial strains have equal ability to cause gastrointestinal inflammation; (3) anaerobic bacteria, especially *B. vulgatus*, have a key role in initiating colitis in B27 transgenic rats, and that other strains, although they cannot initiate colitis, have an important role in mediating inflammation in remote organs such as the stomach. One may hypothesize that the bacterial concentration and composition of the caecum is important not only in inducing local colitis, but also in stimulating remote inflammation, including the stomach. Luminal bacteria prime caecal lymphocytes in the lymphoid aggregates of the caecal tip, which then circulate systemically and home to remote mucosal organs where they are activated if they are exposed to the same bacterial antigens present in the caecum. This hypothesis would explain: (1) the lack of gastritis in rats monoassociated with *B. vulgatus*, since this obligate anaerobe is not present in the partially aerobic stomach in high concentrations; (2) the lack of gastritis in rats monoassociated with *E. coli*, since *E. coli* does not initiate chronic inflammation in the caecum; and (3) the presence of gastritis in DESEP-B rats, since *B. vulgatus* initiates the caecal inflammation, which enhances bacterial antigens from facultative anaerobes present in the caecum as well as in the stomach. This hypothesis is supported by our own observations that HLA-B27 transgenic nude rats in a specific pathogen-free environment develop colitis and gastritis after transfer of lymphocytes from transgenic rats with colitis, while germ-free transgenic rats fail to develop intestinal inflammation after receiving the same T cells (unpublished observations).

The HLA-B27/β_2 microglobulin transgenic rat is an animal model for investigating the influence of commensal luminal bacteria on spontaneous chronic gastrointestinal disease and extraintestinal manifestations.

Acknowledgements

Most of the work described above was carried out at the laboratories of Dr R. Balfour Sartor, University of North Carolina at Chapel Hill, NC, and was supported by United States Public Health Service grants DK 34989, DK 40249, the Crohn's and Colitis Foundation of America (Dr Sartor) and the Deutsche Forschungsgemeinschaft Ra 671/1-1. The author gratefully acknowledges the supervision of Dr Sartor, the collaborators Hans H. Herfarth, MD; Jack S. Ikeda, PhD; Michael Schultz, MD; Leo A. Dieleman, MD; Kenneth H. Wilson, MD; Edward Balish, PhD; and Joel D. Taurog, MD; the technical support of Lisa C. Holt, Wetonia B. Grenther, Diane E. Bender, Roger Brown, Sanjib Mohanty, Ram Janardaham, Julie Vorobiov and Rhonda Blitchington, and the editorial support of Krishna Mondal, PhD.

References

1. Abbas AK, Lichtman AH, Pober JS. The Major Histocompatibility Complex. In: Abbas AK, Lichtman AH, Pober JS, editors. Cellular and Molecular Immunology, 2nd edn. Philadelphia: WD Saunders, 1994.96–114.

2. Inman RD, Scofield RH. Etiopathogenesis of ankylosing spondylitis and reactive arthritis. Curr Opin Rheumatol. 1994;6:360–70.
3. Linssen A. B27+ disease versus B27– disease. Scand J Rheumatol. Suppl. 1990;87:111–18 (discussion 118–19).
4. Sartor RB, Lichtman SN. Mechanisms of systemic inflammation associated with intestinal injury. In: Targan SR, Shanahan F, editors. Inflammatory Bowel Disease: From bench to bedside. Baltimore: Williams & Wilkins; 1993:210–29.
5. Hammer RE, Maika SD, Richardson JA, Tang JP, Taurog JD. Spontaneous inflammatory disease in transgenic rats expressing HLA-B27 and human beta 2m: an animal model of HLA-B27-associated human disorders. Cell. 1990;63:1099–112.
6. Hammer RE, Richardson JA, Simmons WA, White AL, Breban M, Taurog JD. High prevalence of colorectal cancer in HLA-B27 transgenic F344 rats with chronic inflammatory bowel disease. J Invest Med. 1995;43:262–8.
7. Taurog JD, Maika SD, Simmons WA, Breban M, Hammer RE. Susceptibility to inflammatory disease in HLA-B27 transgenic rat lines correlates with the level of B27 expression. J Immunol. 1993;150:4168–78.
8. Rath HC, Herfarth HH, Ikeda JS et al. Normal luminal bacteria, especially *Bacteroides* species, mediate chronic colitis, gastritis, and arthritis in HLA-B27/human beta2 microglobulin transgenic rats. J Clin Invest. 1996;98:945–53.
9. Keith JC, Jr, Albert L, Sonis ST, Pfeiffer CJ, Schaub RG. IL-11, a pleiotropic cytokine: exciting new effects of IL-11 on gastrointestinal mucosal biology. Stem Cells (Dayt). 1994;12 (Suppl. 1):79–89.
10. Aiko S, Grisham MB. Spontaneous intestinal inflammation and nitric oxide metabolism in HLA-B27 transgenic rats. Gastroenterology. 1995;109:142–50.
11. Breban M, Hammer RE, Richardson JA, Taurog JD. Transfer of the inflammatory disease of HLA-B27 transgenic rats by bone marrow engraftment. J Exp Med. 1993;178:1607–16.
12. Khare SD, Hansen J, Luthra HS, David CS. HLA-B27 heavy chains contribute to spontaneous inflammatory disease in B27/human beta2-microglobulin (beta2m) double transgenic mice with disrupted mouse beta2m. J Clin Invest. 1996;98:2746–55.
13. Sartor RB. Current concepts of etiology and pathogenesis of ulcerative colitis and Crohn's disease. Gastro Clin N Am. 1995;24:475–506.
14. Sartor RB. Microbial factors in the pathogenesis of Crohn's disease, ulcerative colitis and experimental intestinal inflammation. In: Kirsner JB, Shorter RG, editors. Inflammatory Bowel Disease. 4th edn. Baltimore: Williams & Wilkins; 1995:96–124.
15. Taurog JD, Richardson JA, Croft JT et al. The germfree state prevents development of gut and joint inflammatory disease in HLA-B27 transgenic rats. J Exp Med. 1994;180:2359–64.
16. Rath HC, Ikeda JS, Wilson KH, Sartor RB. Varying cecal bacterial loads influences colitis and gastritis in HLA-B27 transgenic rats. Gastroenterology. 1997;112:A1068 (abstract).
17. Rath HC, Schultz M, Grenther WB et al. Colitis, gastritis and antibacterial lymphocyte response in HLA-B27 transgenic rats monoassociated with *Bacteroides vulgatus* or *Escherichia coli*. Gastroenterology. 1997;112:A1068 (abstract).
18. Rath HC, Schultz M, Dieleman LA et al. Selective vs. broad spectrum antibiotics in the prevention and treatment of experimental colitis in two rodent models. Gastroenterology. 1998 (abstract).

Section III
Basic Concepts of Mucosal Immunology

9
Mucosal immune system: an overview

J. MESTECKY and C. O. ELSON

INTRODUCTION: MUCOSAL BARRIER

Mucosal surfaces represent by far the largest surface area (~400 m^2) of the host. Thus, it is not surprising that most pathogens invade through or infect mucosal tissues[1]. Furthermore, mucosal surfaces are colonized by an estimated 10^{14} bacteria that belong to more than 50 different species[2]. To defend such large areas continuously stimulated by resident or transient microbiota, and by the multitude of antigens present in ingested food and inhaled air, the host has developed innate and adoptive immune mechanisms consistent with the antigen burden (Figure 1). The mucosal immune system is quantitatively the largest

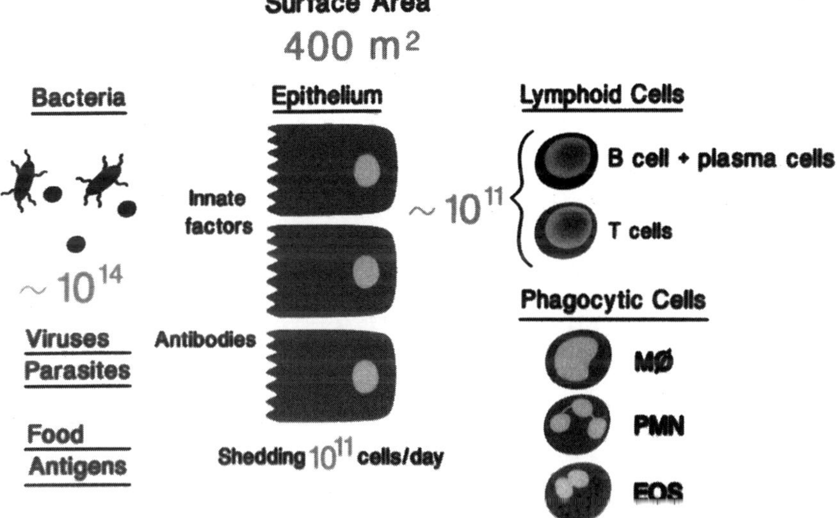

Figure 1 Defence mechanisms in mucosal tissues

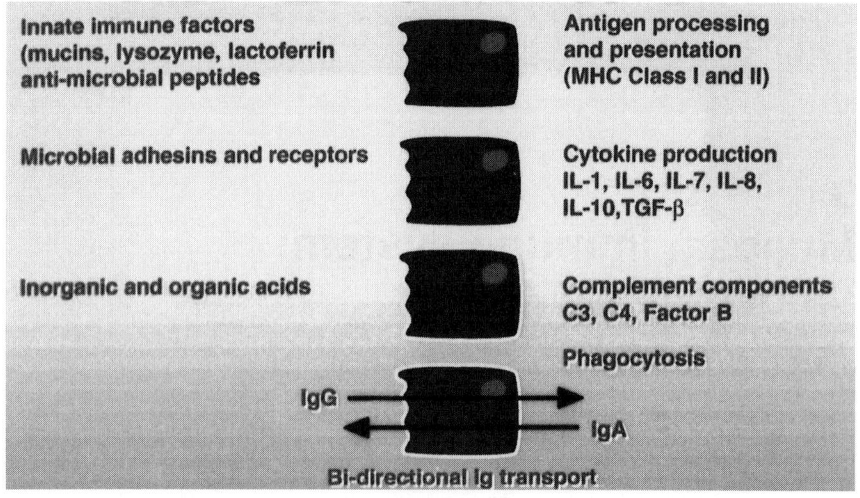

Figure 2 Functions of epithelial cells in mucosal defence

compartment of the immune system containing the majority of all lymphoid cells in the body[3]. Not surprisingly, it is the mucosal tissues, particularly the intestine, which are the sites of most antibody production in the body[4,5]. Mucosal epithelial cells also play a crucial role in mucosal defence[6,7] (Figure 2).

In addition to providing a mechanical barrier, epithelial cells remove inhaled antigens through their ciliary movement and, in the intestine, the large numbers of desquamated epithelial cells ($\sim10^{11}$ cells/day in the small intestine) retain receptor-bound bacteria (several hundred bacteria/cell) on their surfaces which are ultimately eliminated in the stool. Furthermore, epithelial cells are an important source of innate immune factors, such as mucins, lactoferrin, lactoperoxidase, lysozyme, and various antibacterial peptides. Considering their numbers, and the spectrum of pro- and anti-inflammatory and immunoregulatory cytokines (e.g. interleukin 6 (IL-6), IL-7, IL-8, IL-10, transforming growth factor beta (TGF-β), tumour necrosis factor alpha (TNF-α), MIP-1α and others) that they produce, the conclusion that the epithelial cells are essential partners in mucosal immunity is inescapable[6–8].

MUCOSAL LYMPHOID COMPARTMENTS

Lymphoid cells in the mucosal tissues are found in three histologically and functionally distinct compartments, Peyer's patches (PP), lamina propria lymphocytes, and intraepithelial lymphocytes.

Lymphoepithelial inductive sites

PP are organized lymphoid aggregates with one or more lymphoid follicles that extend from the epithelial layer into the lamina propria. Although PP are visible, macroscopic structures clustered in certain regions such as the ileum, structurally and functionally analogous small lymphoid follicles are dispersed abundantly throughout the intestine in humans and some other species[9–11]. PP and these small follicles together comprise gut-associated lymphoid tissue (GALT). PP differ from other peripheral lymphoreticular tissues by the lack of afferent lymphatics, but do have efferent lymphatics. Instead of afferent lymphatics, they have a specialized epithelium that actively takes up material present in the intestinal and luminal respiratory tracts and delivers it via transcytosis and exocytosis into the lymphoid follicle. Distinguishing features of this specialized follicle-associated epithelium (FAE) include a relative lack of goblet cells and the presence of M or microfold cells that lack polymeric immunoglobulin receptor (pIgR) (see below)[7,9,10]. The M cell serves as an important first step in the initiation of mucosal immune responses, but relatively little is known about the factors determining selectivity of the antigen uptake. Soluble proteins, viruses, bacteria, protozoa, and inert particles (e.g. liposomes and microspheres) are all taken up by M cells[9]. Some organisms such as *Salmonella* and poliovirus exploit this feature, using M cells as a portal of entry into the body. M cell uptake of *Salmonella* and particles such as microspheres is being exploited to deliver vaccine antigens into GALT.

Consistent with this active antigen uptake by the specialized dome epithelium, PP and related lymphoid follicles serve as sites for the induction of mucosal immune responses (Figure 3)[11]. It is now recognized that these lymphoepithelial structures contain all the cells needed for induction of immune responses, i.e. B cells, T cells, and antigen-processing and -presenting cells (macrophages, dendritic cells, and follicular dendritic cells)[12]. These cell types

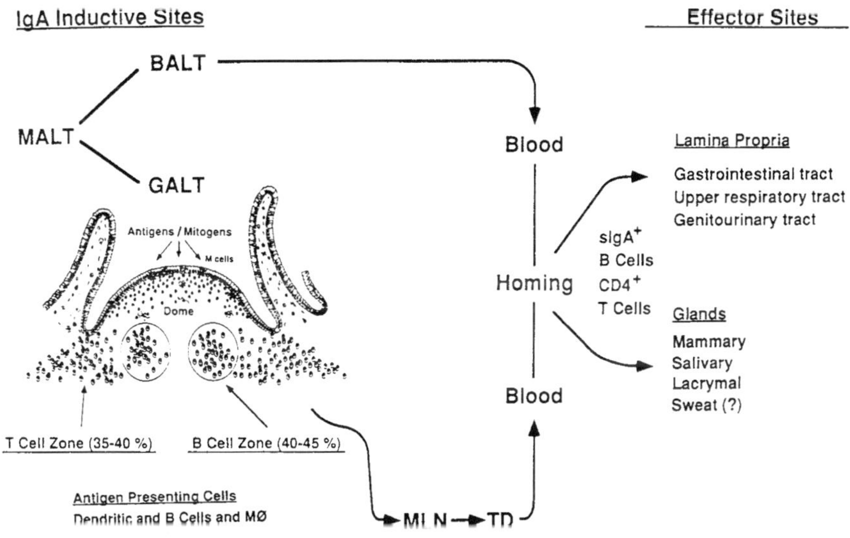

Figure 3 The common mucosal immune system. MALT, BALT, GALT – mucosa-, bronchus-, and gut associated lymphoepithelial tissues; MLN – mesenteric lymph nodes; TD – thoracic duct

are structured in B-cell-dependent and T-cell-dependent areas similar to other peripheral lymphoid tissues. B cells predominate in the lymphoid follicles, whereas T cells predominate in the interfollicular areas and beneath the dome epithelium; dendritic cells appear to be scattered both beneath the dome epithelium and in the follicles[9,10]. Quantitatively, B cells predominate in the PP of adult animals constituting some 60–70% of total cells, while T cells, including both CD4+ and CD8+ cells, comprise about 20% of the total. An important feature of PP cells is that they consist of precursor rather than effector cells[11]. For example, although the PP contains many B cells, few plasma cells are present, even after extensive immunization[9]. The same appears to be true for cytotoxic T cells (CTL). One explanation is that differentiating B cells and T cells leave PP and migrate to the gut and other lymphoid tissues (see below). A second important feature of PP is that the induction of immune responses there is highly dependent on the route of antigen exposure. PP respond predominantly, if not exclusively, to antigen present on the mucosal surface, that is, antigen transported by M cells; systemic immunization does not induce immune responses in PP.

GALT[12] are sites in which there is preferential induction of IgA responses[11], an important function considering that IgA is the major immunoglobulin at mucosal surfaces[4,5]. PP cells are enriched for B cell precursors of IgA-producing plasma cells relative to other lymphoid tissues[6], particularly for IgA B cell precursors recognizing antigens present in the intestine. The mechanism for this preferential expression of IgA by PP B cells is not clear, but microenvironmental-B-cell interactions, the influence of a specialized dendritic cell, or the expression of cytokines such as TGF-β in PP are possible explanations. Furthermore, T cells present in PP regulate B-cell differentiation by secreting a variety of cytokines[13,14].

The discovery that antigen-stimulated GALT or BALT are the source of antigen-sensitized and IgA-committed plasma cell precursors that populate remote mucosal tissues and glands has led to the concept of a *common mucosal immune system* (CMIS)[11],[12] in which an antigen exposure at one mucosal surface contributes cells to help protect remote mucosal sites also (Figure 3). For example, immunization of the gut or nasal mucosa can generate a mucosal response in tears, milk, saliva, and genital tract secretions. This had led to a renewed interest in the development of mucosally delivered vaccines to protect non-intestinal mucosal sites. Although priming for a mucosal response is convenient and effective, an optimal immunity at distant mucosal sites may also require local exposure of that mucosal surface to the antigen. In fact, the CMIS may contain certain subcompartments so that, for example, optimal vaginal immune responses may occur after rectal immunization, whereas optimal upper respiratory immune responses may occur after nasopharyngeal or bronchial immunization[15].

Lamina propria lymphocytes

The lamina propria of most mucosal tissues contains an abundance of B cells, plasma cells, T cells, and macrophages, as well as a smaller number of other cell types such as eosinophils, mast cells and dendritic cells[16–18]. The intestinal lamina propria is the only site in the body where large numbers of plasma cells are present continuously. Approximately 70–90% of the plasma cells in the

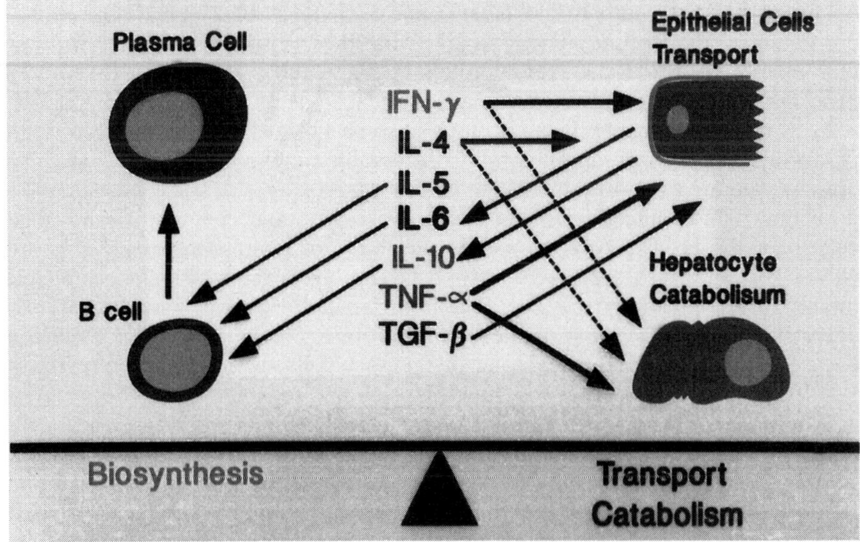

Figure 4 Regulation of IgA biosynthesis, transport and catabolism by cytokines

intestine produce IgA. In humans, the next most common isotype produced is IgM, representing 5–15%, followed by IgG, representing only 3–5%. IgE and IgD plasma cells are infrequent[17]. Plasma cells are terminally differentiated, end-stage cells whose half-life is approximately 5–10 days, indicating that there must be a dynamic, continuous repopulation of lamina propria B cells. The proliferation and differentiation of B cells appears to be regulated by cytokines produced by a broad spectrum of resident cell types, particularly T cells, but also macrophages and epithelial cells[6,13,14] (Figure 4). With respect to differentiation

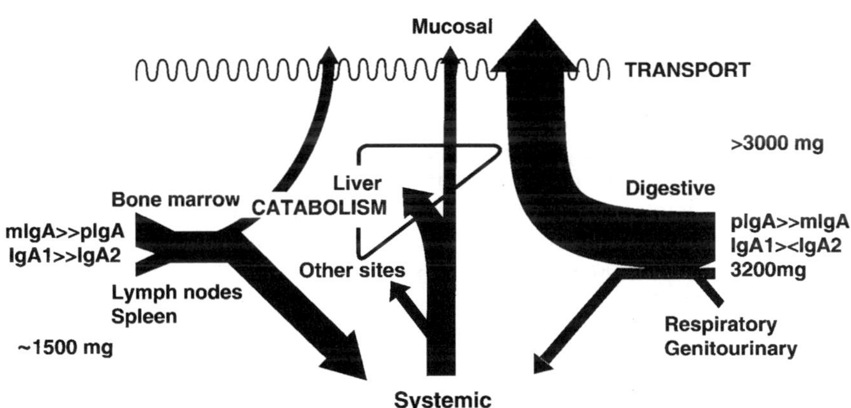

Figure 5 Production and distribution of IgA in humans

of mucosal B cells into IgA plasma cells, IL-5, IL-6, IL-10 and TGF-β play prominent roles. Recent studies suggest that these cytokines are derived not only from T cells, but also from epithelial cells which can produce IL-6, IL-10 and TGF-β[6,13,14].

Cells of B lymphocyte lineage comprise some 15–40% of the total cells, with IgA-producing cells predominating. Considerable numbers of T cells[16] are also present, ranging from 40% to 90% in lamina propria digests. Macrophages make up about 10% of intestinal lamina propria isolates, and eosinophils and mast cells from 1% to 3%. Approximately two-thirds of lamina propria T cells are CD4+ and one-third are CD8+, which is similar to their ratio in peripheral blood. However, lamina propria T cells differ in substantial ways from peripheral blood T cells. Most of the lamina propria T cells have the CD45RO+ CD45RA– phenotype characteristic of memory cells, whereas the converse is true for peripheral blood T cells. Lamina propria T cells are in a higher state of activation based on expression of IL-2Rα chain, HLA-DR molecules, transferrin receptors, and CD98. Lamina propria as well as intraepithelial T cells produce greater amounts of cytokines such as IL-2, IL-4, IL-5 and interferon-gamma (IFN-γ), which is consistent with their increased helper activity for B cell responses[15,16]. Nevertheless, lamina propria T cells do not appear to be actively producing such cytokines in the normal intestine.

Intraepithelial lymphocytes (IEL)

Lymphocytes that are physically located within the epithelial layer, or IEL, comprise some 6–10% of cells in the epithelium[19]. The cellular composition of this compartment is different from that in either the PP or the lamina propria. Plasma cells are not present, and B cells are absent or infrequent. The predominant cell type in small intestinal IEL is the CD8+ T cell. Analysis of human IEL T cell antigen receptor (TCR) gene expression shows evidence of pauciclonality. In contrast to mice or chickens, T$\gamma\delta$ cells are a minor component in human IEL, most of which are TCR$\alpha\beta$+, CD8+, CD45RO+. Most existing data on IEL come from studies done on small intestinal isolates. It is interesting therefore that mouse colon IEL have been found to consist mainly of CD4+, TCR$\alpha\beta$+ T cells, revealing previously unsuspected regional differences within the intestinal immune system. IEL T$\alpha\beta$ cells appear to originate in the PP and traffic to the epithelium via the lamina propria, but there is also evidence for a thymic-independent lineage of T cells in small intestinal IEL.

The function of IEL in host defence remains unclear[19]. First, IEL have full cytotoxic capabilities including natural killer (NK), antibody-dependent cell-mediated cytotoxicity (ADCC), and T cell cytotoxicity[18], and may serve a cytotoxic function, e.g. against parasites. Second, IEL may be a marker for cell-mediated immune responses in the intestine. Third, IEL might defend the epithelium against viral infections by local secretion of IFN-γ, and perhaps by direct cytotoxicity. They may produce other cytokines that may influence enterocyte functions[20]. Although we know little about their precise function *in vivo* IEL are situated in a site that would render them exposed to a variety of antigenic stimuli and thus they probably play an important role in mucosal host defence.

Mucosal lymphocyte trafficking

Lymphocytes stimulated with environmental antigens in the inductive sites exit via efferent lymphatics and enter into regional lymph nodes where they may undergo further division and differentiation[21,22]. From there they travel via the thoracic duct into the circulation and are dispersed widely in the body[22]. However, these cells selectively accumulate back (or 'home') to the tissues of their origin (e.g. gut), as well as other mucosal sites such as the lactating breast, salivary and lacrimal gland and perhaps genitourinary tissues, i.e. tissue of CMIS[15]. In order to populate the lamina propria of the intestine or remote secretory glands, such cells must exit the circulation. Numerous studies suggest that specific sequential interactions between receptors on lymphocytes and their ligands on endothelial cells regulate the selective distribution of lymphocytes to secondary lymphoid tissues[21,22], including the intestine. A number of molecules important in cell migration into the intestine have been identified to date. Recent biochemical characterization of one mucosal vascular addressin that is selectively expressed on high endothelial venules (HEV) of mucosal lymphoid organs and on lamina propria venules reveals that this receptor displays features common to members of the immunoglobulin supergene family. This receptor, designated the mucosal addressin cell adhesion molecule (MAdCAM-1), is composed of three immunoglobulin domains and a 37-amino-acid region localized between the second and third domains. This region is rich in serine and threonine, which are potential glycosylation sites for O-linked carbohydrates. Interestingly, the first and second domains display sequences homologous to the human VCAM-1 molecule and the third domain to the CH2 domain of human IgA1; the intervening serine/threonine-rich region exhibits structural features characteristic of mucins. The receptor on lymphocytes that binds to MAdCAM–1 in endothelial cells is $\alpha4\beta7$ integrin.

MUCOSAL IMMUNOGLOBULINS AND THEIR CONTRIBUTION TO DEFENCE MECHANISMS

Approximately 8 g of immunoglobulins (Ig) are produced per day in a 75 kg human. When individual isotypes are considered, roughly 60% of all Ig produced is IgA, 30% is IgG, 7% is IgM, and 10% is IgD and IgE[4,5]. However, human sera contain relatively low levels of IgA as compared to IgG, because more than half of the IgA produced is selectively transported by a receptor-mediated mechanism into external secretions[5,7]. Furthermore, the half-life of human serum IgA is considerably shorter due to its fast catabolism (5–6 days for IgA and 20–24 days for IgG).

In contrast to other species that produce IgA, human IgA molecules are more heterogeneous: there are two subclasses (IgA1 and IgA2) as well as two characteristically distributed molecular forms – monomeric (m) and polymeric (p) IgA[23,24]. In serum, mIgA1 predominates over mIgA2 while in external secretions equal proportions of pIgA1 and pIgA2 are found (Figure 5). The different molecular forms of human IgA display different biological activities including different interactions with IgA receptors and antigens[23,24].

The cells that produce IgA1 or IgA2 also display a characteristic tissue distribution[4,17,23,24]. In the bone marrow, approximately 90% of the cells are

IgA1-positive and thus mirror the intravascular distribution of this subclass; on the other hand, mucosal tissues and glands contain variable proportions of IgA1 and IgA2 cells, depending on the anatomical site of the tissue. Although IgA1 cells predominate in most of these mucosal tissues, the relative contribution of IgA2 cells is more pronounced in the large intestine and the female genital tract where IgA2 cells outnumber IgA1 cells. Although the reason for this typical tissue distribution of IgA1 and IgA2 cells is not known, it is possible that environmental antigens present in a given locale may be responsible for the IgA subclass-specific expansion of cells (see below).

In pIgA, an additional small glycoprotein, J chain, is attached to the penultimate cysteine residues of two α chains[25]. pIgA is principally produced by plasma cells distributed in the mucosal tissues and glands where almost all of the IgA-positive cells express J chain. In contrast, IgA-positive plasma cells in normal human bone marrow secrete almost exclusively mIgA lacking J chain.

Receptors involved in the distribution of IgA molecules and their functional significance

IgA interacts with surface membrane receptors on a broad spectrum of morphologically and functionally different cell types[23,26]. As a consequence of these interactions, a variety of biologically important phenomena occur, including the selective transport of pIgA through epithelial cells and hepatocytes into external secretions and bile, removal of IgA-containing immune complexes (IgA-IC) by hepatocytes and Kupffer cells, hepatic catabolism of IgA, enhanced phagocytosis of IgA-coated bacteria by mucosal polymorphonuclear leukocytes and macrophages, and degranulation of eosinophils[5,26] (also see below). The receptors involved in IgA binding by various cells have been only partially characterized with respect to their properties, distribution, and relative biological importance.

The best characterized receptor, pIgR, is expressed on human and animal epithelial cells covering mucosal surfaces, and on ductal and acinar cells of external secretory glands[5,7]. pIgR displays Ig domain-like structure and plays a key role in the selective epithelial transport of IgA and IgM[5,7]. After synthesis in the rough endoplasmic reticulum and heavy glycosylation in the Golgi complex, pIgR reaches and is inserted into the basolateral membrane of epithelial cells and, in some species, hepatocytes. After the initial interactions of pIgA with pIgR on epithelial cells through non-covalent binding, the pIgR first domain binds to the Cα3 domain, and the fifth pIgR domain binds covalently to the Cα2 domain. J chain is essential for polymeric IgA to interact with pIgR, probably by inducing conformational changes in IgA that permit binding to pIgR. Following these molecular events, the membrane pIgR–pIgA complex is internalized and transported in vesicles towards the apical surface of the epithelial cells. Once there, these vesicles fuse with the apical membrane. Proteolytic cleavage of pIgR–IgA complex releases the assembled molecule of secretory IgA (S-IgA) into external secretions. pIgR-mediated transport of pIgA represents a unique system of interaction between a receptor and its ligand: pIgR is produced by epithelial cells regardless of the presence of its ligand and is not recycled[7]. Those molecules that do bind to IgA remain permanently attached to it, conferring an increased resistance of S-IgA to proteolytic enzymes in the intestinal tract. The magnitude of selective IgA transport is enormous, comprising 3–5 g S-IgA produced and transported each day into the human intestine[5].

The synthesis and expression of both J chain and SC is regulated by cytokines and hormones: IL-5, IL-2 and possibly IL-6 up-regulate J chain synthesis while IL-4, IFN-γ, TNF-α, TGF-β and oestrogens significantly enhance pIgR expression[5,7]. Thus, the synthesis of all component chains of S-IgA is regulated by cytokines that are locally produced in the intestinal microenvironment.

From a functional point of view, S-IgA can neutralize biologically active antigens (e.g. viruses and toxin), interfere with the absorption of protein antigens from the gut lumen, and inhibit the adherence of microorganisms to epithelial cells[27]. As a result, and in contrast to the function of other isotypes of Ig that can be easily demonstrated by dramatic biological reactions (antibody-dependent killing and lysis of prokaryotic and eukaryotic cells, promotion of phagocytosis, anaphylaxis, etc.), the consequences of the union of IgA antibodies with corresponding antigens are more subtle. Generally, this is due to the restricted ability of IgA to use ancillary effector mechanisms such as activation of complement, phagocytosis, and binding to other effector cells[26]. As a result, and in contrast to IgM and IgG, IgA antibodies are essentially non-inflammatory, a property that is probably of great importance for the maintenance of the integrity of mucosal surfaces as well as internal tissues[26,27].

INDUCTION OF MUCOSAL IMMUNE RESPONSES VS. TOLERANCE

The antigenic challenge to the mucosal immune system is so enormous that it could easily overwhelm the entire immune system. To prevent such a potentially disastrous situation, the mucosal immune system has developed a unique mechanism – mucosal tolerance – to down-regulate specific immune responses to frequently encountered antigens from relatively constant mucosal microbiota and ingested food[8] (Figure 3).

The feeding of an antigen prior to parenteral immunization can induce an immune response manifested in the humoral (Ig) as well as cellular (CTL) compartments and/or a state of systemic unresponsiveness or 'mucosal (formerly oral) tolerance'[8,28,29]. The factors determining whether immunity or tolerance result from an antigen encounter in mucosal tissues are not well understood, but presumably the answer lies in complex regulatory cell interactions within the inductive sites. Mucosal tolerance has been demonstrated in animals after the feeding of a variety of antigens including proteins, contact allergens, heterologous erythrocytes, and viral glycoproteins. Multiple mechanisms of tolerance have been demonstrated, including deletion, clonal anergy, and the induction of regulatory cells producing inhibitory cytokines such as TGF-β, IL-10 and IL-4[8,28]. There seems to be differential cellular susceptibility to oral tolerance induction, with Th1 cells being most sensitive, followed by Th2 cells and possibly B cells. Feeding autoantigens has been used to successfully abrogate or treat experimental autoimmune diseases, and trials are under way in humans. A recent study has shown that the feeding of a previously unencountered foreign protein antigen to human volunteers did result in T cell but not B cell tolerance, establishing that oral tolerance can be induced in humans[29]. It is unclear whether protein antigens of bacterial origin can induce oral tolerance. Bacterial lipopolysaccharide or cholera toxin B subunit given together with a non-bacterial protein antigen increased the degree of oral tolerance to the latter, so the presence of highly stimulatory adjuvant molecules in microbes does not necessarily shift the mucosal response away from a tolerizing one. There have been very few studies in which bacterial antigens have been tested for their ability to induce oral tolerance and to explain the lack of elimination of our own microbiota by immune mechanisms[30]. Therefore, the factors which determine whether tolerance or immunity occurs after a mucosal encounter with such microbial antigens need to be defined. This is clearly an important consideration both for the outcome of any encounter with an intestinal pathogen, as well as for the possible development of oral vaccines against such infectious agents.

References

1. McGhee JR, Mestecky J. In defense of mucosal surfaces. Development of novel vaccines for IgA responses protective at portals of entry for microbial pathogens. Infect Dis Clin N Am. 1990;4:315–41.
2. Savage D. Mucosal microbiota. In: Ogra PL, Mestecky J, Lamm ME, Strober W, Bienenstock J, McGhee JR, editors. Mucosal Immunology. San Diego: Academic Press; 1999:19–30.
3. Ogra PL, Mestecky J, Lamm ME, Strober W, Bienenstock, J, McGhee JR, editors. Mucosal Immunology. San Diego: Academic Press; 1999.
4. Conley ME, Delacroix DL. Intravascular and mucosal immunoglobulin A: two separate but related systems of immune defense? Ann Intern Med. 1987;206:892–9.
5. Mestecky J, Lue C, Russell MW. Selective transport of IgA: cellular and molecular aspects. Gastroenterol Clin N Am. 1991;20:441–71.
6. Chist AD, Blumberg RS. The intestinal epithelial cell: immunological aspects. Springer Semin Immunopathol. 1997;18:449–61.
7. Mostov K, Kaetzel C. Immunoglobulin transport and positive polymeric immunoglobulin receptor. In: Ogra PL, Mestecky J, Lamm ME, Strober W, Bienenstock J, McGhee JR, editors. Mucosal Immunology. San Diego: Academic Press; 1999:181–211.
8. Weiner HL. Oral tolerance: immune mechanisms and treatment of autoimmune diseases. Immunol Today. 1997;18:335–43.
9. Bockman DE, Boydston WR, Beezhold DH. The role of epithelial cells in gut-associated immune reactivity. Ann NY Acad Sci. 1983;409:129–43.
10. Owen RL, Davis IC. The immunopathology of M cells. Springer Semin Immunopathol. 1997;18:421–48.
11. Craig SW, Cebra JJ. Peyer's patches: an enriched source of precursors for IgA-producing immunocytes in the rabbit. J Exp Med. 1971;134:188–200.
12. Croitoru K, Bienenstock J. Characteristics and functions of mucosa-associated lymphoid tissue. In: Ogra PL, Mestecky J, Lamm ME, Strober W, McGhee JR, Bienenstock J, editors. Handbook of Mucosal Immunology. San Diego: Academic Press; 1994:141–9.
13. McGhee JR, Mestecky J, Elson CO, Kiyono H. Regulation of IgA synthesis and immune response by T cells and interleukins. J Clin Immunol. 1989;9:175–99.
14. Beagley KW, Elson CO. Cells and cytokines in mucosal immunity and inflammation. Gastroenterol Clin N Am. 1992;21:347–66.
15. McGhee JR, Czerkinsky C, Mestecky J. Mucosal vaccines: an overview. In: Ogra PL, Mestecky J, Lamm ME, Strober W, Bienenstock J, McGhee JR, editors. Mucosal Immunology. San Diego: Academic Press; 1999:741–57.
16. James SP. Mucosal T-cell function. Gastroenterol Clin N Am. 1992;20:97–112.
17. Brandtzaeg P. Distribution and characteristics of mucosal immunoglobulin-producing cells. In: Ogra PL, Mestecky J, Lamm ME, Strober W, McGhee JR, Bienenstock J, editors. Handbook of Mucosal Immunology. San Diego: Academic Press; 1994:251–62.
18. London SD. Cytotoxic lymphocytes in mucosal effector sites. In: Ogra PL, Mestecky J, Lamm ME, Strober W, McGhee JR, Bienenstock J, editors. Handbook of Mucosal Immunology. San Diego: Academic Press; 1994:325–32.

19. Lefrancois L. Basic aspects of intraepithelial lymphocyte immunobiology. In: Ogra PL, Mestecky J, Lamm ME, Strober W, Bienenstock J, McGhee JR, editors. Mucosal Immunology, San Diego: Academic Press; 1999:413–28.

20. Boismenu R, Havran WL. Modulation of epithelial cell growth by intraepithelial $\gamma\delta$ T cells. Science. 1994;266:1253–5.

21. Picker LJ, Butcher EC. Physiological and molecular mechanisms of lymphocyte homing. Annu Rev Immunol. 1992;10:561–91.

22. Phillips-Quaggliata JM, Lamm ME. Lymphocyte homing to mucosal effector sites. In: Ogra PL, Mestecky J, Lamm ME, Strober W, McGhee JR, Bienenstock J, editors. Handbook of Mucosal Immunology. San Diego: Academic Press; 1994:225–34.

23. Underdown BJ, Mestecky J. Mucosal immunoglobulins. In: Ogra PL, Mestecky J, Lamm ME, Strober W, McGhee JR, Bienenstock J, editors. Handbook of Mucosal Immunology. San Diego: Academic Press; 1994:79–97.

24. Mestecky J, Russell MW. IgA subclasses. Monogr Allergy. 1986;19:277–301.

25. Mestecky J, Schrohenloher RE, Kulhavy R, Wright R, Wright GP, Tomana M. Site of J chain attachment to human polymeric IgA. Proc Natl Acad Sci USA. 1974;71;544–48.

26. Russell MW, Sibley DA, Nikolova EB, Tomana M, Mestecky J. IgA antibody as a non-inflammatory regulator of immunity. Biochem Soc Trans. 1997;25:466–70.

27. Kilian M, Russell MW. Microbial evasion of IgA functions. In: Ogra PL, Mestecky J, Lamm ME, Strober W, Bienenstock J, McGhee JR, editors. Mucosal Immunology. San Diego: Academic Press; 1999:241–51.

28. Elson CO. Induction and control of the gastrointestinal immune system. Scand J Gastroenterol. 1985;114:1–15.

29. Husby S, Mestecky J, Moldoveanu Z, Holland S, Elson CO. Oral tolerance in humans. T cell but not B cell tolerance after antigen feeding. J Immunol. 1994;152:4663–70.

30. Kroese FGM, de Waard R, Bos NA. B-1 cells and their reactivity with the murine intestinal microflora. Semin Immunol. 1996;8:11–18.

10
Effector mechanisms in intestinal immunity and inflammation

H. TLASKALOVÁ-HOGENOVÁ, R. ŠTĚPÁNKOVÁ,
L. TUČKOVÁ, B. CUKROWSKA, T. HUDCOVIČ,
F. BENDJELLOUL, P. MALÝ, M. JIRKOVSKÁ, V. MANDYS,
O. KOFRONOVÁ, E. F. VERDÚ, P. BERČIK, M. FARRE,
L. PROKEŠOVÁ, D. P. FUNDA, H. KOZÁKOVÁ, P. MICHETTI
and J. CEBRA

INTRODUCTION

Each organism lives in a continuous interaction with its environment. Exchange of nutritional compounds, export products and waste components takes place in the interface between the organism and the outside world. The interface must be selectively permeable; at the same time it must constitute a barrier equipped by local defence mechanisms against environmental threats such as invading pathogens. The intestinal epithelium covers the largest and most critical area of the body, which is in contact with the external environment. In humans the mucosal surface has an extension of 200–300 m^2 and the lymphoid tissue associated with gut mucosa comprises more than 50% of lymphoid tissues in the body. Daily production of IgA prevails over the production of other isotypes[1–3]. The mucosal immune system consists of inductive sites, which are regions of organized lymphoid tissue where processing and presentation of antigens and activation of lymphocytes occur. It also consists of effector sites, which are formed by lamina propria cells present in the gastrointestinal, respiratory and genitourinary tracts and their mucosal epithelium. Other effector regions include mammary, lacrimal and salivary glands[4].

The main effector mechanisms of intestinal immunity are aimed at: (1) ensuring mucosal barrier function (preventing penetration of bacteria and antigens from lumen to circulation); (2) developing a state of non-reactivity to non-pathogenic luminal antigens (oral tolerance induction); (3) mediating communication between different regions of the mucosal system ('common mucosal system'); and (4) protecting the epithelial cell layer characterized by a high cell turnover against malignant transformation (immunosurveillance function). All these functions arc performed by the complex of non-specific and immunologically specific factors represented by the epithelial layer and immune cells present in the mucosal compartment (Figure 1).

It has recently been found that epithelial cells are directly involved in immune processes, in addition to their absorptive, digestive and secretory functions[5]. Epithelial cells play a role in the transfer of polymeric immunoglobulins, produced by lamina propria B lymphocytes, to the luminal content of the mucosals (secretory Ig). Epithelial cells have been found to perform various other immunological functions which involve interaction with other cells of the immune system and an efficient inflammatory response to microbial invasion. Specifically, they have a role in enzymatic processing of dietary antigens, expression of class I and II MHC antigens, presentation of antigens to lymphocytes, expression of adhesive molecules mediating interaction with intraepithelial lymphocytes and components of extracellular matrix, production of cytokines and probably in extrathymic T cell development of intraepithelial lymphocytes[5]. All these functions have been suggested to influence substantially the mucosal immune system and its responses. The epithelial layer of polarized cells, interconnected by desmosomes and tight junctions, is separated from the connective and supporting tissue surrounding lymphocytes, macrophages and dendritic cells in the lamina propria by the basal membrane. This membrane is composed of collagen, laminin, fibronectin and proteoglycans, and regulates epithelial cell differentiation and properties[2]. The thin epithelial layer contains two different kinds of cells: intestinal epithelial cells and the so-called intraepithelial lymphocytes (IEL) which are intercalated among the basolateral parts of enterocytes and form a population differing substantially from other lymphocyte populations in phenotype, ontogeny and repertoire[3,4,6]. Antigen presentation in the gut may involve non-classical, non-polymorphic class I-like molecules expressed by epithelial cells. Lamina propria compartments from conventionally reared organisms are characterized by the presence of thymically derived, highly activated memory lymphocytes of the Th2 cell phenotype[7].

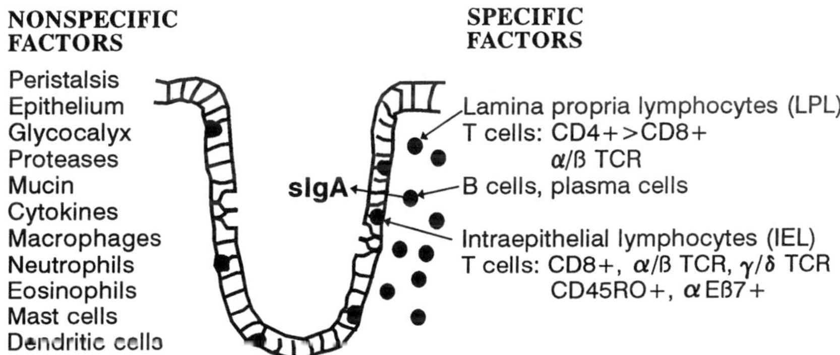

Figure 1 Components of intestinal effector mechanisms

ANALYSIS OF EFFECTOR MECHANISMS PARTICIPATING IN INTESTINAL INFLAMMATION

The integrity of the mucosal surface is the basic prerequisite for its perfect functioning. Coeliac disease and inflammatory bowel disease (IBD) are two examples of pathological situations where immune factors play a crucial role in affecting the gut mucosa. Coeliac disease is the only autoimmune condition affecting the gut mucosa where gluten, the environmental inducing agent, is defined. Intestinal epithelial cells have been found to react with autoantibodies present in the sera of patients with coeliac disease and in media from cultured jejunal biopsy specimens[8]. We found that structures shared by enterocyte molecules and gliadin are recognized by one of our antigliadin monoclonal antibodies and by antigliadin antibodies isolated from patients with coeliac disease. Further findings led us to propose that enterocyte calreticulin could be one of the target structures for autoimmune reactions occurring in this disease[9,10]. The use of animal models for the study of human diseases with immunological pathogenesis has provided new insights into the influence of environmental, genetic and immunoregulatory factors involved in the development of intestinal inflammation[11] (Table 1). Moreover, the use of experimental models may help develop new therapeutic strategies. Recently we have developed an experimental model of coeliac disease in which a defined food antigen (gliadin) is responsible for autoimmune reactions occurring in the intestinal mucosa. Prolonged feeding with gliadin to the AVN strain of rats during the first 2 months after birth triggers morphological changes in rat gut mucosa similar to those observed in human coeliac disease[12].

An approach which enables direct evaluation of the intestinal effector mechanisms consists of testing various factors in an experimental system of surgically prepared jejunal loops. We used this system to analyse the effector mechanism playing a role in gluten-induced enteropathy of AVN rats. The fate of intraepithelial T cells isolated from the jejunum of rats fed with gliadin, labelled with fluorescein and injected into the lumen of loops prepared in germ-free recipients, differed significantly from the fate of intraepithelial cells isolated from control, albumin-fed rats. Briefly, gliadin-activated cells were able to pass through the epithelial cell layer and cause impairment of the intestinal mucosa (Figure 2). Injection of medium from cultivated mesenteric lymph-node cells of rats treated with gliadin into the loop, exerted morphological impairment of the intestinal mucosa. The direct *in-vivo* effect of various cytokines administered into the

Table 1   Effector mechanisms in mucosal inflammation

Epithelial cell activation
Cytokines, nitric oxide, proteases

Macrophage and neutrophil activation
Cytokines (IL-1, IL-6, IL-8, TNF-α, etc.), reactive oxygen metabolites, nitric oxide, arachidonic acid metabolites, proteases

Lymphocyte activation
Cytokines, immunoglobulins

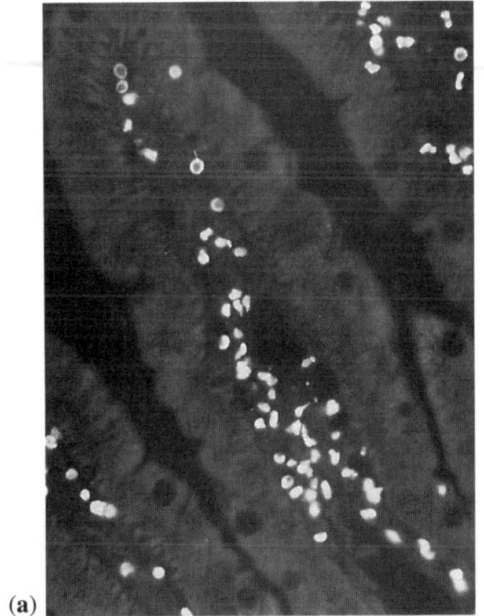
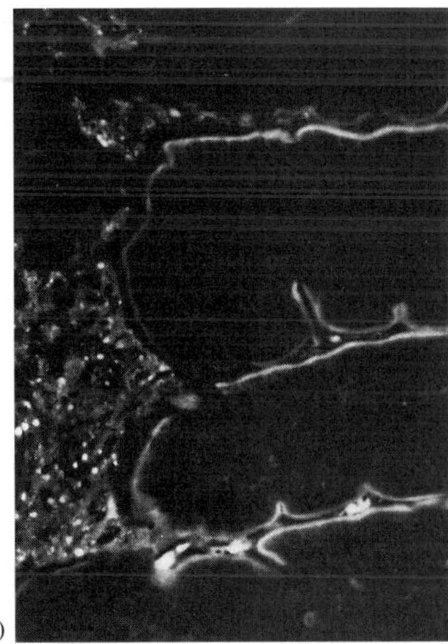

(a)   **(b)**

Figure 2   Immunofluorescence of jejunal mucosa after transfer of fluorescein isothiocyanate-labelled intraepithelial lymphocytes into intestinal loops of inbred 1-month-old germ-free rats. Sampling after 1 h. (**a**) Lymphocytes isolated from jejunum of inbred germ-free rats after 2 months feeding with gliadin penetrated through the intestinal wall and appeared in the lamina propria of the recipient's loop. (**b**) Lymphocytes from control rats remained in the intestinal lumen of the loop[12]

lumen of jejunal loops of germ-free rats can be evaluated. Administration of interferon gamma (IFN-γ) or tumour necrosis factor alpha (TNF-α) into the lumen of surgically prepared jejunal loops of germ-free rats led to dose-dependent morphological changes in mucosal structure detected within 6 h after application (Figures 3 and 4).

Adhesion molecules are known to participate in the development of an inflammatory reaction by mediating cell interactions, migration and homing. The role of adhesion molecules in intestinal inflammation was studied using mice with deleted gene for ICAM-1 in comparison with genetically corresponding wild-type controls. Acute and chronic colitis was induced after a 7-day application of dextran sodium sulphate (DSS) in drinking water[11]. Only minor changes were found in ICAM-1 deficient mice: in contrast the wild-type controls exhibited severe changes with ulcerations, suggesting direct involvement of ICAM-1 molecules in the development of the inflammatory reaction (Table 2).

INTESTINAL INFLAMMATION AS A SENSITIVE INDICATOR OF IMMUNOREGULATORY DEFECTS IN MUCOSAL RESPONSE TO LUMINAL MICROFLORA

The interaction of microorganisms with the macroorganism taking place at the mucosal surface is characterized by the active participation of both counterparts. Normal flora profoundly influences host mucosal structure and function, as well

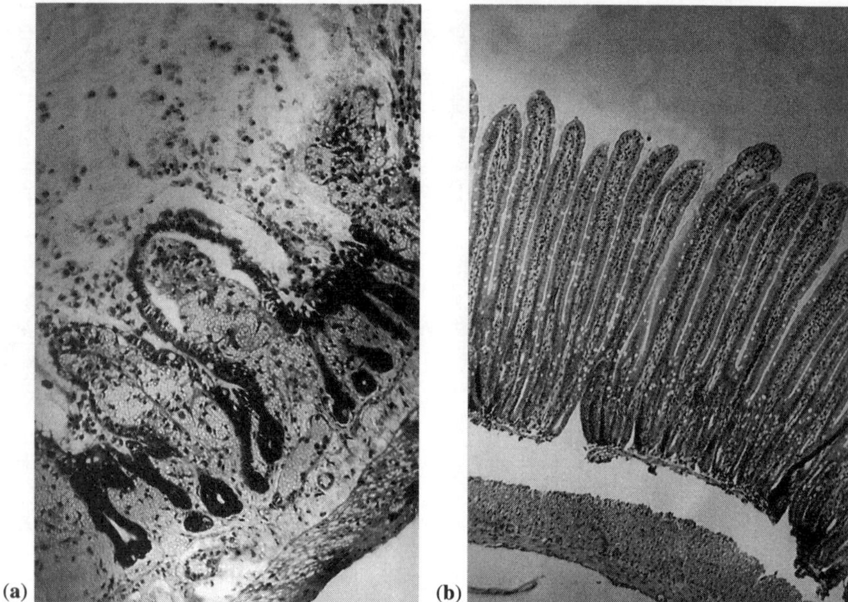

Figure 3 Histopathology of jejunal mucosa of intestinal loops 6 h after application of interferon gamma or PBS. (**a**) Changes in the structure of intestinal mucosa after injection of 600 U of IFN-γ. (**b**) Structure of control loop with injected PBS

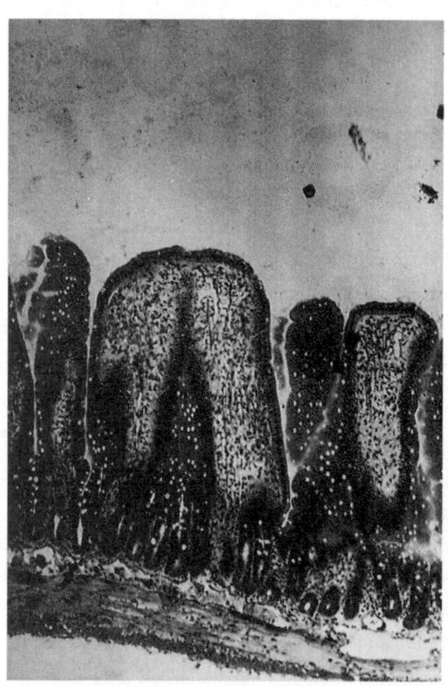

Figure 4 Histopathology of jejunal mucosa of intestinal loop 6 h after luminal application of tumor necrosis factor (60 000 pg)

Table 2 ICAM-1-Deficient mice do not develop severe forms of experimental colitis. Clinical symptoms and histopathological findings in ICAM-1-deficient and control wild-type mice on day 7 after administration of dextran sodium sulphate.

	ICAM-1 knockout mice	*Controls (wild-type)*
Mortality (%)	8	28
Prolapsus recti (%)	0	50
Rectal bleeding (%)	0	100
Diarrhoea (%)	0	100
Length of colon (cm)	7.0	5.6
Oedema	±	+
Erosions	±	+++
Ulcers	±	+
Infiltration	±	++

as the development of the whole immune system[13–16]. This is best appreciated when comparing animals reared in germ-free and conventional conditions[17]. Physiological intestinal inflammation occurring after colonization of germ-free animals or newborn humans with non-pathogenic flora is characterized by heavy cellular infiltration of the gut mucosa, by an increase in epithelial cell turnover and by a rapid development of non-specific and specific immune responses positively influencing the overall immunological reactivity[18–21]. After a few days the stimulatory effect of luminal antigens on mucosal and systemic immunity is replaced by a suppressive effect[22].

One of the most striking conclusions arising from contemporary work with genetically engineered immunodeficient mouse models is the existence of a high level of redundancy of the components of the immune system[23]. However, when genes encoding molecules involved in T cell immunoregulatory functions are deleted, spontaneous chronic inflammation of the gut mucosa develops[24]. Alterations in T cell subpopulations have been reported to affect the regulatory role of T cells and to result in chronic intestinal inflammation. For example, T cell receptor (TCR) alpha chain-deficient mice, TCR beta chain-deficient mice and MHC class II-deficient mice, cytokine knockout mice lacking interleukin 2 (IL-2), IL-10 and transforming growth factor beta (TGF-β) develop chronic inflammation affecting various parts of the gut to a different extent[24]. Another experimental model of IBD directly evidencing the participation of T cell subpopulations in gut immunoregulation has been described in severe combined immunodeficiency (SCID) mice. In this model, SCID mice restored with unique CD4 T cell subpopulation (CD45RB^{hi}) from conventional BALB/c mice develop colitis. However, colitis is prevented by simultaneous transfer of the CD45RB^{lo} subpopulation of CD4 T cell[25]. Surprisingly, when such compromised animals were placed into a germ-free environment, most of the inflammatory reactions did not develop[24]. Also, SCID mice remained healthy after transfer of a pathogenic T cell subpopulation when reared in germ-free conditions (Powrie, personal communication). The finding that there is an abnormal T cell responsiveness against indigenous microflora in human IBD and its experimental models, awakened interest in the possibility that commensals may initiate and/or maintain IBD lesions. Under conditions of an immunoregulatory disorder the common intestinal flora is obviously capable of evoking stimulation leading to a chronic intestinal or systemic inflammation[26]. From the fact of the regular development of pathological changes in the gastrointestinal system it could be concluded that the gut mucosa is extremely sensitive and responds by inflammation to lack of individual factors participating in immunoregulatory mechanisms which control the reactivity of the mucosal immune system to components of normal luminal microflora. Impairment of the intestinal immune response to the normal bacterial flora has been proposed to play a crucial role in the pathogenesis of chronic intestinal inflammation. A loss of physiological, regulatory mechanisms of the local immune system, or a lack of induction or breakdown of oral tolerance to commensal gut bacteria, could be involved[27–29]. It should be pointed out that the lymphatic system in the gut is permanently activated by microflora components and is in a state of 'physiological' inflammation[14,18,20].

Colitis induced by DSS in immunodeficient mouse models was used to study the environmental and immunological factors involved in pathogenetic mechanisms of intestinal inflammation. Mice with SCID were used to analyse the role of microflora in development of intestinal inflammation. SCID mice reared in conventional conditions (colonized by microflora) developed signs of colitis after 7 days feeding with DSS (colonic bleeding, epithelial erosions, increase in the number of inflammatory cells in lamina propria and submucosa, reduction of the number of goblet cells, etc.). The intestinal mucosa of SCID mice reared in germ-free conditions showed only minor changes after DSS feeding (Table 3, Figure 5). These experiments suggest that in DSS-induced colitis of severely immunodeficient mice, the presence of microflora augments the development of the inflammatory reaction which occurs in the absence of specific components of the immune system.

The possible role of breakdown of oral tolerance to microflora antigens was suggested to play a role in the development of intestinal inflammation. We therefore addressed the question whether oral administration of an intestinal microflora sonicate could affect experimentally induced intestinal inflammation. We showed that severity of DSS-induced intestinal inflammation in Balb/c mice is reduced by orally administered microflora sonicate[30]. We hypothesize that induction of oral tolerance, as achieved by repetitively feeding the sonicate, affects intestinal immunity against microflora and protects against DSS-induced colitis in mice. The higher anti-flora antibody levels in the sonicate, compared with the control group, suggest that tolerance may be T cell-mediated rather than associated with a B cell anergy.

Table 3 Effect of the presence of microflora on development of acute colitis induced by dextran sodium sulphate (DSS) feeding. Histopathological analysis of the colon of SCID mice (mice with severe combined immunodeficiency) reared in germ-free or conventional conditions and fed for 7 days with DSS.

Germ-free SCID mice	*Conventional SCID mice*
Minor changes	Erosions, ulcers, oedema, cellular infiltration, reduction of goblet cells

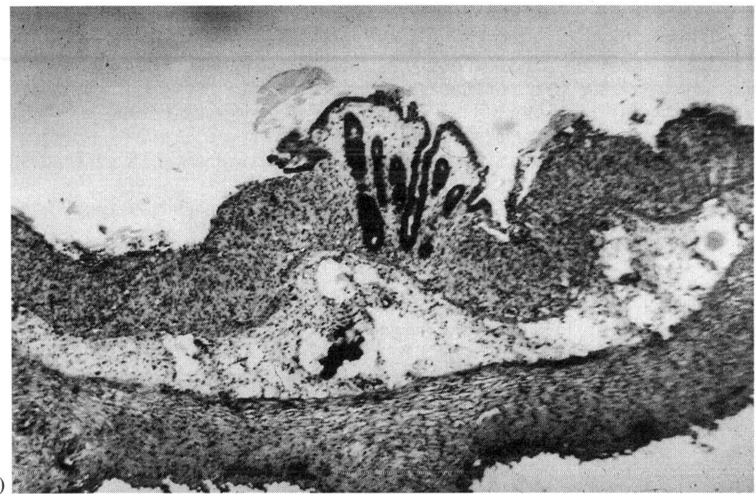

(a)

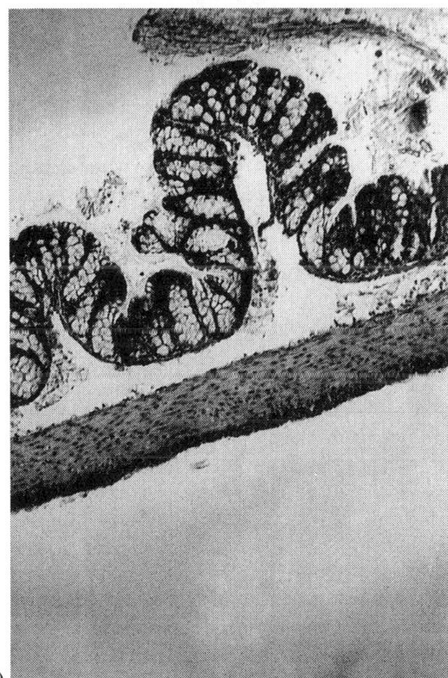

(b)

Figure 5 Histopathology of colonic wall of SCID mice after ingestion of dextran sodium sulphate for 7 days (acute colitis). (**a**) Severe infiltration of inflammatory cells and crypt abscesses were observed in conventional SCID mice colonized by microflora. (**b**) Minor changes were present in colon of germ-free SCID mice

Acknowledgements

Experimental work was supported by grants: FIRCA, 5R01 AI35936-03 (NIH), 7020716 (Grant Agency of the Academy of Science of the Czech Republic), 310/96/1366, 310/96/0516, 303/96/1256, 311/97/0784, 306/98/0433 (Grant Agency of the Czech Republic), 3761-3, 2158 (Ministry of Health), VS 96149 (Ministry of Education, Youth and Sports).

References

1. Mestecky J, Mc Ghee J. Immunoglobulin A (IgA): molecular and cellular interaction involved in IgA biosynthesis and immune response. Adv Immunol. 1987;40:153–245.
2. Ogra PL, Mestecky J, Lamm ME, Strober W, McGhee J, Bienenstock J. Handbook of Mucosal Immunology. San Diego: Academic Press; 1994.
3. Mestecky J, Russell MW, Jackson S, Michalek SM, Tlaskalová-Hogenová H, Šterzl J. Advances in Mucosal Immunology. New York: Plenum Press; 1995.
4. Brandtzaeg P. Molecular and cellular aspects of the secretory immunoglobulin system. APMIS 1995;103:1–19.
5. Kagnoff MF, Eckmann L, Yang SK *et al*. Intestinal epithelial cells: an integral component of the mucosal immune system. In: Kagnoff MF, Kiyono H, editors. Essentials of Mucosal Immunology. New York: Academic Press; 1996:63–72.
6. Blumberg RS, Balk SP. Intraepithelial lymphocytes and their recognition of non-classical MHC molecules. Int Rev Immunol. 1994;11:15–23.
7. Abreu-Martin MT, Targan SR. Lamina propria lymphocytes. A unique population of mucosal lymphocytes. In: Kagnoff MF, Kiyono H, editors. Essentials of Mucosal Immunology. New York: Academic Press; 1996:63–72.
8. Tlaskalová-Hogenová, Štěpánková R, Tučková L *et al*. Autoimmune reactions induced by gliadin. Adv Exp Med Biol. 1995;371:1191–8.
9. Karská K, Tučková L, Steiner L, Tlaskalová H, Michalak K. Calreticulin – the potential autoantigen in coeliac disease. Biochem Biophys Res Commun. 1995;209:597–605.
10. Tučková L, Karska K, Walters JRF *et al*. Anti-gliadin antibodies in patients with celiac disease cross-react with enterocytes and human calreticulin. Clin Immunol Immunopathol. 1997; 85:289–96.
11. Elson Ch, Sartor RB, Tennyson G, Ridell RH. Experimental models of inflammatory bowel disease. Gastroenterology. 1995;109:1344–67.
12. Štěpánková R, Tlaskalová-Hogenová H, Šinkora J, Jodl J, Frič P. Changes of jejunal mucosa after longterm feeding of germfree rats with gluten. Scand J Gastroenterol. 1996;31:551–7.
13. Šterzl J, Mandel L, Štěpánková, R. The use of gnotobiological models for the studies of immune mechanisms. Die Nahrung. 1997;31:599–608.
14. Tlaskalová-Hogenová H, Šterzl L, Štěpánková R *et al*. Development of immunological capacity under germfree and conventional conditions. Ann NY Acad Sci. 1983;409:96–113.
15. Kramer DR, Cebra JJ. Early appearance of 'natural' mucosal IgA responses and germinal centers in suckling mice developing in the absence of maternal antibodies. J Immunol. 1995;154:2051–62.
16. Cebra JJ, Jiang HQ, Šterzl J, Tlaskalová-Hogenová H. The role of mucosal microbiota in the development and maintenance of the mucosal immune system. In: Ogra PL, Mestecky J, Lamm ME, Strober W, McGhee JR, Bienenstock J, editors. Mucosal Immunology. New York: Academic Press: 1998 (In press).
17. Tlaskalová-Hogenová H. Gnotobiology as a tool. In: Lefkovits I, editor. Manual of Immunological Methods. New York: Academic Press; 1997;1524–9.
18. Tlaskalová H, Kamarýtová V, Mandel L *et al*. The immune response of germ-free piglets after peroral monocontamination with living *Escherichia coli* strain 086. I. The fate of antigen, dynamics and site of antibody formation, nature of antibodies and formation of heterohaemagglutinins. Folia Biol. 1970;16:177–87.
19. Tlaskalová-Hogenová H, Černá J, Mandel L. Peroral immunization of germfree piglets: appearance of antibody-forming cells and antibodies of different isotypes. Scand J Immunol. 1980;13:467–72.
20. Tlaskalová-Hogenová H, Štěpánková R. Development of antibody formation in germ-free and conventionally reared rabbits: the role of intestinal lymphoid tissue in antibody formation to *E. coli* antigens. Folia Biol. 1980;26:81–93.
21. Lodinová-Žádniková R, Slaviková M, Tlaskalová-Hogenová H *et al*. The antibody response in breast-fed and non-breast-fed infants after artificial colonisation of the intestine with *Escherichia coli* 083. Ped Res. 1991:29:396–9.
22. Tlaskalová-Hogenová H, Tucková L, Větvicka V. Development of immunological memory and inhibition of immune response after long-term feeding with antigen. In: Hraba T, Hašek M, editors. Cellular and Molecular Mechanisms of Immunological Tolerance. New York: Marcel Dekker; 1981:267–73.

23. Rajewsky K. A phenotype or not: targeting genes in the immune system. Science. 1992;256:483.
24. Strober W, Ehrhardt RO. Chronic intestinal inflammation: an unexpected outcome in cytokine or T cell receptor mutant mice. Cell. 1993;78:203–95.
25. Powrie F. T cells in inflammatory bowel disease: protective and pathogenic roles. Immunity. 1995;3:171–4.
26. Sartor RB. Current concepts of etiology and pathogenesis of ulcerative colitis and Crohn's disease. Gastroenterol Clin N Am. 1995;24:475–506.
27. MacDonald TT. Breakdown of tolerance to the intestinal bacteria flora in inflammatory bowel disease (IBD). Clin Exp Immunol. 1995;102:445–7.
28. Podolsky DK. Regulatory peptides and integration of the intestinal epithelium in mucosal responses. In: Kagnoff MF, Kiyono H, editors. Essentials of Mucosal Immunology. New York: Academic Press; 1996:101–10.
29. Tlaskalová-Hogenová H, Štěpánková R, Tučková L *et al*. Autoimmunity, immunodeficiency and mucosal infections: chronic intestinal inflammation as a sensitive indicator of immunoregulatory defects in response to normal luminal microflora. Folia Microbiol. 1998:43 (In press).
30. Verdú EF, Michetti P, Farré MA *et al*. Oral administration of intestinal flora sonicate reduces severity of DSS-induced acute colitis in BALB/c mice. Gastroenterology. 1998;114:A1109.

11
Homing of mucosally activated lymphocytes in humans

A. KANTELE

INTRODUCTION

Mucosal surfaces constitute the major interface between host and environment. At these sites the body needs to deal with an enormous variety of different food antigens, bacteria, viruses, etc. Almost all pathogens use mucosal surfaces as a site of entry to the body. In addition to numerous non-specific defence mechanisms, mucosal surfaces are guarded by a local mucosal immune system[1]. This immune system is believed to function quite independently from its conventional systemic counterpart. It contains more lymphocytes than any other tissue in the body, and it has some unique characteristics related to its specialized role as a first defence line of the body. One of these features is the preferential production, transport and secretion of immunoglobulin A, a molecule that has been shown to function, for example, by preventing the attachment of bacteria, neutralizing viruses and limiting the absorption of protein antigens[1].

Since the classic studies of Gowans and Knight[2], who demonstrated that large lymphocytes from rat thoracic duct home preferably to the gut, several studies in animals have confirmed and extended the notion of circulation and homing of mucosa-derived lymphocytes to mucosa[3–6]. In this cycle lymphocytes activated by an antigen at the mucosa migrate to regional lymph nodes, and later return via lymphatics and blood back to the mucosa. Consistently, in humans, it has been shown that antigen-specific lymphocytes appear in the blood after intestinal immunization[7–9]. It has been suggested that stimulation at one mucosal site can lead to a distribution of the activated lymphocytes to all mucosal surfaces of the body. This migration of lymphocytes from one mucosal site to another underlies the concept of the common mucosal immune system (CMIS)[1], which implies that the various mucosal surfaces of the body are interconnected or communicate via circulating lymphocytes. Indeed, immunization at one mucosal site (e.g. intestinal Peyer's patches) has been shown to induce an antibody response at other, anatomically remote, mucosal sites (e.g. saliva or genital tract secretions)[1]. However, recent data suggest that some degree of compartmentalization occurs within the CMIS[10];

therefore the general routes of lymphocyte homing from each mucosal site remain to be explored.

LYMPHOCYTE TRAFFICKING IN THE BODY

Recent reviews have dealt with the trafficking and homing of lymphocytes in the body[11–14]. Naive lymphocytes originating from bone marrow or thymus patrol the body in search of their specific antigen. These cells are capable of recirculating through all secondary lymphoid tissues (Peyer's patches, lymph nodes, tonsils and spleen), presumably with the same capability within a given lymphocyte subset. Naive cells are believed to continue this recirculation until they either die or meet their specific antigen. Secondary lymphoid tissues are known to collect antigen from the surrounding epithelial surfaces, various tissues and the circulating blood, and present it to the naive lymphocytes in the context of the specialized lymphoid microenvironment. An encounter with the right antigen initiates the differentiation of the cells into blasts and finally effector and memory cells. Most effector and memory cells probably also circulate through secondary lymphoid tissues but, unlike naive cells, they can also recirculate through tertiary lymphoid tissues (intestinal lamina propria, pulmonary interstitium, inflamed skin and joints). Another distinguishing property of the effector and memory cells is that they are no longer homogeneous in their homing behaviour, but have taken on tissue-selective homing properties. This is believed to function in the targeting of the immune responses to sites where they are most likely to re-encounter their specific antigen. The tissue-selectivity of the homing event is regarded to be regulated at the molecular level in lymphocyte extravasation.

HOMING OF LYMPHOCYTES INTO TISSUES

The extravasation of lymphocytes in the lymph nodes takes place in postcapillary high endothelial venules (HEV)[15,16]. Currently, the lymphocyte–endothelial cell interaction during the process of extravasation is regarded to be a multistep process[14] consisting of four distinct yet overlapping steps (Figure 1): (a) initial transient interactions (tethering and rolling), (b) activation, (c) arrest and (d) diapedesis. The first contact between the lymphocyte and the endothelium may involve separable contact formation (tethering) with a loose rolling of the lymphocyte along the vessel wall, and a gradual slackening of the speed of rolling. This slackening provides the lymphocyte with sufficient time to react with the pro-adhesive factors, soluble or endothelial, of the microenvironment.

The tissue-selectivity of lymphocyte migration is believed to be largely based on an interaction of complementary pairs of adhesion molecules (Table 1)[12–14]. Lymphocyte surface homing receptors (HR) bind to the vascular addressins expressed by the endothelial cells of the postcapillary venules. These addressins are distributed in a tissue-selective manner in the body and, therefore, a tissue-selective homing of lymphocytes expressing the corresponding HR ensues. Some homing receptor–vascular addressin pairs have been identified: lymphocyte

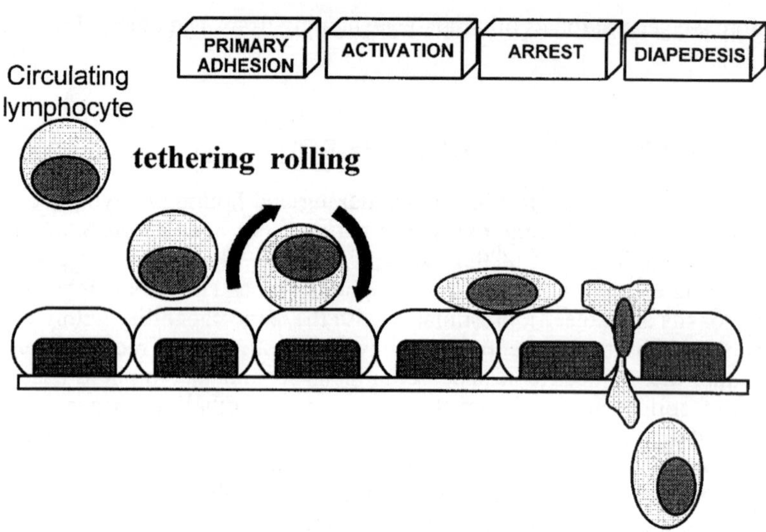

Figure 1 Homing of lymphocytes into tissues: multistep adhesion model consisting of four distinct, yet overlapping, steps of primary adhesion, activation, arrest and diapedesis

Table 1 Some adhesion molecules involved in lymphocyte–endothelial recognition.

Lymphocyte homing receptor	Predominant endothelial cell ligand	Primary homing pathway
L-selectin	PNAd	Peripheral lymph node
$\alpha4\beta7$	MAdCAM-1	Naive lymphocyte to Peyer's patch; effector lymphocyte to intestinal lamina propria
CLA	E-selectin	Skin

PNAd, peripheral lymph node addressin; MAdCAM-1, mucosal addressin cell adhesion molecule; CLA, cutaneous lymphocyte-associated antigen (modified from ref. 14).

surface $\alpha4\beta7$ binds to mucosal addressin cell adhesion molecule-1 (MAdCAM-1) in the intestinal mucosa[17], L-selectin binds to PNAd in the peripheral lymph nodes (PLN)[18] and cutaneous lymphocyte antigen (CLA) to E-selectin in the skin tissue[19]. The respiratory tract has been suggested to have its own, still-unidentified HR–vascular addressin pair.

Tissue-selective homing is believed to target the immunoblasts to sites where they are most likely to re-encounter their specific antigen. Investigation of the expression of homing receptors on the surface of antigen-specific lymphocytes provides a useful model for examining the targeting of immune responses from/to different sites of the body.

Homing of antigen-specific intestinal B cells in humans

Homing of antigen-specific intestinal B cells has been the subject of recent research. Quiding-Järbrink *et al.* showed, with volunteers immunized orally with cholera toxin B-subunit or parenterally with tetanus toxoid that, as compared to the parenterally activated cells, a lower proportion of the mucosally induced B cells express L-selectin, the PLN HR[20]. In a comparable experimental design, with patients suffering from bacterial diarrhoea or volunteers parenterally immunized with tetanus toxoid, we confirmed this finding and showed that, as compared to parentally induced cells, a significantly higher proportion of the mucosally activated cells express $\alpha 4\beta 7$, the gut homing receptor[21]. As both of these experimental designs used different antigens for oral and parenteral priming, we confirmed the findings by giving the same antigen, *Salmonella typhi* Ty21a, orally and parenterally to previously non-immunized volunteers, and found that, as compared to the parenterally activated cells, a higher proportion of the mucosally activated cells express $\alpha 4\beta 7$ and a smaller proportion of them express L-selectin[22]. All the mucosally activated cells expressed $\alpha 4\beta 7$[22]. In conclusion, these results show that the site of antigen encounter determines the expression of homing receptors. Moreover, it shows that B cells activated at the gut mucosa are highly committed to homing back to the gut.

Homing of antigen-specific intestinal T cells in humans

The expression of homing receptors on antigen-specific intestinal T cell has been studied less than that of B cells. Paronen *et al.*[23] found, in patients with diabetes, that T cells specific to a pancreatic islet cell antigen, GAD65, express $\alpha 4\beta 7$, the gut HR, more frequently than T cells specific to tetanus toxoid. Rott *et al.* showed that T cells specific to rotavirus, an intestinal antigen, express $\alpha 4\beta 7$ more frequently than T cells specific to tetanus toxoid, a parenteral antigen[24]. We have recently investigated the homing receptor-expression of newly recruited antigen-specific T cells after administration of the same antigen, keyhole limpet haemocyanin (KLH) via the oral vs. parenteral route. As compared to parenterally induced T cells a significantly higher proportion of the mucosally activated cells were found to express the gut homing receptor $\alpha 4\beta 7$ (Kantele *et al.*, unpublished data). These data imply that mucosally activated T cells have homing potentials favouring their homing back to the mucosa. Moreover, the data provide evidence for recirculation of mucosal T cells in humans.

HOMING OF LYMPHOCYTES INTO TISSUES IN INFLAMMATORY BOWEL DISEASE

A typical feature of the pathology of IBD is the infiltration of lymphocytes in the bowel mucosa[25,26]. Lymphocyte homing both to normal tissues and to sites of inflammation is, in part, regulated by differential expression of cell surface homing receptors and their interactions with tissue-selective vascular addressins at sites of lymphocyte recruitment from the blood. Recent studies on lamina propria lymphocytes isolated from normal and inflamed tissue show that blasts from the inflamed gut have lost their selectivity of HEV binding[27]. It is suggested that lymphocytes not physiologically migrating to the mucosa-associated lymphatic tissue gain entrance to the mucosa. The aberrant selectivity of homing in the inflamed tissue seems to be caused by inflammation-related alterations in the adhesion molecule pattern expressed on the endothelial cells. Salmi *et al.* have found that the peripheral lymph node addressin, PNAd, which is recognized by L-selectin, is absent in the normal gut but abundantly present on mucosal epithelial cells in the inflamed bowel[27].

Recently Briskin *et al.*[28] examined, in human tissues, the expression of MAdCAM-1, the vascular addressin recognized by $\alpha4\beta7$. It was found to be selectively expressed on the endothelium of venules in the intestinal lamina propria. As compared to normal tissues, the proportion of lamina propria venular endothelium expressing MAdCAM-1 was found to be increased at inflammatory foci associated with ulcerative colitis and Crohn's disease.

Prevention of inflammation by modulating the adhesion molecule function has been suggested as a strategy for modulating IBD activity. One of the approaches could be using the lymphocyte recirculatory pathway defined by MAdCAM-1/$\alpha4\beta7$ as a tissue-specific therapeutic target[28].

References

1. Mestecky J. The common mucosal immune system and current strategies for induction of immune responses in external secretions. J Clin Immunol. 1987;7:265–76.
2. Gowans JL, Knight EJ. The route of recirculation of lymphocytes in rat. Proc R Soc Lond B Biol Sci. 1964;159:257–82.
3. Griscelli C, Vassalli P, McClusky RT. The distribution of large dividing lymph node cells in syngeneic recipient rats after intravenous injection. J Exp Med. 1969;130:1427–42.
4. Craig SW, Cebra JJ. Peyer's patches: an enriched source of precursors for IgA-producing immunocytes in the rabbit. J Exp Med. 1971;134:188–200.
5. Husband AJ, Gowans JL. The origin and antigen-dependent distribution of IgA-containing cells in the intestine. J Exp Med. 1978;148:1146–59.
6. Weisz-Carrington P, Roux ME, McWilliams M, Phillips-Quagliata JM, Lamm ME. Organ and isotype distribution of plasma cells producing specific antibody after oral immunization: evidence for a generalized secretory immune system. J Immunol. 1979;123:1705–8.
7. Kantele A, Arvilommi H, Jokinen I. Specific immunoglobulin-secreting human blood cells after peroral immunization against *Salmonella typhi.* J Infect Dis. 1986;153:1126–31.
8. Czerkinsky C, Prince SJ, Michalek SM *et al.* IgA antibody-producing cells in peripheral blood after antigen ingestion: evidence for a common mucosal immune system in humans. Proc Natl Acad Sci USA. 1987;84:2449–53.
9. Wenneras C, Svennerholm A-M, Czerkinsky C. Vaccine-specific T cells in human peripheral blood after oral immunization with an inactivated enterotoxigenic *Escherichia coli* vaccine. Infect Immun. 1994;62:874–9.
10. Moldoveanu Z, Russell MW, Wu H-Y, Mestecky J. Compartmentalization within the mucosal immune system. Adv Exp Med Biol. 1995;371A:97–101.
11. Butcher EC. The regulation of lymphocyte traffic. Curr Top Microbiol Immunol. 1986;128:85–122.
12. Springer TA. Adhesion receptors of the immune system. Nature. 1990;346:425–34.
13. Yednock TA, Rosen SD. Lymphocyte homing. Adv Immunol. 1989;44:313–78.
14. Butcher EC, Picker LJ. Lymphocyte homing and homeostasis. Science. 1996;272:60–6.
15. Marchesi VT, Gowans JL. The migration of lymphocytes through the endothelium of venules in lymph nodes: an electron microscope study. Proc R Soc Lond B Biol Sci. 1964;159:283–95.
16. Schoefl GI. The migration of lymphocytes across the vascular endothelium in lymphoid tissue. J Exp Med. 1972;136:568–88.
17. Berlin C, Berg EL, Briskin MJ *et al.* $\alpha4\beta7$ integrin mediates lymphocyte binding to the mucosal vascular addressin MAdCAM-1. Cell. 1993;74:185–95.
18. Kansas GS. Structure and function of L-selectin. APMIS. 1992;100:287–93.

19. Berg EL, Yoshino T, Rott LS *et al.* The cutaneous lymphocyte antigen is a skin lymphocyte homing receptor for the vascular lectin endothelial cell-leukocyte adhesion molecule 1. J Exp Med. 1991;174:1461–6.
20. Quiding-Järbrink M, Lakew M, Nordström I *et al.* Human circulating specific antibody-forming cells after systemic and mucosal immunizations: differential homing commitments and cell surface differentiation markers. Eur J Immunol. 1995;25:322–7.
21. Kantele JM, Arvilommi H, Kontiainen S *et al.* Mucosally activated circulating human B cells in diarrhoea express homing receptors directing them back to the gut. Gastroenterology. 1996;110:1061–7.
22. Kantele A, Kantele JM, Savilahti E *et al.* Homing potentials of circulating lymphocytes in humans depend on the site of activation: oral, but not parenteral, typhoid vaccination induces circulating antibody-secreting cells that all bear homing receptors directing them to the gut. J Immunol. 1997;158:574–9.
23. Paronen J, Klemetti P, Kantele JM *et al.* Glutamate decarboxylase-reactive peripheral blood lymphocytes from patients with IDDM express gut-specific homing receptor $\alpha4\beta7$-integrin. Diabetes. 1997;46:583–8.
24. Rott LS, Rosé JR, Bass D, Williams MB, Greenberg HB, Butcher EC. Expression of mucosal homing receptor $\alpha4\beta7$ by circulating CD4$^+$ cells with memory for intestinal rotavirus. J Clin Invest. 1997;100:1204–9.
25. Kirsner JB, Shorter RG. Recent developments in nonspecific inflammatory bowel disease. N Engl J Med. 1982;306:837–48.
26. Selby WS, Janossy G, Bofill M, Jewell DP. Intestinal lymphocyte subpopulations in inflammatory bowel diseases: an analysis by immunohistochemical techniques. Gut. 1984;C25:32–40.
27. Salmi M, Granfors K, MacDermott R, Jalkanen S. Aberrant binding of lamina propria lymphocytes to vascular endothelium in inflammatory bowel disease. Gastroenterology. 1994;106:596–605.
28. Briskin M, Winsor-Hines D, Shyjan A *et al.* Human mucosal addressin cell adhesion molecule-1 is preferentially expressed in intestinal tract and associated lymphoid tissue. Am J Pathol. 1997;151:97–110.

12
Principles of oral tolerance

J. H. ZIVNY, H. L. VU, M. W. RUSSELL, Z. MOLDOVEANU,
J. MESTECKY and C. O. ELSON

GENERAL CONCEPTS

The mucosal immune system is stimulated every day by antigens from food and microbiota and plays an essential role in the regulation and maintenance of the normal balance between immunity and tolerance[1]. Oral tolerance is an antigen-specific immune hyporesponsiveness induced by the oral administration of antigen. Antigen administration to other mucosal surfaces has a similar effect; thus, the term mucosal tolerance may be more appropriate than oral tolerance. However, the majority of studies have been done after the oral administration of antigen so most of our knowledge applies to this route of tolerance induction.

Important parameters for the induction of oral tolerance

A number of important parameters for the induction of oral tolerance have been defined in animal models (Table 1). The type of antigens that have induced oral tolerance include various eukaryotic protein antigens, contact allergens, heterologous red blood cells and certain killed viruses. A common feature of tolerogenic antigens is that most of them induce T-cell-dependent immune response and are good immunogens when given parenterally. T-cell-independent antigens do not appear to induce oral tolerance[2]. Another important parameter for the induction of oral tolerance is the dose of antigen, in that the mechanism of toler-

Table 1 Important parameters for the induction of oral tolerance

Type of antigen
Dose of antigen
Frequency of feeding
Mucosal route
Immunogenicity of the antigen
Species
Genetic background of individual
Age
Delivery system/adjuvant

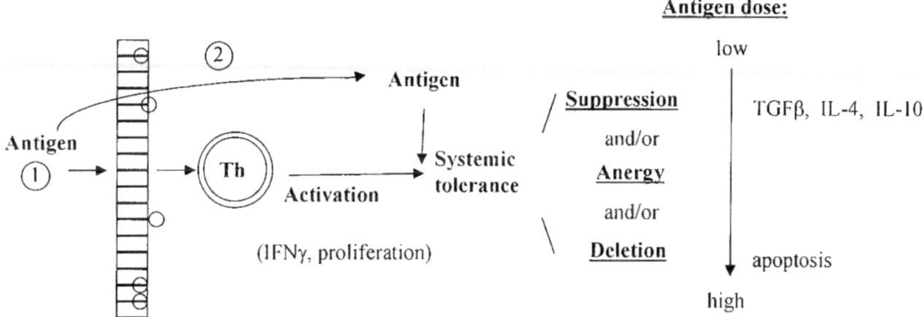

Figure 1 Induction of oral tolerance. ① Antigen exposure at the mucosal surface results in activation of CD4 helper T cells which is manifested by some cell cycling and cytokine production. ② A further dose of antigen affects T cells that had been partially activated. The exact site of induction of tolerance and the cells, cytokines, and other molecules involved remain to be defined. The systemic tolerance that follows antigen feeding is the net result of a number of mechanisms. The predominant mechanism may be related to the dose of antigen fed, with regulatory cells producing inhibitory cytokines generated at low doses and anergy or deletion occurring at high doses

ance induced by antigen feeding is related to the dose of antigen fed. Regulatory cells producing inhibitory cytokines appear to be generated at lower doses and anergy or deletion occur at higher doses[3] (Figure 1). Also several other important parameters have been defined: the mucosal route of antigen delivery, the age of an animal[4,5], genetic background, and species of the host[6,7].

Little is known about the modulation of oral tolerance in animals and even less in humans. Recent studies in experimental animals have shown that oral tolerance can be enhanced or the effective tolerogenic dose can be reduced by varying the delivery vehicle or incorporating the immunomodulator with the fed antigen. Khoury *et al.* showed that feeding of antigen along with bacterial lipopolysaccharide enhanced oral tolerance to myelin basic protein[8]. Sun *et al.* have demonstrated that the feeding of recombinant cholera toxin B subunit (rCTB) covalently linked to antigen can enhance tolerance for DTH responses[9] and protect against EAE[10] more effectively than does the feeding of unconjugated antigens. Oral antigen delivery by way of a multiple emulsion system enhanced oral tolerance induction to bovine serum albumin, ovalbumin, and a bacterial protein (PhoA)[11]. These studies show that oral tolerance can be enhanced and usage of these delivery and immunomodulatory systems may result in marked reduction of the antigen doses required to induce tolerance.

Important features of oral tolerance

A number of important features have been defined. First, cellular and humoral immune tolerance is antigen specific. Second, immune tolerance is partial with no more than 80–90% reduction in measured responses that occur without the feeding. Third, tolerance wanes with time, lasting several months in mice. Fourth, feeding of antigen abrogates the induction of response better than it reduces an established response. However, established immune responses can be reduced by the feeding of antigen, suggesting the possible use of oral tolerance for the treatment of autoimmune diseases[1].

Treatment of experimental autoimmune (AI) diseases

The induction of immune tolerance by antigen feeding has been shown to have a beneficial effect on the prevention and treatment of several experimental auto-immune diseases (Table 2)[12].

Arthritis

Oral administration of Type II collagen abrogates the induction of arthritis in several models, including collagen-induced arthritis, adjuvant arthritis, pristane arthritis and antigen-induced arthritis. Nasal administration of collagen has also suppressed arthritis.

Experimental autoimmune encephalomyelitis (EAE)

Several studies have demonstrated the effectiveness of orally administered myelin basic protein (MBP) and proteolipid protein (PLP) in both rat and mouse models of EAE.

Diabetes

Oral insulin and glutamic acid decarboxylase (GAD) have been shown to delay and, in some instances, prevent the onset of diabetes in young non-obese diabetic (NOD) mice.

Uveitis

Oral administration of S-antigen and interphotoreceptor binding protein (IRBP) prevented and markedly diminished the clinical appearance of S-antigen-induced and IRBP-induced disease, respectively.

Myasthenia

Although myasthenia gravis is an antibody-mediated disease, oral and nasal administration of the acetylcholine receptor to Lewis rats prevented or delayed the onset of disease. Large doses of antigen were required.

Table 2 Oral tolerance as a therapy for experimental models of disease

Model	*Antigen fed*
EAE	MBP, PLP
Uveitis	S-antigen, IRBP
Arthritis	Collagen type II
Diabetes (NOD mice)	Insulin, GAD protein
Myasthenia gravis	Acetylcholine receptor
Thyroiditis	Thyroglobulin
Transplantation	Alloantigen, MHC peptides
Experimental colitis	TNBS, TNP-intestinal proteins

Transplantation models

Significant reduction in delayed-type hypersensitivity (DTH) can be achieved by the feeding of allogeneic cells or synthetic allogeneic MHC antigens. The feeding of such antigens has extended the graft survival in several models.

Chronic intestinal inflammation

Administration of the contact sensitizing agent, trinitrobenzene sulphonic acid (TNBS) in 50% ethanol, into the mouse colon results in transmural inflammation. Feeding of TNBS prior to the induction of colonic disease reduced the histological severity of disease and abolished the antibody response[13]. Neurath *et al.* induced similar protection against TNBS-induced colitis by feeding TNBS-haptenized colonic proteins[14]. The protection was associated with increased mucosal production of TGF-β, IL-4, and IL-10 and with reduced production of IL-12. Administration of recombinant IL-12 or antibodies to TGF-β were both able to abrogate the protection. These studies represent the first demonstration that mucosal tolerance might be exploited to prevent chronic inflammatory disease of the mucosa itself. Whether this approach should be used in the treatment of chronic inflammatory bowel diseases in humans is yet to be seen because they may involve defects in mucosal tolerization.

In the majority of animal models of autoimmune disease, the antigen being fed is the same as that used to induce the disease by parenteral immunization. In contrast, the antigens mediating disease in humans are not known and thus the challenge of applying this approach to the treatment of human disease is greater.

MECHANISMS OF ORAL TOLERANCE

The most common mechanisms of immune tolerance to orally administered antigens in animal models appear to be clonal anergy, clonal deletion, and T-cell-mediated suppression[15]. So far, clonal deletion has been observed only in ovalbumin T-cell-receptor transgenic mice fed huge bolus doses of antigen[6].

T cells having an anergic phenotype have been detected in orally tolerized animals fed with relatively large doses of antigen[3,17–19]. Anergy is characterized by reduced proliferation of antigen-specific T cells after stimulation with antigen and functional antigen-presenting cells caused by an induced defect in IL-2 transcription and production. Reactivity of T cells can be restored by incubation with IL-2 for several days[20].

T cell-mediated suppression has been described using various transfer models of immune tolerance[21,22]. The mechanisms of suppression are not fully understood. Two current concepts are proposed. First, preferential induction of suppressive cytokines produced by antigen-specific T cells, such as IL-4, IL-10 and TGF-β, inhibit immune responses by bystander suppression[18,23,24]. In several experimental models of autoimmune diseases, oral tolerance induced to a third-party antigen expressed within the affected organ ameliorated the outcome of the experimentally-induced organ-specific autoimmune disease[25–27]. Importantly, such cytokines do not require cell contact and can inhibit T cells activated within the same microenvironment. Second, the antigen-specific anergic T cells suppress other T cells through competition for cytokines, such as IL-2, and for antigen-presenting cell ligands[28]. This mechanism of suppression requires direct contact of involved cells. Mechanisms of oral tolerance are probably not mutually exclusive and more than one of them could be operative simultaneously.

Potential adverse effects of immune deviation

Experiments on non-human primates have indicated that the stimulation of antibody responses by parenterally-induced immune tolerance may be harmful[29]. The feeding of autoantigen induced a cytotoxic T lymphocyte response that could lead to the onset of autoimmune diabetes[30] in a transgenic model. These results suggest that caution should be used when applying immune deviation to the treatment of human autoimmune diseases.

HUMAN STUDIES

Oral tolerance has been extensively studied in various animals[1,12,26] but there have been only a few attempts to explore oral tolerance in humans[31–36]. Based on the impressive results of oral tolerance induction in animal models of autoimmunity, clinical trials with the oral administration of the potential autoantigens have been initiated in multiple sclerosis[37], rheumatoid arthritis[38,39]; uveitis[40] and juvenile rheumatoid arthritis[41].

Short-term feeding of antigen in humans

Oral tolerance can be induced in humans by short-term feeding (10 doses) of the protein antigen keyhole limpet haemocyanin (KLH). However, the unresponsiveness occurred only in T cells, manifested by reductions in delayed-type hypersensitivity (DTH) and *in-vitro* proliferative responses, whereas antibody responses appeared to be primed[34]. Subsequent experiments have shown that the response to such short-term feeding is variable, with some individuals becoming tolerant while no evident effect is observed in others. These data suggest that the short-term feeding of autoantigens to humans could be useful for treatment in T cell-mediated autoimmunity but not in antibody-mediated autoimmunity. In additional studies, human volunteers were fed KLH alone or KLH plus recombinant CTB (rCTB) in 10 equal feeds. After feeding, each volunteer was parenterally immunized with KLH. KLH ingestion alone or with rCTB did not induce significant levels of serum IgG and IgA anti-KLH, nor did it induce significant levels of secretory IgA (S-IgA) anti-KLH in the intestinal secretions in most of the volunteers. However, antigen-specific S-IgA in the intestinal secretions, as well as serum IgG and IgA anti-CTB, were elevated in the group fed KLH plus rCTB. After parenteral immunization, the serum IgG anti-KLH was significantly greater in the group fed KLH alone than in the group fed KLH plus rCTB ($p = 0.02$). Feeding of KLH alone or KLH plus rCTB suppressed equally the DTH responses compared with the non-fed group given only parenteral immunization. Recombinant CTB, free of toxic A subunit, stimulated immune response to itself but did not stimulate active immunity to co-administered antigen. Instead, rCTB inhibited the priming effect to the co-administered antigen and thus may enhance immune tolerance toward other mucosally co-administered antigens.

Long-term feeding of antigen in humans

Humans are exposed naturally to large quantities of food antigens but little is known about the immune response to them. Using food antigens would represent the ideal way to explore the effects of long-term feeding of antigen on immune response and the mechanism of oral tolerance in humans.

Food antigens, such as ovalbumin (OVA) and bovine γ-globulin (BGG) are present in large quantities in the normal human diet, whereas soy bean protein (SBP) is present in lower quantities in the typical North American diet. It is known that small amounts of these dietary antigens are not digested and are detectable as intact antigen in the systemic circulation within an hour after a test meal[42]. Low levels of dietary antigen-specific IgG, IgM, and IgA have been detected in sera, as well as in secretions[43,44]. Parenteral immunization of human volunteers with bovine serum albumin (BSA) induced little or no response to BSA in sera[31]. These observations suggest the presence of active natural immune tolerance to common food antigens in humans but the mechanisms involved remain unknown.

We measured the systemic and mucosal immune responses and the mechanisms of oral tolerance to common dietary antigens, such as BGG, OVA, and SBP, in normal human volunteers. The T-cell proliferative response to these antigens was relatively low with mean stimulation indexes (SI) of BGG = 3.9 ± 0.6, OVA = 4.6 ± 0.6, SBP = 5.7 ± 1.4, which are close to the borderline of responsiveness, SI > 3. Serum IgG, IgA, and IgM and parotid saliva (IgA) antibody levels to these dietary antigens were measurable but also low. Individuals with higher proliferative responses or high titres of antibodies to BGG in serum and saliva tend to have higher responses to OVA. However, no significant correlation was observed between the systemic and mucosal immune responses to these antigens, suggesting mutual independence of the systemic and mucosal immune compartments.

Peripheral blood mononuclear cells (PBMC) stimulated with BGG or OVA did not express IL-2 mRNA, but they did express IL-2 receptor α-chain (IL-2Rα) mRNA, whereas PBMC stimulated with tetanus toxoid (TT), a parenteral immunogen, upregulated both IL-2 and IL-2Rα mRNA. Incubation with exogenous IL-2 alone did not restore T-cell proliferation to BGG or OVA, although incubation with exogenous rhIL-2 plus antigen did. Co-culture with BGG and OVA repeatedly suppressed the T-cell proliferative response to TT and purified protein derivative from *Mycobacterium tuberculosis* (PPD) in some of the individuals while, in others, there was no significant inhibition of proliferative responses. The BGG- and OVA-induced inhibition required cell contact and could be reversed with a low dose of rhIL-2 added at the beginning of the culture. These data show that human T cells specific for dietary antigens have properties compatible with anergic cells: low proliferation, no IL-2 expression, and expression of IL-2Rα-chain after the antigenic stimulus. Furthermore, dietary antigen-specific T cells can inhibit *in-vitro* proliferative responses and the cell contact is essential for this to occur. We propose that oral tolerance is mediated by several mechanisms acting simultaneously and that anergic antigen-specific T cells may also play a role in immune inhibition.

Trials of oral tolerance in human disease

Phase I trials

Phase I safety trials of oral tolerance in humans have been reported for patients with multiple sclerosis and rheumatoid arthritis. In a double-blind study, patients with multiple sclerosis were fed bovine myelin basic protein (300 mg/day) or placebo for one year[37]. No significant toxicity and some reduction of major attacks, as compared with those fed placebo, were observed in patients fed myelin. A marked increase in TGF-β secreting myelin basic protein- and proteo-lipid protein-specific *in vitro* derived short-term T cell lines from a myelin-fed group was reported as compared with non-fed individuals[45]. There were no significant differences in TGF-β-secreting cells found in the control tetanus toxoid T-cell lines between the groups. These data suggest that TGF-β regula-tory cells can be generated by the feeding of antigens in humans.

Patients with severe active rheumatoid arthritis were fed chicken type II colla-gen at 0.1–0.5 mg/day for three months. Again, no significant toxicity and the reduction in some parameters of disease activity were observed[38]. Both of these studies involved relatively small numbers of patients and no firm conclusions on efficacy can be derived.

Phase II trials

Several multicentre randomized controlled clinical trials have been completed in the United States and Germany. In Germany, 90 patients with early rheumatoid arthritis from 5 centres were treated with oral bovine collagen type II at 0.1 and 10 mg per day for 12 weeks in a double-blind randomized study[39]. Response was assessed by standard American College of Rheumatology (ACR) criteria. No statistically significant differences were found between the groups fed colla-gen and those fed placebo, although a trend toward improvement was observed in the groups given collagen. In a second multicentre randomized trial on rheumatoid arthritis in the United States, 274 patients resistant to disease-modifying anti-rheumatic drugs (DMARDS) were randomized into 4 treatment groups plus a placebo group. Groups were fed with 0, 0.2, 0.1, 0.5 and 2.5 mg of chicken type II collagen per day for 24 weeks. The criteria were >30% improve-ment in ACR and Paulus criteria[46]. No treatment-related adverse effects were detected. A positive effect was observed only at the lowest dose of collagen tested.

Other multicentre dose-ranging controlled trials are underway in a number of human autoimmune diseases (Table 3). The dose of the antigen fed and the patients selected for testing are a critical variable. Since antigen feeding has been shown to be safe in patients, it would be reasonable to target patients early in their disease course. The results from these clinical trials demonstrated that the mucosal administration of potential autoantigen is safe, does not exacerbate disease, and may have a positive clinical effect by decreasing T-cell autoreactiv-

Table 3 Controlled trials of oral tolerance as a therapy for human diseases

Disease	*Antigen fed*
Rheumatoid arthritis	Collagen type II (bovine/chicken)
Multiple sclerosis	Myelin (bovine)
Type I diabetes mellitus	Insulin (human)
Uveoretinitis	Retinal S-antigen (bovine)

ity in some of the patients[45]. However, the parameters involved in the induction, modulation and maintenance of different mechanisms of tolerance in humans are far from understood.

References

1. Mowat AM. Oral tolerance and regulation of immunity to dietary antigens. In: Ogra PL, Mestecky J, Lamm ME, Strober W, McGhee JH, Bienenstock J, editors. Handbook of Mucosal Immunology. San Diego: Academic Press; 1994:185–98.
2. Titus RG, Chiller JM. Orally induced tolerance. Definition at the cellular level. Int Arch Allergy Appl Immunol. 1981;65:323–38.
3. Friedman A, Weiner HL. Induction of anergy or active suppression is determined by antigen dosage. Proc Natl Acad Sci USA. 1993;91:6688–92.
4. Strobel S, Ferguson A. Immune responses to fed protein antigens in mice. 3. Systemic tolerance or priming is related to age at which antigen is first encountered. Pediatr Res. 1984;18:558–94.
5. Faria AM, Garcia G, Rios MJ, Michalaros CL, Vaz NM. Decrease in susceptibility to oral tolerance induction and occurrence of oral immunization to ovalbumin in 20–38-week-old mice. The effect of interval between oral exposures and rate of antigen intake in the oral immunization. Immunology. 1993;78:147–51.
6. Miller CC, Cook ME. Evidence against the induction of immunological tolerance by feeding the antigens to chickens. Poult Sci. 1994;73:106–12.
7. Peri BA, Rothberg RM. Circulating antitoxin after ingestion of diphtheria toxoid. Infect Immun. 1981;32:1148–54.
8. Khoury SJ, Lider O, al-Sabbagh A, Weiner HL. Suppression of experimental autoimmune encephalomyelitis by oral administration of myelin basic protein. III. Synergistic effect of lipopolysaccharide. Cell Immunol. 1990;131:302–10.
9. Sun JB, Holmgren J, Czerkinsky C. Cholera toxin B subunit: an efficient transmucosal carrier-delivery system for induction of peripheral immunological tolerance. Proc Natl Acad Sci USA. 1994;91:10795–9.
10. Sun JB, Rask C, Olsson T, Holmgren J, Czerkinsky C. Treatment of experimental autoimmune encephalomyelitis by feeding myelin basic protein conjugated to cholera toxin B submit. Proc Natl Acad Sci USA. 1996;93:7196–201.
11. Elson CO, Tomasi M, Dertzbaugh MT, Thaggard G, Hunter R, Weaver C. Oral-antigen delivery by way of multiple emulsion system enhances oral tolerance. Ann NY Acad Sci. 1996;778:156–62.
12. Weiner HL, Friedman A, Miller A *et al*. Oral tolerance: immunologic mechanisms and treatment of animal and human organ-specific autoimmune diseases by oral administration of autoantigens. Annu Rev Immunol. 1994;12:809–37.
13. Elson CO, Beagley KW, Sharmanov AT *et al*. Hapten-induced model of murine inflammatory bowel disease: mucosa immune responses and protection by tolerance. J Immunol. 1996;157:2174–85.
14. Neurath MF, Fuss I, Kelsall BL, Presky DH, Waegell W, Strober W. Experimental granulomatous colitis in mice is abrogated by induction of TGF-beta-mediated oral tolerance. J Exp Med. 1996;183:2605–16.
15. Weiner HL. Oral tolerance: immune mechanisms and treatment of autoimmune diseases. Immunol Today. 1997;18:335–43.

16. Chen Y, Inobe J, Marks R, Gonnella P, Kuchroo VK, Weiner HL. Peripheral deletion of antigen-reactive T cells in oral tolerance. Nature. 1995;376:177–80.
17. Melamed D, Friedman A. Direct evidence for anergy in T lymphocytes tolerized by oral administration of ovalbumin. Eur J Immunol. 1993;23:935–42.
18. Miller A, Lider O, Weier HL. Antigen-driven bystander suppression after oral administration of antigens. J Exp Med. 1991;174:791–8.
19. Whitacre CC, Gienapp IE, Orosz CG, Bitar DM. Oral tolerance in experimental autoimmune encephalomyelitis. III. Evidence for clonal anergy. J Immunol. 1991;147:2155–63.
20. Schwartz RH. Models of T cell anergy: is there a common molecular mechanism? J Exp Med. 1996;184:1–8.
21. Richman LK, Chiller JM, Brown WR, Hanson DG, Vaz NM. Enterically induced immunologic tolerance. I. Induction of suppressor T lymphocytes by intragastric administration of soluble proteins. J Immunol. 1978;121(6):2429–34.
22. MacDonald TT. Immunosuppression caused by antigen feeding II. Suppressor T cells mask Peyer's patch B cell priming to orally administered antigen. Eur J Immunol. 1983;13:138–42.
23. Tanaka T, Hu-Li J, Seder RA, Fazekas de St Groth B, Paul WE. Interleukin 4 suppresses interleukin 2 and interferon gamma production by naive T cells stimulated by accessory cell-dependent receptor engagement. Proc Natl Acad Sci USA. 1993;90:5914–18.
24. de Waal Malefyt R, Yssel H, de Vries JE. Direct effects of IL-10 on subsets of human CD4+ T cells clones and resting T cells. Specific inhibition of IL-2 production and proliferation. J Immunol. 1993;150:4754–65.
25. von Herrath MG, Dyrberg T, Oldstone MB. Oral insulin treatment suppresses virus-induced antigen-specific destruction of beta cells and prevents autoimmune diabetes in transgenic mice. J Clin Invest. 1996;98:1324–31.
26. al-Sabbagh A, Miller A, Santos LM, Weiner HL. Antigen-driven tissue-specific suppression following oral tolerance: orally administered myelin basic protein suppresses proteolipid protein-induced experimental autoimmune encephalomyelitis in the SJL mouse. Eur J Immunol. 1994;24:2104–9.
27. Zhang ZY, Lee CS, Lider O, Weiner HL. Suppression of adjuvant arthritis in Lewis rats by oral administration of type II collagen. J Immunol. 1990;145:2489–93.
28. Lombardi G, Sidhu S, Batchelor R, Lechler R. Anergic T cells as suppressor cells *in vitro*. Science. 1994;264:1587–9.
29. Genain CP, Abel K, Belmar N *et al*. Late complications of immune deviation therapy in a non-human primate. Science. 1996;274:2054–7.
30. Blanas E, Carbone FR, Allison J, Miller JF, Heath WR. Induction of autoimmune diabetes by oral administration of autoantigen. Science. 1996;274:1707–9.
31. Korenblat PE, Rothberg RM, Minden P, Farr RS. Immune responses of human adults after oral and parenteral exposure to bovine serum albumin. J Allergy. 1968;41:226–35.
32. Bierme SJ, Blanc M, Abbal M, Fournie A. Oral Rh treatment for severely immunized mothers. Lancet. 1979;1:604–5.
33. Gold WR Jr, Queenan JT, Woody J, Sacher RA. Oral desensitization in Rh disease. Am J Obstet Gynecol. 1983;146:980–1.
34. Husby S, Mestecky J, Moldoveanu Z, Holland S, Elson CO. Oral tolerance in humans. T cell but not B cell tolerance after antigen feeding. J Immunol. 1994;152:4663–70.
35. Waldo FB, van den Wall Bake AW, Mestecky J, Husby S. Suppression of the immune response by nasal immunization. Clin Immunol Immunopathol. 1994;72:30–4.
36. Thompson HS, Staines NA. Could specific oral tolerance be a therapy for autoimmune disease? Immunol Today. 1990;11:396–9.
37. Weiner HL, Mackin GA, Matsui M *et al*. Double-blind pilot trial of oral tolerization with myelin antigens in multiple sclerosis. Science. 1993;259:1321–4.
38. Trentham DE, Dynesius-Trentham RA, Orav EJ *et al*. Effects of oral administration of type II collagen on rheumatoid arthritis. Science. 1993;261:1727–30.
39. Sieper J, Kary S, Sorensen H *et al*. Oral type II collagen treatment in early rheumatoid arthritis. A double-blind, placebo-controlled, randomized trial. Arthritis Rheum. 1996;39:41–51.
40. Nussenblatt RB, Whitcup SM, de Smet MD. Intraocular inflammatory disease (uveitis) and the use of oral tolerance: a status report. Ann NY Acad Sci. 1996;778:325–37.
41. Barnett ML, Combitchi D, Trentham DE. A pilot trial of oral type II collagen in the treatment of juvenile rheumatoid arthritis. Arthritis Rheum. 1996;39:623–8.

42. Husby S, Jensenius JC, Svehag SE. Passage of undegraded dietary antigen into the blood of healthy adults. Quantification, estimation of size distribution, and relation of uptake to levels of specific antibodies. Scand J Immunol. 1985;22:83–92.
43. O'Mahony S, Arranz E, Barton JR, Ferguson A. Dissociation between systemic and mucosal humoral immune responses in coeliac disease. Gut. 1991;32:29–35.
44. Russell MW, Mestecky J, Julian BA, Galla JH. IgA-associated renal diseases: antibodies to environmental antigens in sera and deposition of immunoglobulins and antigens in glomeruli. J Clin Immunol. 1986;6:74–86.
45. Fukaura H, Kent SC, Pietrusewicz MJ, Khoury SJ, Weiner HL, Hafler DA. Induction of circulating myelin basic protein and proteolipid protein-specific transforming growth factor-betal-secreting Th3 T cells by oral administration of myelin in multiple sclerosis patients. J Clin Invest. 1996;98:70–7.
46. Barnett ML, Kremer JM, St Clair EW *et al.* Treatment of rheumatoid arthritis with oral type II collagen. Results of a multicenter, double-blind, placebo-controlled trial. Arthritis Rheum. 1998;41:290–7.

13
Immunological tolerance in IBD

R. DUCHMANN

INTRODUCTION

Immunological tolerance describes a state in which specific antigen either does not elicit a T or B cell response or leads to the induction of immunoregulatory cells which effectively suppress the immune response against it. First of all, and this relates to the gut as it does to other organs, tolerance is important to prevent unwanted immune responses towards tissue-expressed self-antigens. Second, and this is rather unique to the gut, the intestinal immune system must also be tolerant to 'beneficial non-self-antigens' in the form of dietary antigens and antigens from the intestinal flora (Figure 1). When any of the mechanisms that regulate these various forms of immunological tolerance become perturbed, chronic intestinal inflammation may be induced.

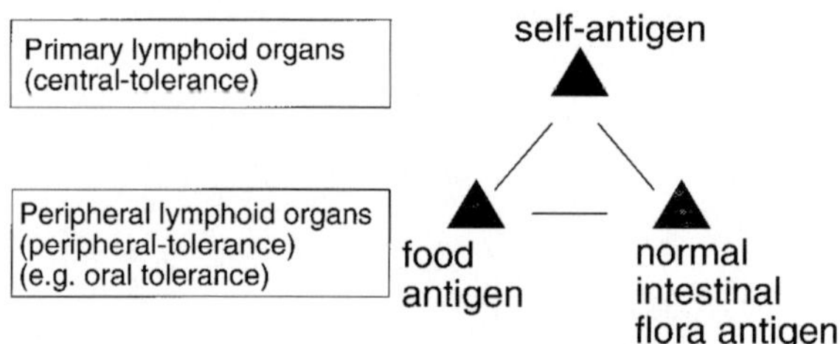

Figure 1 *Tolerance*. Immunological tolerance (IT) describes a state in which specific antigen either does not elicit a T or B cell response or leads to the induction of immunoregulatory cells which effectively suppress the immune response against it. IT is actively acquired and maintained throughout life as a result of several mechanisms. These include events in primary lymphoid organs (central tolerance) which lead to the clonal deletion of immature lymphocytes bearing receptors specific for self-antigens expressed in the thymus (T cells) and bone marrow (B cells); they also include events in peripheral lymphoid organs (peripheral tolerance) which act on more mature lymphocytes and involve clonal deletion, anergy, suppression, and/or clonal ignorance. In the gut, IT is important to prevent unwanted immune responses towards tissue expressed self antigens and 'beneficial non-self antigens' in the form of dietary antigens and antigens from the intestinal flora. When any of the mechanisms that regulate these various forms of immunological tolerance become perturbed, chronic intestinal inflammation may result

TOLERANCE TO SELF-ANTIGENS

Immunological self-tolerance is necessary to avoid autoimmune diseases. It requires the efficient elimination or silencing of lymphocytes with antigen receptors specific for the host's own antigens, and is in great part based on the expression of unique antigen receptors on T and B lymphocytes (TCR/immunoglobulin) generated through genetic recombination events. Immunological self-tolerance is actively acquired and maintained throughout life as a result of several mechanisms. These include events in primary lymphoid organs (central tolerance) which lead to the clonal deletion of immature lymphocytes bearing receptors specific for self-antigens expressed in the thymus (T cells) and bone marrow (B cells); they also include events in peripheral lymphoid organs (peripheral tolerance) which act on more mature lymphocytes and involve clonal deletion, anergy, suppression, and/or clonal ignorance (Figure 1). In the intestinal immune system, for which a role as a primary lymphoid organ has been suggested, the situation may be even more complex and include the fascinating but little-explored possibility that self-reactive lymphocytes generate and need to be controlled locally. Abnormal regulation of central and/or peripheral tolerance mechanisms might induce lymphocytes with reactivity to self-intestine and thus cause or contribute to chronic inflammatory bowel disease (IBD).

AUTOIMMUNE PHENOMENA IN IBD

Autoimmune cytotoxicity, mediated by cytotoxic T cells, natural killer (NK) cells or antibody-dependent cellular cytotoxicity (ADCC) may result in the destruction of intestinal epithelial cells and therefore constitutes a potential mechanism of IBD pathogenesis (Figure 2).

Early studies demonstrated decreased cell-mediated cytotoxicity of IBD peripheral blood and intestinal cells[1] and seemed to argue against the involvement of such mechanisms in IBD pathogenesis. More recent investigations found that cytotoxicity of peripheral blood mononuclear cells was not different from controls but significantly reduced in Crohn's disease (CD) in the TCRVβ8 subset[2] and thus provided evidence for a selective defect in cytotoxic T cell function in CD. Using allogeneic peripheral blood lymphocytes from CD and ulcerative colitis

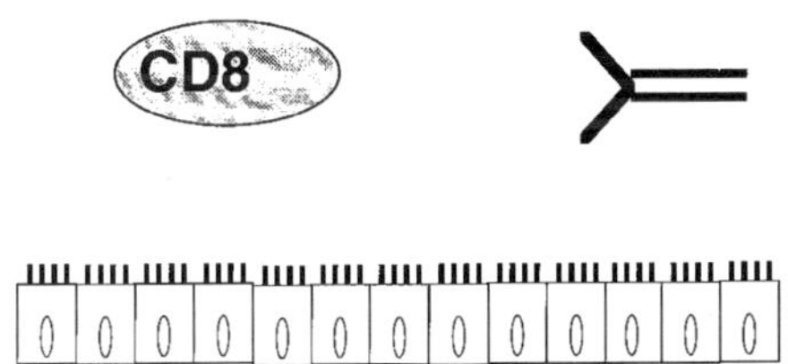

Figure 2 *Cytotoxicity.* Autoimmune cytotoxicity, mediated by cytotoxic T cells, NK cells or antibody dependent cellular cytotoxicity (ADCC) may result in the destruction of intestinal epithelial cells and therefore constitutes a potential mechanism of IBD pathogenesis

(UC) patients another group reported that these were not more cytotoxic to epithelial cells than those of controls[3], whereas in another study using a more relevant experimental design it was found that cytotoxic T lymphocyte (CTL) activity of peripheral blood mononuclear cells for autologous colonic target cells was increased compared with allogeneic target cells[4]. Due to the different experimental systems used, present data on cellular autoimmune cytotoxicity in IBD remain inconclusive. Further studies in IBD, especially those which investigate cell-mediated cytotoxicity towards intestinal epithelium in an autologous system, will hopefully be forthcoming to resolve this issue.

With regard to humoral autoimmune phenomena, a plethora of autoantibodies, including anti-erythrocyte antibodies, pancreatic antibodies, antineutrophilic cytoplasmic antibodies (ANCA), lymphocytotoxic antibodies and antibodies to epithelial cell components have been described in IBD patients[5]. Of these, due to their target and functional activity, antibodies reactive with intestinal epithelial cells[6], antibodies reactive with epithelial cell components purified from mouse epithelial cells (ECAC) and shown to mediate antibody-dependent cytotoxicity using antigen-coated red cell targets[7] and antibodies involved in epithelial deposition of activated complement[8] are candidates for mediating mucosal injury and thus IBD pathogenesis. Another antibody reactive with a 40 kDa protein of the tropomyosin family[9] was initially identified in extracts of resected UC tissue[10]. This antibody was found in virtually all UC patients but not in patients with CD or normal individuals, indicating a disease-specific abnormality.

ANCA are present in both CD and UC patients and seem to be useful to identify subgroups of IBD patients. Thus, it was shown that most of the 10–30% of CD patients with serum ANCA exhibit cytoplasmic binding patterns[11]. In contrast, perinuclear binding (pANCA) in CD, which is the predominant binding pattern in UC, has been reported to be associated with a rare allele (R241) of the intracellular adhesion molecule-1 (ICAM-1) gene and was suggested to characterize a subgroup of CD patients with UC-like clinical phenotype[12].

TOLERANCE TO BENEFICIAL NON-SELF-ANTIGENS

In addition to tolerance to self-antigens, tolerance to beneficial non-self-antigens in the form of food antigens or antigens from the normal intestinal flora is required to avoid deleterious immune stimulation by these permanently present antigens. Non-responsiveness to food antigens is achieved and maintained by oral tolerance. Oral tolerance is by now a well-established form of peripheral tolerance induced through prior oral administration of the same antigen, and its scope has recently been widened to therapeutic applications for the treatment of autoimmune diseases[13–15]. Non-responsiveness to antigens from the normal intestinal flora, in contrast, despite growing evidence that it exists and that it is abnormally regulated in chronic intestinal inflammation[16–19], has hardly been studied. In theory, immunological consequences of the exposure to normal intestinal flora, which co-develops in its host and stays permanently, can be expected to differ substantially from the immunological consequences that result from the exposure to food antigens, which is by chance repetitive and more transient in nature. This and the apparent influence of genetic factors on the selection of the normal intestinal flora[17,20,21] make it quite likely that tolerance to normal flora antigens is even more complex than oral tolerance and may also include features of self-tolerance.

At present, clinical studies convincingly demonstrate that the inflammatory stimulus causing early lesions of recurrent CD is within the faecal stream[22,23] and overwhelming data from various animal models incriminate the normal intestinal flora as the pivotal endogenous stimulus driving chronic intestinal inflammation[24,25]. Mounting evidence that these abnormal immune responses involve antigen-specific responses and an abnormal regulation of tolerance by T cells is discussed below.

Food antigens

Oral tolerance to food antigens involves mechanisms of clonal deletion, anergy and the induction of regulatory cells producing inhibitory mediators such as interleukin 4 (IL-4), IL-10 or transforming growth factor beta (TGF-β)[13–15]. It is known that the choice of mechanism of oral tolerance is influenced by factors such as the type of antigen, duration and dose of feeding. Oral tolerance is well established in animal models but has hardly been studied in humans[26]. Since there are no data on the status of oral tolerance in patients with IBD, it cannot be excluded that abnormal tolerance to food antigens contributes to IBD pathogenesis. Elevated levels of food antibodies[27] and a beneficial influence of exclusion diets observed in CD patients[28] would indeed suggest that this may be the case. Animal models of IBD discussed below at present, however, incriminate bacterial antigens rather than food antigens in the pathogenesis of chronic intestinal inflammation[24,25,29–31]. This has also become evident in a model of spontaneous colitis in C3H-HeJBir mice, where it could be shown that colitic CD4+ T cells are strongly reactive towards enteric bacterial flora but not to epithelial or food antigens[32].

Normal flora antigens

Although the bacterial flora is a potent immune stimulus, and drives the development of the mucosal immune system, little is known about how the normal response to antigens from the normal intestinal flora is regulated[24]. Colonization of the intestinal tract by the normal flora during infancy is not random, and has led to the concept of an autochthonous intestinal flora, common to all members of an animal species[33], to which the immune system is supposed to be tolerant. In addition, there is evidence for genetically controlled selection of an individual 'self' flora during colonization[21], as well as cross-tolerization between self-antigens and antigens from normal intestinal flora[17], indicating that tolerance to normal intestinal flora may also share aspects of individual self-tolerance[24].

Relating to IBD pathogenesis, it has been mentioned above that overwhelming evidence has accrued from a large variety of different animal models of IBD which all incriminate the normal intestinal flora as the relevant endogenous stimulus driving the chronic inflammatory process[24,25,30]. Unfortunately, the initial studies did not address the question of whether the bacterial stimulus is mediated through antigen or polyclonal activators and whether abnormal tolerance to enteric bacterial antigens is involved. In the meantime, however, human intestinal bacteria-reactive T cells have been shown to respond to discrete antigens[34], to be increased in involved IBD intestine[34], and, as discussed below, dysregulated T cells reactive to enteric bacterial antigens have been shown to mediate colitis[32]. In addition, abnormal T cell tolerance to intestinal flora[18,19] and both thymic dysregulation[35] and peripheral dysregulation of T cells[36–38] have been described in IBD or animal models of IBD which require an intestinal flora as endogenous stimulus to generate inflammation.

Central (thymic) dysregulation

Experiments in gene-targeted mice lacking the IL-2 gene (IL-2 –/– mice) demonstrate that thymic maturation defects (Figure 3) need to be included in the list of candidate defects which might cause hyperresponsiveness to normal luminal bacteria and thus IBD[35]. IL-2 –/– mice[39] develop lymphoid hyperplasia and anaemia when maintained under germ-free conditions and develop colitis in a conventional environment[40]. It was further shown that colitis in IL-2 –/– mice can be induced in a conventional environment by intraperitoneal administration of 2,4,6-trinitrophenol-keyhole limpet haemocyanin (TNP-KLH) and that intestinal inflammation in this model is dependent on peripheral CD4+ T cells producing high levels of interferon gamma (IFN-γ) under the influence of IL-12[38]. Interestingly, intraperitoneal challenge of IL-2 –/– mice with TNP-KLH not only led to the appearance of dysregulated peripheral T cells but also induced an IL-12-dependent increase of CD4+ CD8+ double-positive (DP) thymocytes, capable of inducing colitis upon transfer into IL-2 +/+ mice[35]. In this model, antigen stimulation in the absence of IL-2 thus induces an IL-12-directed abnormal maturation of thymocytes which mediate colitis when stimulated by luminal bacteria in the periphery.

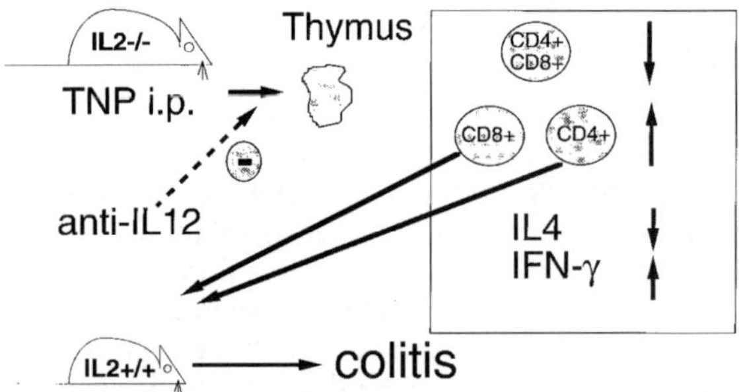

Figure 3 *Central (thymic) dysregulation in IL-2 –/– mice with chronic colitis.* IL-2 –/– mice develop colitis in a conventional environment, but not under germ-free conditions. In addition, colitis can be induced in IL-2 –/– mice by intraperitoneal (i.p.) administration of TNP-KLH. Investigating the mechanisms of colitis induction, it was shown that (i.p.) administration of TNP-KLH to IL2 –/– mice leads to an IL-12-dependent increase of CD4+ CD8+ double-positive (DP) thymocytes producing high levels of IFN-γ and low levels of IL-4. These abnormal thymocytes were capable of inducing colitis upon transfer into IL-2 +/+ mice. This indicates that antigen stimulation in the absence of IL-2 induces an IL-12-directed abnormal maturation of thymocytes which mediate colitis when stimulated by luminal bacteria in the periphery[35,38]

Peripheral dysregulation

Dysregulation of the peripheral T cell response to enteric bacteria as a common principle of colitis pathogenesis emerges from the observations that colitis can be induced by T cells from C3H/HeJBir mice stimulated with enteric bacterial antigens and transferred into SCID mice[32], by CD45RB[hi] CD4+ T cells transferred into SCID mice maintained in a conventional environment[29,37] and the transfer experiments using T cells from IL-2 –/– mice discussed above[35]. In addition, addressing more closely the issue of immune tolerance, it was shown that mononuclear cells from inflamed IBD intestine have an abnormal loss of tolerance to antigens from own intestinal flora[18]. This loss of tolerance to own intestinal flora was also observed in mice with trinitrobenzenesulphonic acid (TNBS) colitis and could be restored by treatment with IL-10 or antibodies to IL-12[19]. Although mechanisms of tolerance induction to antigens from the normal intestinal flora are still unclear, the finding that antibodies to IL-12 restore tolerance to self-intestinal flora in experimental murine colitis indicates that IL-12 is not only an important counterregulator of TGF-β-mediated oral tolerance[41,42], but also counterregulates tolerance to normal intestinal flora. In summary (Figure 4), current data suggest that the immune response to normal intestinal flora involves CD4+ T cell responses to discrete bacterial antigens. Under normal circumstances these responses seem to result in some form of immune tolerance. In chronic intestinal inflammation, however, CD4+ T cells seem to be dysregulated.

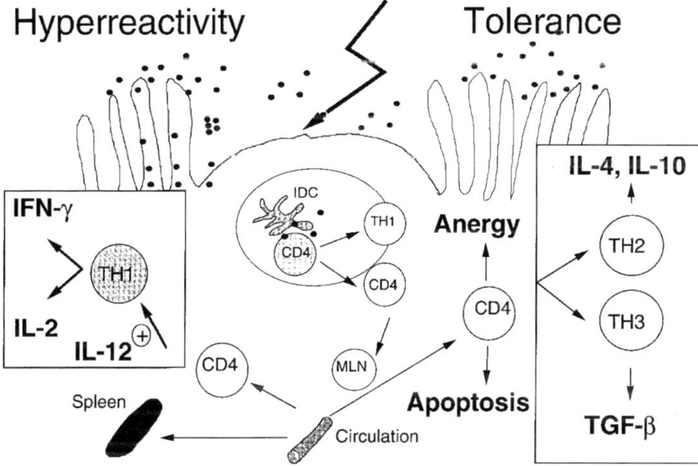

Figure 4 *Loss of tolerance to normal intestinal flora.* Current data suggest that the immune response to normal intestinal flora involves CD4+ T cell responses to discrete bacterial antigens. Under normal circumstances, these responses seem to result in some form of immune tolerance which may be mediated by T cell anergy, apoptosis or the induction of T cells producing regulatory cytokines like IL-4, IL-10 and TGF-β. In chronic intestinal inflammation, however, CD4+ T cells seem to be dysregulated. Many different causes of immune dysregulation seem to be able to induce such changes, and IL-12-mediated induction of high IFN-γ producing CD4+ T cells may be a common pathway, leading to immune hyperactivity to normal intestinal flora and ultimately chronic intestinal inflammation

Many different causes of immune dysregulation seem to be able to induce such changes, and IL-12-mediated induction of high IFN-γ producing CD4+ T cells may be a common pathway, leading to immune hyperreactivity to normal intestinal flora and ultimately chronic intestinal inflammation.

CONCLUSION

The formation of autoantibodies in IBD patients has clearly been demonstrated. Whether it reflects a primary abnormality of immune tolerance or is secondary to, e.g., an increased exposure to environmental antigens, antigens from the normal intestinal flora and inflammation itself, is unclear.

Clinical studies convincingly demonstrate that the decisive immune stimulus contributing to IBD inflammation rests within the faecal stream. Animal models demonstrate that alterations of a variety of immunoregulatory molecules involved in immune tolerance may lead to chronic intestinal inflammation. It emerges from these studies that hyperresponsiveness, i.e. a loss of tolerance to normal flora bacterial antigens mediated by dysregulated T cells, may be a common denominator driving chronic intestinal inflammation. Further studies in patients with IBD, which prove that these individuals have an abnormal regulation of tolerance, explore their potential immunological heterogeneity and help to device new treatment strategies will be necessary to ultimately determine the pathogenetic relevance of this concept.

References

1. MacDermott RP, Bragdon MJ, Kodner IJ, Bertovich MJ. Deficient cell-mediated cytotoxicity and hyporesponsiveness to interferon and mitogenic lectin activation by inflammatory bowel disease peripheral blood and intestinal mononuclear cells. Gastroenterology. 1986;90:6–11.
2. Baca EM, Wong DK, Croitoru K. Cytotoxic activity of V beta 8+ T cells in Crohn's disease: the role of bacterial superantigens. Clin Exp Immunol. 1995;99:398–403.
3. Gibson PR, van de Pol E, Pullman W, Doe WF. Lysis of colonic epithelial cells by allogeneic mononuclear and lymphokine activated killer cells derived from peripheral blood and intestinal mucosa: evidence against a pathogenic role in inflammatory bowel disease. Gut. 1988;29:1076–84.
4. Okazaki K, Morita M, Nishimori I et al. Major histocompatibility antigen-restricted cytotoxicity in inflammatory bowel disease. Gastroenterology. 1993;104:384–91.
5. Seibold F, Weber P, Scheurlen M. Autoantibodies in IBD patients and their families. In: Tytgat GNJ, Bartelsman JFWM, van Deventer SJH, editors. Inflammatory Bowel Diseases. Dordrecht: Kluwer; 1995:239–43.
6. Broberger O, Perlmann P. Experimental studies of ulcerative colitis. I. Reactions of serum from patients with human fetal colon cells in tissue culture. J Exp Med. 1963;117:705–15.
7. Fiocchi C, Roche JK, Michener WM. High prevalence of antibodies to intestinal epithelial antigens in patients with inflammatory bowel disease and their relatives. Ann Intern Med. 1989;110:786–94.
8. Halstensen TS, Mollnes TE, Fausa O, Brandtzaeg P. Deposits of terminal complement complex (TCC) in muscularis mucosae and submucosal vessels in ulcerative colitis and Crohn's disease of the colon. Gut. 1989;30:361–6.
9. Das KM, Dasgupta A, Mandal A, Geng X. Autoimmunity to cytoskeletal protein tropomyosin: a clue to the pathogenetic mechanism of ulcerative colitis. J Immunol. 1993;150:2487.
10. Das KM, Dubin R, Nagai T. Isolation of characterization of colonic tissue-bound antibodies from patients with idiopathic ulcerative colitis. Proc Natl Acad Sci USA. 1978;75:4528–32.
11. Duerr RH, Targan SR, Landers CJ, Sutherland LR, Shanahan F. Anti-neutrophil cytoplasmic antibodies in ulcerative colitis. Comparison with other colitides/diarrheal illnesses. Gastroenterology. 1991;100:1590–6.

12. Targan SR, Murphy LK. Clarifying the causes of Crohn's. Nat Med. 1995;1:1241–3.
13. Strobel S, Mowat A. Immune responses to dietary antigens: oral tolerance. Immunol Today. 1998;19:173–81.
14. Mowat AM. The regulation of immune responses to dietary protein antigens. Immunol Today. 1987;8:93–8.
15. Weiner H. Oral tolerance: immune mechanisms and treatment of autoimmune diseases. Immunol Today. 1997;7:335–43.
16. Berg RD, Savage DC. Immune response of specific pathogen-free and gnotobiotic mice to antigens of indigenous and non-indigenous microorganisms. Infect Immun. 1975;11:320–9.
17. Foo MC, Lee A. Antigenic cross-reaction between mouse intestine and a member of the autochthonous microflora. Infect Immun. 1974;9:1066–9.
18. Duchmann R, Kaiser I, Hermann E, Mayet W, Ewe K, Meyer zum Büschenfelde KH. Tolerance exists towards resident intestinal flora but is broken in active inflammatory bowel disease. Clin Exp Immunol. 1995;102:448.
19. Duchmann R, Schmitt E, Knolle P, Meyer zum Büschenfelde KH, Neurath M. Tolerance towards resident intestinal flora in mice is abrogated in experimental colitis and restored by treatment with interleukin-10 or antibodies to interleukin-12. Eur J Immunol. 1996;26:934–8.
20. Van de Merwe JP, Schroder AM, Weinsinck F, Hazenberg MP. The obligate anaerobic faecal flora of patients with Crohn's disease and their first-degree relatives. Scand J Gastroenterol. 1988;23:1125–31.
21. Van de Merwe JP, Stegeman JH, Hazenberg MP. The resident faecal flora is determined by genetic characteristics of the host. Implications for Crohn's disease? Antonie van Leeuwenhoek. 1983;49:119–24.
22. D'Haens GR, Geboes K, Peeters M, Baert F, Penninckx F, Rutgeerts P. Early lesions of recurrent Crohn's disease caused by the infusion of intestinal contents in excluded colon. Gastroenterology. 1998;114:262–8.
23. Sartor RB. Postoperative recurrence of Crohn's disease: the enemy is within the fecal stream. Gastroenterology. 1998;114:398–400.
24. Duchmann R, Neurath MF, Meyer zum Büschenfelde KH. Responses to self and non-self intestinal microflora in health and inflammatory bowel disease. Res Immunol. 1997;148:589–601.
25. Sartor RB. The influence of the microbial flora on the development of chronic mucosal inflammation. Res Immunol. 1997;148:567–76.
26. Husby S, Mestecky J, Moldoveanu Z, Holland S, Elson CO. Oral tolerance in humans. T cell but not B cell tolerance to antigen feeding. J Immunol. 1994;152:4663–70.
27. Lochs H, Genser D, Bühner S. Role of nutrition in IBD. In: Tytgat GNJ, Bartelsman JFWM, van Deventer SJH, editors. Inflammatory Bowel Diseases. Dordrecht: Kluwer; 1995:498–50.
28. Riordan AM, Hunter JO, Cowan RE et al. Treatment of active Crohn's disease by exclusion diet: East Anglian Multicentre Controlled Trial. Lancet. 1993;343:1131–4.
29. Aranda R, Sydora BC, McAllister PL et al. Analysis of intestinal lymphocytes in mouse colitis mediated by transfer of CD4+, CD45Rbhigh T cells to SCID recipients. J Immunol. 1997;158:3464–73.
30. Strober W, Ehrhardt RO. Chronic intestinal inflammation: an unexpected outcome in cytokine or T cell receptor mutant mice. Cell. 1993;75:203–5.
31. Rath HC, Herfarth HH, Ikdeda JS et al. Normal luminal bacteria, especially *Bacteroides* species, mediate chronic colitis, gastritis, and arthritis in HLA-B27/human $\beta2$ microglobulin transgenic rats. J Clin Invest. 1996;98:945–53.
32. Cong Y, Brandwein SL, McCabe RP et al. CD4+ T cells reactive to enteric bacterial antigens in spontaneously colitic C3H/HeJBir mice: increased T helper cell type I response and ability to transfer disease. J Exp Med. 1998;187:855–64.
33. Berg RD. The indigenous gastrointestinal microflora. Trends Microbiol. 1996;4:430–5.
34. Duchmann R, Märker-Hermann E, Meyer zum Büschenfelde KH. Bacteria-specific T-cell clones are selective in their reactivity towards different Enterobacteria or *H. pylori* and increased in inflammatory bowel disease. Scand J Immunol. 1996;44:71–9.
35. Ludviksson BR, Gray B, Strober W, Ehrhardt RO. Dysregulated intrathymic development in the IL-2-deficient mouse leads to colitis-inducing thymocytes. J Immunol. 1997;158:104–11.
36. Neurath M, Fuss I, Kelsall BL, Stüber E, Strober W. Antibodies to IL-12 abrogate established granulomatous colitis in mice. J Exp Med. 1995;182:1281–90.
37. Powrie F, Mauze S, Coffman RL. CD4+ T-cell subsets in the regulation of inflammatory responses in the intestine. Res Immunol. 1997;148:576–82.

38. Ehrhardt RO, Ludviksson BR, Gray B, Neurath M, Strober W. Induction and prevention of colonic inflammation in IL-2-deficient mice. J Immunol. 1997;158:566–73.
39. Sadlack B, Merz H, Schorle H, Schimpl A, Feller AC, Horak I. Ulcerative colitis-like disease in mice with a disrupted interleukin-2 gene. Cell. 1993;75:253–61.
40. Contractor NV, Bassiri H, Reya T *et al.* Lymphoid hyperplasia, autoimmunity, and compromised intestinal intraepithelial lymphocyte development in colitis-free gnotobiotic IL-2 deficient mice. J Exp Med. 1998;160:385–94.
41. Marth T, Strober W, Kelsall BL. High dose oral tolerance to ovalbumin TCR-transgenic mice: systemic neutralization of IL-12 augments TGF-beta secretion and T cell apoptosis. J Immunol. 1996;157:2348–57.
42. Neurath MF, Fuss I, Kelsall B, Pretsky DH, Waegell W, Strober W. Experimental granulomatous colitis in mice is abrogated by induction of TGF-β-mediated oral tolerance. J Exp Med. 1996;183:2605–16.

Section IV
IBD and Immunology

14
Intestinal macrophages

G. ROGLER, T. ANDUS, J. SCHÖLMERICH and V. GROSS

INTRODUCTION

Macrophages play a key role during inflammation in many different tissues. Intestinal macrophages represent one of the largest compartments of the mononuclear phagocyte system in the body[1]. They are localized preferentially in the subepithelial region of the mucosa and constitute 10–20% of the mononuclear cells in the intestinal lamina propria[2,3]. A number of studies dealing with phenotypic and functional characteristics of intestinal macrophages suggest that they differ markedly from blood monocytes, from macrophages found in other tissues, and from *in-vitro* differentiated macrophages. In this chapter the phenotypic characteristics of intestinal macrophages in comparison with other mononuclear phagocyte populations will be described.

PHENOTYPE OF INTESTINAL MACROPHAGES

Experiments to determine the phenotype of intestinal macrophages were performed by immunohistology as well as by fluorescence-activated cell sorter (FACS) analysis.

Immunohistology

Most studies to determine the phenotype of intestinal macrophages were performed by immunohistological techniques. Mahida *et al.*[4] found that the monocyte-specific surface marker CD16 (Fc-γ_3 receptor) was almost absent in normal intestinal mucosa. In inflammatory bowel disease (IBD) CD16 was present in the mucosa and on isolated cells. The typical macrophage marker CD11b (complement receptor 3, CR3, a member of the integrin family) was present on less than 5% of intestinal macrophages of the normal mucosa[5]. Less than 15% of the macrophages expressed CD11a (LFA1), and less than 40% CD11c (complement receptor 4, CR4). CD54 (ICAM-1) was found to be present in 7% of the intestinal macrophages of normal mucosa. CD54 expression was increased to 70% in ulcerative colitis and to 46% in Crohn's disease. CD25 (interleukin-2-receptor) was only expressed in ulcerative colitis, but not in controls or in Crohn's disease[6,7]. Rugtveit *et al.* described an increase of a macrophage subset expressing CD68 and cal-protectin (L1) close to small vessels in IBD[8]. When the expression of the cos-timulatory molecules B7.1 (CD80) and B7.2 (CD86) was analysed on sections of uninflamed bowel specimens from patients with IBD and normal controls only a selective subepithelial accumulation of B7.2 positive cells was found. In inflamed IBD mucosa, however, subsets appeared consisting of both B7.2[hi] and B7.1[hi] cells as well as CD14[hi] macrophages[9].

FACS analysis

Grim and co-workers recently described a low expression of CD14 by normal intestinal mononuclear cells but a high expression by mononuclear cells in IBD mucosa[10]. In order to characterize distinct macrophage populations by simulta-neously detecting several surface markers we applied triple fluorescence flow cytometry. We first identified CD33 as a useful recognition marker for intestinal macrophages in flow cytometric analysis and then determined further macro-phage markers: CD14 (LPS receptor), CD16 (Fc-γ3 receptor), HLA-DR, CD44 (hyaluronic acid receptor), CD11b (complement receptor 3), CD11c (comple-ment receptor 4), as well as the costimulatory molecules CD80 (B7.1) and CD86 (B7.2).

CD33 as recognition marker for intestinal macrophages

CD33 is a 67 kDa glycoprotein. It is a member of the Ig superfamily and its expression is restricted to myelomonocytic blood cells. Recently it has been demonstrated that CD33 is the fourth member of the sialoadhesin family of sialic acid-dependent cell adhesion molecules[11]. The binding to CD33 can be modulated by endogenous sialoglycoconjugates when CD33 is expressed on plasma membranes.

We isolated human intestinal macrophages according to a modification of the method of Bull and Bookman[12]. Flow cytometric forward-to-side scatter charac-teristics of isolated colonic lamina propria mononuclear cells did not allow us to identify clearly the macrophage population (Figure 1A). After CD33 labelling a positive cell population could be easily distinguished from the other cells (Figure 1B). The gating of the CD33 positive cells showed forward-to-side scatter characteristics typical for monocytes/macrophages. To ensure that no lymphocytes were analysed we performed a FACS triple fluorescence technique, which allowed us to exclude CD3 and CD19 positive cells for each measure-ment. For the determination of the other macrophage surface markers only CD33 positive, CD3/CD19 negative cells were used. Less than 10% of the cells analysed showed double expression of the macrophage marker CD33 and the lymphocyte markers CD3 and CD19. This might be due either to lymphocytes attached to macrophages or to incomplete or insufficient compensation.

To further establish CD33 as a marker of intestinal macrophages we performed double staining for intracellular CD68. CD68 is a well-established intracellular marker for macrophages which has been widely used in immunohistochemical studies. As shown in Figure 2 more than 95% of the analysed cells coexpressed CD68 and CD33. Permeabilization of the cells which was needed to perform the CD68 stain, however, increased the amount of cell debris.

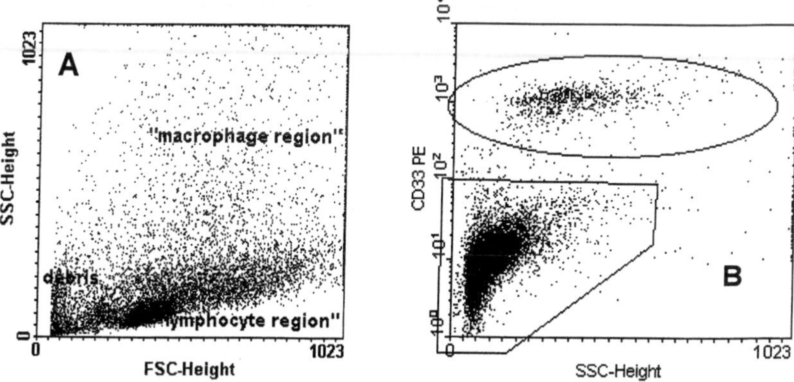

Figure 1 FACS analysis of intestinal macrophages. **A**: Forward/side scatter characteristics of mononuclear cells from normal colon. Isolated mononuclear cells from normal colon were analysed by FACS (10 000 cells each). It is almost impossible to discriminate clearly between the lymphocyte and the macrophage region. **B**: Flow cytometric detection of CD33 positive cell from colonic mucosa. Dot plot of side-scatter characteristics versus CD33 fluorescence. Ten thousand cells were analysed. CD33 positive cells are easily discriminated from the other cells, which are mainly lymphocytes

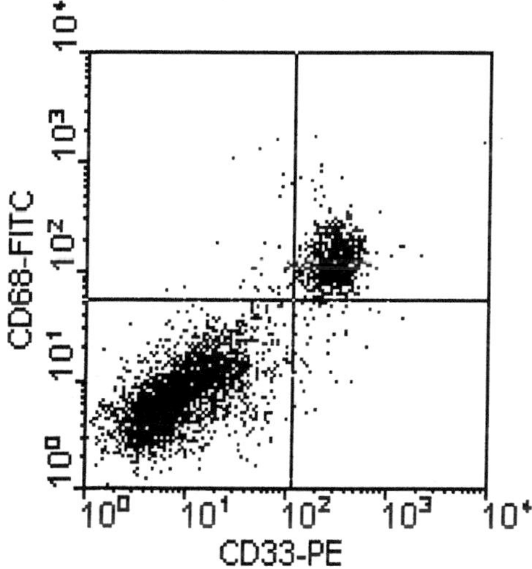

Figure 2 FACS analysis of the co-expression of CD68 and CD33. Co-expression of CD68 and CD33: upper right quadrant. The cells expressing both antigens have optical characteristics of macrophages. There are almost no cells expressing either CD33 (lower right quadrant) or CD68 (upper left quadrant) alone

Phagocytosis assays showed that 83 ± 5% of the CD33 positive cells were able to phagocytose latex beads. On the other hand, 81 ± 5% of the phagocytosing cells were positive for CD33. These results confirmed that the CD33 positive cells isolated from the intestinal mucosa represent macrophages.

Further characterization of the phenotype of intestinal macrophages and its alterations in IBD

Macrophages of the normal colonic mucosa show a low expression of the typical macrophage markers CD14, CD16, CD11b, CD11c, as well as HLA-DR. Figure 3A–F shows the expression of CD14 (A), CD16 (B), HLA-DR (C), CD44 (D), CD11b (E), and CD11c (F) versus CD33. To discover whether the finding of a very low number of colonic macrophages expressing typical macrophage markers was due to digestion of the antigens during the isolation procedure we analysed, in addition, peripheral blood monocytes after applying the same isolation conditions as for colonic mononuclear cells. In addition, we analysed *in-vitro* differentiated macrophages. It is obvious that *in-vitro* differentiated macrophages show a substantially higher expression of CD14, CD16, HLA-DR, CD11b, and CD11c when compared with macrophages isolated from intestinal mucosa (Table 1).

In contrast to colonic macrophages from normal mucosa there was a significantly higher expression of CD14, CD16, HLA-DR, CD11b, and CD11c in IBD, indicating additional macrophage populations in the inflamed mucosa. This may reflect either a recruitment of immune cells from the circulation or a change in the phenotype of resident cells (Table 2).

When the expression of the costimulatory molecules CD80 and CD86 was determined on colonic macrophages from the normal mucosa their expression was found to be low (9.2 ± 4.2% for CD80 (Figure 4A), 15.2 ± 7.3% for CD86 (Figure 4B)). When *in-vitro* differentiated dendritic cells were used as a positive control for the expression of the CD80 and CD86, almost all of these cells were positive. On colonic macrophages from patients with IBD there was a significant increase in the expression of CD80 (33.8 ± 8.9% positive cells (Figure 4C)) and CD86 (39.9 ± 8.8% positive cells (Figure 4D)). There was no significant

Table 1 Phenotypic characterization of monocytes and macrophages of various origin

	CD14+ (percentage of total CD33+ cells)	*CD16+ (percentage of total CD33+ cells)*	*HLA-DR+ (percentage of total CD33+ cells)*	*CD44+ (percentage of total CD33+ cells)*	*CD11b+ (percentage of total CD33+ cells)*	*CD11c+ (percentage of total CD33+ cells)*
Normal mucosa	10.5 ± 3.8	10.1 ± 3.9	27.6 ± 9.3	90.9 ± 6.9	17.4 ± 6.8	17.9 ± 10.4
Blood monocytes	84.1 + 8.7	25.1 ± 23.4	89.0 ± 7.8	97.1 ± 2.6	93.1 ± 4.6	21.2 ± 20.1
In vitro differentiated macrophages	92.0 ± 3.1	29.2 ± 33.5	91.7 ± 8.5	85.7 ± 10.4	69.1 ± 12.1	56.9 ± 42.8

Data represent percentage of CD33 positive, CD3/CD19 negative cells positive for the indicated surface antigen (mean ± standard deviation). The expression of CD14, CD16, HLA-DR, CD11b, and CD11c is low in macrophages from normal human colonic mucosa. In blood monocytes and in *in-vitro* differentiated macrophages the expression of the surface antigens is positive in a large number of cells. CD44 is positive in almost all cells in all macrophage populations.

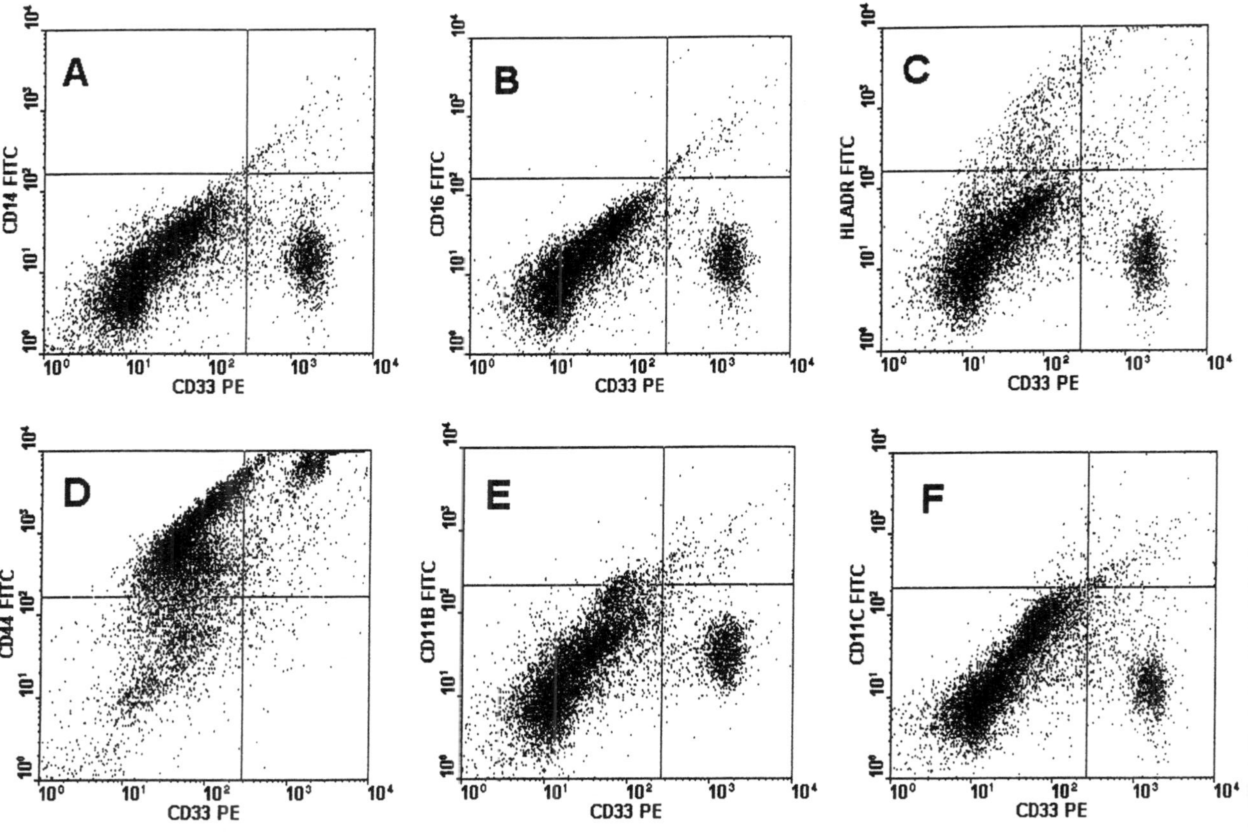

Figure 3 Phenotype of mononuclear cells isolated from normal colonic mucosa. **A**: Dot plot of CD33 (PE-) fluorescence versus CD14 (FITC-) fluorescence. CD33 positive/CD14 negative cells are easily discriminated from the other cells. **B**: Dot plot of CD33 (PE-) fluorescence versus CD16 (FITC-) fluorescence. **C**: Dot plot of CD33 (PE-) fluorescence versus HLA-DR (FITC-) fluorescence. **D**: Dot plot of CD33 (PE-) fluorescence versus CD44 (FITC-) fluorescence. **E**: Dot plot of CD33 (PE-) fluorescence versus CD11b (FITC-) fluorescence. **F**: Dot plot of CD33 (PE-) fluorescence versus CD11c (FITC-) fluorescence. Ten thousand cells were analysed. There was only a low number of CD14, CD16, HLA-DR, CD11b, and CD11c positive macrophages (CD33+)

Table 2 Phenotypic characterization of intestinal macrophages from normal mucosa or from mucosa from IBD patients

	CD14+ (percentage of total CD33+ cells)	CD16+ (percentage of total CD33+ cells)	HLA-DR+ (percentage of total CD33+ cells)	CD44+ (percentage of total CD33+ cells)	CD11b+ (percentage of total CD33+ cells)	CD11c+ (percentage of total CD33+ cells)
Normal mucosa	10.5 ± 3.8	10.1 ± 3.9	27.6 ± 9.2	90.0 ± 6.9	17.4 ± 6.8	17.9 ± 10.4
IBD	36.0 ± 13.2	28.6 ± 10.3	53.1 ± 15.9	90.3 ± 8.5	42.8 ± 14.2	35.1 ± 15.9
Crohn's disease	33.6 ± 14.7	29.4 ± 13.7	53.0 ± 17.5	86.9 ± 9.9	40.5 ± 13.8	38.8 ± 16.7
Ulcerative colitis	38.3 ± 12.0	27.8 ± 5.8	53.2 ± 15.2	93.8 ± 5.3	45.1 ± 15.0	31.4 ± 15.1

Percentage of positive cells for the indicated surface antigens of all CD33 positive cells. Data are given as means ± standard deviation. The expression of CD14, CD16, HLA-DR, CD11b, and CD11c is low in macrophages from normal human mucosa. The number of positive cells for these antigens is significantly increased in IBD with minor differences between Crohn's disease and ulcerative colitis. CD44 is positive in almost all cells in all subgroups.

difference between Crohn's disease and ulcerative colitis in the expression in CD80 (Crohn's disease 31.3 ± 6.7%, ulcerative colitis 34.4 ± 3.3%) and CD86 (Crohn's disease 41.9 ± 3.8%, ulcerative colitis 35.6 ± 13.8%). Interestingly, more than 90% of the CD86/CD80 positive cells of the inflamed mucosa were positive for CD14, indicating that a new macrophage population is found with high expression of costimulatory molecules presumably responsible for the perpetuated immune response.

In conclusion, normal colonic macrophages exhibit a characteristic phenotype (CD33, CD44, CD14–, CD16–, CD11b–, CD11c–, HLA-DR^{low}, CD80–, CD86–. In the inflamed mucosa a new macrophage population with significantly higher expression of CD14, CD16, CD11b, CD11c, HLA-DR, CD80, and CD86 appears.

Similar results as for intestinal macrophages have been found for alveolar macrophages. These cells show a low level of expression of CD14 and CC11b[13]. Only during inflammatory lung diseases is the number of CD14 and CD11b positive macrophages increased[14–18]. Ziegler-Heitbrock and co-workers described a correlation between the expression of CD14 on alveolar macrophages and the impairment of lung function in pulmonary sarcoidosis[17]. In addition, similar results were obtained for liver macrophages. In an immunohistochemical characterization using intracellular CD68 as a recognition marker most liver macrophages were negative for CD14[19,20]. In rats CD14 and CD11b were not expressed in normal liver macrophages whereas an increase in expression of both antigens was observed in cholestatic animals[21].

Compared with intestinal macrophages *in-vitro* differentiated macrophages show a different phenotype with high expression of CD14, CD16, HLA-DR, and CD11b. No *in-vitro* incubation conditions are known to lower the expression of CD14 to the level observed in colonic macrophages. After culture of the monocyte-like cell line U937 with lipopolysaccharide CD14 expression was even

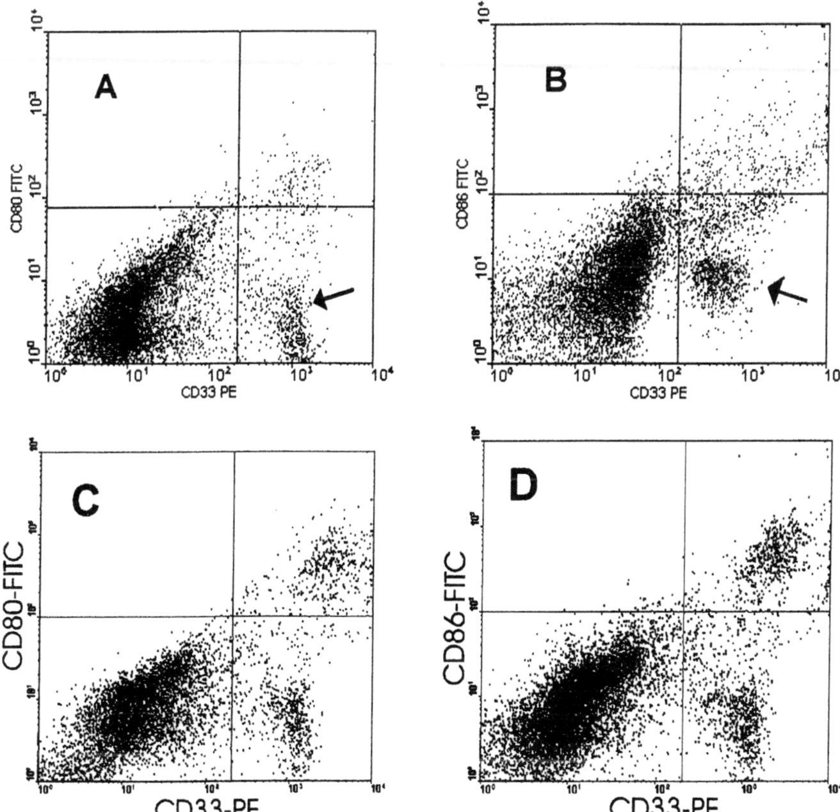

Figure 4 Expression of CD80 (B7-1) and CD86 (B7-2) on colonic macrophages from normal and inflamed mucosa. **A**: Dot plot of CD33 (PE-) fluorescence versus CD80 (FITC-) fluorescence of LPMNC from normal mucosa. **B**: Dot plot of CD33 (PE-) fluorescence versus CD86 (FITC-) fluorescence of LPMNC from normal mucosa. The majority of the population of colonic macrophages lacks CD80 and CD86 expression (arrows). Only a small number of cells is positive for CD80 or CD86 (upper right quadrant). **C**: Dot plot of CD33 (PE-) fluorescence versus CD80 (B7-1) fluorescence on colonic macrophages from inflamed mucosa. A population of intestinal macrophages expression CD80 is found during intestinal inflammation (upper right quadrant). **D**: Dot plot of CD33 (PE-) fluorescence versus CD86 (B7-2) fluorescence on colonic macrophages from inflamed mucosa (CD). As shown for CD80 a population of intestinal macrophages expression CD86 is found during intestinal inflammation (upper right quadrant)

induced[22]. The same phenomenon could be observed with blood monocytes[23]. Under conditions found in the intestine with high levels of lipopolysaccharide (LPS) a high expression of CD14 on macrophages would have been expected. On the other hand, there may be only a low contact to LPS when the mucosal barrier is intact.

An interesting finding is the low expression of the costimulatory molecules B7.1 and B7.2 on colonic macrophages. A lack of these molecules could lead to antigen desensitization and anergy[24]. This could be an important mechanism for the induction of oral tolerance to abundant antigens to which the mucosa is continuously exposed. Again, intestinal macrophages resembled alveolar macrophages which do not costimulate T cells CD28 pathway and do not express CD80 or CD86[25]. The increased expression of costimulatory molecules on intestinal macrophages isolated from IBD mucosa might be an important mechanism for breaking the immunological tolerance to luminal antigens.

References

1. Lee SH, Starkey PM, Gordon S. Quantitative analysis of total macrophage content in adult mouse tissues. Immunochemical studies with monoclonal antibody F4/80. J Exp Med. 1985;161:475–89.
2. Pavli P, Doe WF. Intestinal macrophages. In: MacDermott RP, Stenson WF, editors. Inflammatory Bowel Disease. New York: Elsevier; 1992:177–88.
3. Donnellan WL. The structure of the colonic mucosa. The epithelium and subepithelial reticulo-histiocytic complex. Gastroenterology. 1965;49:496–14.
4. Mahida YR, Patel S, Gionchetti P, Vaux D, Jewell DP. Macrophage subpopulations in lamina propria of normal colon and inflamed colon and terminal ileum. Gut. 1989;30:826–34.
5. Malizia G, Calabrese A, Cottone M *et al.* Expression on leukocyte adhesion molecules by mucosal mononuclear phagocytes in inflammatory bowel disease. Gastroenterology. 1991;100:150–9.
6. Mahida YR, Patel S, Wu K, Jewell DP. Interleukin 2 receptor expression by macrophages in inflammatory bowel disease. Clin Exp Immunol. 1988;74:382–6.
7. Choy MY, Walker Smith JA, Williams CD, MacDonald TT. Differential expression of CD25 (interleukin-2 receptor) on lamina propria T-cells and macrophages in the intestinal lesions of Crohn's disease and ulcerative colitis. Gut. 1990;31:1365–70.
8. Rugtveit J, Brandtzaeg P, Halstensen TS, Fausa O, Scott H. Increased macrophage subset in inflammatory bowel disease: apparent recruitment from peripheral blood monocytes. Gut. 1994;35:669–74.
9. Rugtveit J, Bakka A, Brandtzaeg P. Differential distribution of B7.1 (CD80) and B7.2 (CD86) costimulatory molecules on mucosal macrophage subsets in human inflammatory bowel disease (IBD). Clin Exp Immunol. 1997;110:104–13.
10. Grimm MC, Pavli P, van de Pol E, Doe WF. Evidence for a CD14+ population of monocytes in inflammatory bowel disease mucosa – implications for pathogenesis. Clin Exp Immunol. 1995;100:291–7.
11. Freeman SD, Kelm S, Barber EK, Crocker PR. Characterization of CD33 as a member of the sialoadhesin family of cellular interaction molecules. Blood. 1995;85:2005–12.
12. Bull DM, Bookman MA. Isolation and functional characterization of human intestinal mucosal lymphoid cells. J Clin Invest. 1977;59:966–74.
13. Barbosa IL, Gant VA, Hamblin AS. Alveolar macrophages from patients with bronchogenic carcinoma and sarcoidosis similarly express monocyte antigens. Clin Exp Immunol. 1991;86:173–8.
14. Striz I, Wang YM, Teschler H, Sorg C, Costabel U. Phenotypic markers of alveolar macrophage maturation in pulmonary sarcoidosis. Lung. 1993;171:293–303.
15. Perez-Arellano JL, Losa-Garcia JE, Orfao-Matos A *et al.* Comparison of two techniques (flow cytometry and alkaline immunophosphatase) in the evaluation of alveolar macrophage immunophenotype. Diagn Cytopathol. 1993;9:259–65.
16. Wassermann K, Subklewe M, Pothoff G, Banik N, Frederick-Schell E. Expression of surface markers on alveolar macrophages from symptomatic patients with HIV-infection as detected by flow cytometry. Chest. 1994;105:1324–34.
17. Pforte A, Schiessler A, Gais P *et al.* Expression of CD14 correlated with lung function impairment in pulmonary sarcoidosis. Chest. 1994;105:349–54.
18. Pforte A, Schiessler A, Gais P *et al.* Increased expression of the monocyte differentiation antigen CD14 in extrinsic allergic alveolitis. Monaldi Arch Chest Dis. 1993;48:607–12.
19. Tomita M, Yamamoto K, Kobashi H, Ohmoto M, Tsuji T. Immunohistochemical phenotyping of liver macrophages in normal and diseased liver. Hepatology. 1994;20:317–25.
20. Matsuura K, Ishida T, Setoguchi M, Higuchi Y, Akizuki S, Yamamoto S. Upregulation of mouse CD14 expression in Kupffer cells by lipopolysaccharide. J Exp Med. 1994;179:1671–6.

21. Tracy TF, Fox ES. CD14-lipopolysaccharide receptor activity in hepatic monocytes after cholestatic liver injury. Surgery. 1995;118:371–7.

22. Ikewaki N, Tamauchi H, Inoko H. Modulation of cell surface antigens and regulation of phagocytic activity mediated by CD11b in the monocyte-like cell line U937 in response to lipopolysacharide. Tissue Antigens. 1993;42:125–32.

23. Brugger W, Reinhardt D, Galanos C, Andressen R. Inhibition of *in-vitro* differentiation of human monocytes to macrophages by lipopolysaccharide (LPS): phenotypic and functional analysis. Int Immunol. 1991;3:221–7.

24. Thompson CB. Distinct roles for the costimulatory ligands B7-1 and B7-2 in T-helper cell differentiation. Cell. 1995;81:979–82.

25. Chelen CJ, Fang Y, Freeman GJ *et al.* Human alveolar macrophages present antigen ineffectively due to defective expression of B7 costimulatory cell surface molecules. J Clin Invest. 1995;95:1415–21.

15
Role of fibroblasts in inflammatory bowel disease

A. STALLMACH

INTRODUCTION

The aetiology of inflammatory bowel disease (IBD) is unknown. However, the intensive inflammatory response plays a role in the initiation and perpetuation of these diseases. Features of Crohn's disease (CD) include chronic transmural inflammation, fibrosis and fistula formation. The formation of stenoses and strictures is a common phenomenon in this disease, which causes abdominal pain, anorexia and weight loss. Approximately 50% of Crohn's disease patients undergo surgery for this type of complication during a 10-year course of the disease and the recurrence rate after surgery is high. In contrast, ulcerative colitis rarely causes intestinal stenosis. Therefore, fibrosis of the intestinal tract is a relevant complication in CD and its prevention is an important therapeutic goal. However, despite the significant morbidity associated with strictures in Crohn's disease, the inflammatory mechanisms leading to stricturing of the intestinal tract are unknown.

Historically, the fibroblast has been defined as a mesenchymal cell that is flat and elongated, possessing an oval, flat nucleus and the machinery to produce the collagens and other connective tissue components of the surrounding tissue. Fibroblasts were previously considered important connective tissue cells that construct a supporting matrix crucial for tissue integrity and repair. As a result, they were relegated to a minor role in the inflammatory process. Recent data from several laboratories, including our own, have defined a new concept concerning the function of fibroblasts (for review, see Reference 1). First, fibroblasts, even from a single tissue, are not composed of a homogeneous population but rather of subsets of cells, much like lymphocytes. Distinct fibroblast phenotypes may develop from undifferentiated precursor stem cells during development[2] and are observed in the stroma surrounding benign and malignant tumours[3]. Second, fibroblasts from different anatomic regions display characteristic phenotypes. Moreover, regional diversity may reflect the specialized functions of the tissue of origin. These differences among fibroblasts may be the basis for localized susceptibility to disease manifestation. Third, fibroblasts can be activated to display several functions important, for example, in controlling extracellular matrix synthesis, in producing cytokines and chemokines, and in modulating epithelial cell differentiation and cell function. For instance, intestinal electrolyte transport occurring in response to inflammatory mediators is modulated by fibroblast cells[4]. These features are analogous to cells of the immune system, such as macrophages and T cells.

FIBROBLAST HETEROGENEITY AND INFLUENCE OF DIFFERENT TYPES OF MESENCHYMAL CELLS ON EPITHELIAL CELL DIFFERENTIATION

The concept of fibroblast heterogeneity has received strong support from studies of lung, skin and gingivae. Fibroblasts display tissue- and disease-specific characteristics with evidence of adaptation to a particular tissue environment, resulting in differences in morphology, proliferation rates, cytokine production and secretion of matrix components. In pulmonary fibrosis, for example, interferon-γ induces increased expression of MHC Class II molecules in the pulmonary fibroblast subset that is positive for the Thy-1 antigen, suggesting heterogeneity in the capacity of subsets to activate T cells.

The morphogenesis, differentiation and maintenance of intestinal epithelium is dependent on interactions with the underlying mesenchyme. Thus electron microscopic analysis of the developing gut in the rat duodenum documents that the process of maturation of the epithelium starts after the development of close cell–cell contact between surface and subepithelial cells of the mesenchyme[5]. In addition, experiments with recombined tissues grafted under the kidney capsule of adult rats have confirmed the existence of strong inductive influences of the intestinal mesenchyme on the epithelium of the oesophagus and stomach, which lead to a differentiated intestinal epithelium with regular microvilli and typical intestinal brush border enzymes[6,7]. Furthermore, myofibroblasts of duodenal mucosa of suckling rats can induce 'intestinalization' of undifferentiated gastric cells[8]. These results are of particular interest in view of the known instability of the gastric epithelial phenotype in intestinal metaplasia[9]. Previous *in-vitro* results from our own laboratory also suggested a strong organ-specific potential of the fetal intestinal mesenchyme in inducing epithelial cytodifferentiation (see also Figure 1)[10].

In an elegant study, Fritsch and coworkers established two morphologically different clones of cells from a mixed parental line of intestinal fibroblasts[11]. These two clones were distinguished on the basis of different growth responses to cytokines and their expression of cytoskeletal and surface antigens. Using tissue culture and grafting methods, they were able to show that one clone supported differentiation of intestinal epithelial cells and morphogenesis with formation of crypts and villi. In contrast, the second clone was defective in these respects but was able to support proliferation of fetal epithelial cells in co-culture.

It is important to note that the cellular dialogue between epithelial cells and the adjacent mesenchyme during morphogenesis and in diseases involves inductive influences in both directions. Reciprocity in cell interactions is shown by changes in mesenchymal cell properties under the influence of the adjacent epithelium, e.g. expression of tenascin by the fetal mesenchyme or malignant tumour stroma[12,13].

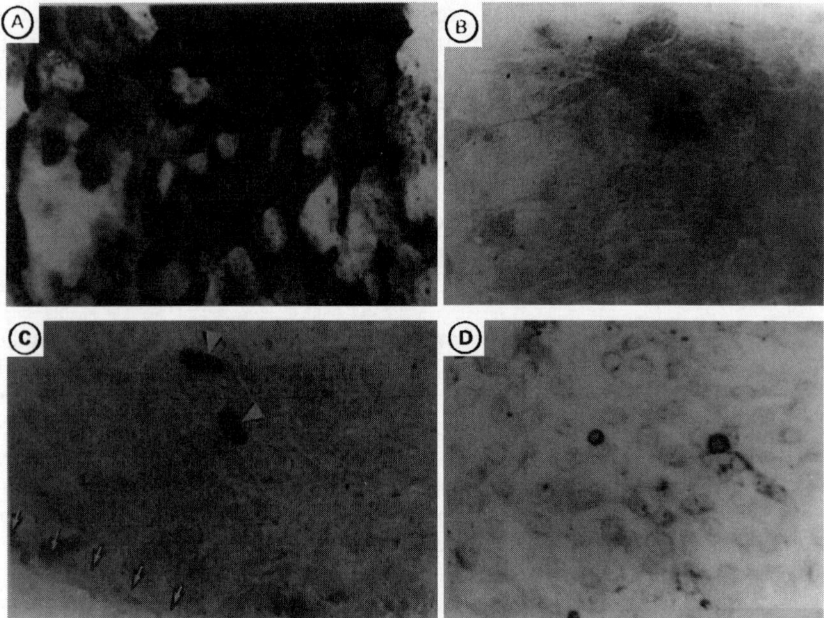

Figure 1 Histochemical demonstration of alkaline phosphatase in epithelial cell cultures derived from 15 day fetal small intestine and co-cultured with Ⓐ intestinal mesenchyme Ⓑ gastric mesenchyme and Ⓒ skin mesenchyme. Ⓓ Identical epithelial colonies cultured on albumin-coated petri dishes. Fetal rat intestinal epithelial cell colonies explanted on the 15th day of gestation, which failed to mature in plain monocultures, were reassociated in co-cultures with three different types of mesenchyme: fetal skin, gastric and intestinal mesenchyme. Only the intestinal mesenchyme gives rise to uniformly alkaline phosphatase expression as a marker of epithelial cell differentiation

FIBROBLASTS AS CYTOKINE-PRODUCING IMMUNOMODULATORY CELLS AND MODULATORS OF T-CELL APOPTOSIS

Several studies demonstrated that mesenchymal cells from normal and inflamed tissues produce various cytokines[14–16], express cytokine receptors[17], and physically interact with immune cells[18], an activity that is in turn modulated by cytokines[19]. Skin, synovial and pulmonary fibroblasts produce granulocyte–macrophage colony-stimulating factor (GM-CSF), granulocyte colony-stimulating factor (G-CSF), IL-1, IL-6 and IL-8 when stimulated with IL-1 or tumour necrosis factor-α (TNF-α)[20–23]. Cytokine secretion is increased by bacterial lipopolysaccharide (LPS) and viruses[24,25]. Similar results have been obtained from murine and human studies using intestinal mesenchymal cells[26,27]. Pang and coworkers demonstrated that fibroblasts grown from histologically normal human duodenal biopsy specimens expressed mRNA genes for GM-CSF, IL-1α, IL-1β, IL-6 and IL-8 in response to IL-1α and LPS[28]. In addition, both IL-1α and LPS upregulated ICAM-1 and VCAM-1 gene expression. Further, proinflammatory cytokines, like IL-1β, IL-6, and TNF-α, induce proliferation of human intestinal mesenchymal cells. Moreover, on exposure to these cytokines, human intestinal cells express gene products for the same cytokine[29]. The type and degree of expression depends on the mediator used, presence of costimulatory cytokines, and responder cell type. Rogler and coworkers demonstrated that activation of NFκb in human colonic fibroblasts by TNF-α results in increases in transcription rate and secretion of proinflammatory cytokines[30]. These findings implicate an important role for intestinal fibroblasts in the initiation and/or regulation of intestinal inflammation.

Another aspect directly relevant to cell–cell interactions during inflammation is the ability of mesenchymal cells to modulate cytokine synthesis in T cells[31]. *In-vitro* results from our own laboratory suggest that fibroblasts can induce or potentiate cytokine synthesis in CD4-positive T cells (see also Figure 2). In addition, fibroblasts can also influence apoptotic reactions of lymphocytes. Several studies demonstrated that T-cell apoptosis induced by cytokine deprivation can be inhibited by the addition of exogenous cytokines or by a fibroblast-derived survival factor. The prevention of cell death is also achieved by conditioned medium from the fibroblasts[32]. Under normal circumstances, fibroblast-mediated T-cell survival may allow persistence of a small number of primed T cells in tissues,

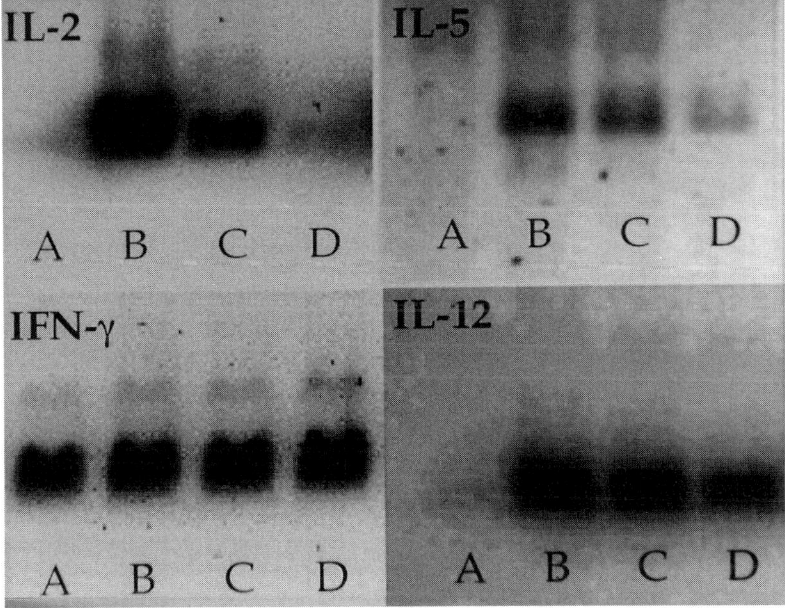

Figure 2 Influence of murine fibroblasts on cytokine gene expression in human CD4+ T cells. 2×10^6 CD4+ T cells (after MACS separation of peripheral blood mononuclear cells) were cultured under different conditions for 3 h. Upper left: IL-2 transcripts, upper right: IL-5 transcripts, lower left: IFN-γ transcripts, lower right: IL-12 transcripts. A, unstimulated cells under basal conditions; B, after addition of 1 μg/ml anti-CD2 antibodies, which activates T cells; C, after addition of 1 μg/ml anti-CD3 antibodies, which activates T cells; D, T cells and fibroblasts in co-culture. As with anti-CD2 or anti-CD3 activation, murine fibroblasts (0.25×10^6 cells) stimulate IL-12 mRNA synthesis. Equivalent loading of each sample was verified by visualization of actin message (not shown)

which can be reactivated to initiate a secondary immune response. In abnormal situations, fibroblast-mediated T-cell survival may lead to the persistence of large numbers of T cells producing a chronic inflammatory state. For example, Burkitt lymphoma cells are highly sensitive to suboptimal *in-vitro* growth conditions and undergo apoptosis when seeded at reduced serum concentration or low cell density. Irradiated fibroblasts can protect lymphoma cells from apoptosis through secretion of a survival- and proliferation-promoting activity which is soluble and labile[33]. Human intestinal fibroblasts also possess this property[34], which, complemented with their adhesiveness for T cells[35], may have profound implications for the duration of an intestinal inflammatory process. This particular aspect, combined with the capacity of mesenchymal cells to produce pro-inflammatory cytokines, raises a provocative question. Which cells are actually responsible for the chronicity of inflammation, immune cells activated by an unknown primary antigen or byproducts of surrounding mesenchymal cells activated by immune cell- or self-derived cytokines, or perhaps both cell types stimulating one another in a perpetuating dysregulated loop? This critical question has still to be answered by ongoing studies.

ROLE OF FIBROBLASTS IN COLLAGEN SYNTHESIS

Biochemical and immunohistological studies have shown increased collagen deposition in Crohn's disease compared with ulcerative colitis. Enhanced expression of type III and type V collagen was demonstrated particularly in intestinal segments altered by fibrosis and stenosis in Crohn's disease[36-38]. However, using immunohistochemical approaches or biochemical analyses, it is not possible to detect the cells which synthesize the gene product. Therefore, we analysed the steady-state levels of collagen transcripts in IBD and control patients using an *in-situ* hybridization technique[39]. Low steady-state levels of the interstitial $\alpha_1(I)$, $\alpha_1(III)$ and $\alpha_2(V)$ procollagen mRNA transcripts were present in histologically normal intestinal tissues. Transcripts of the procollagen genes were primarily present in lamina propria mesenchymal cells located directly beneath the epithelial layer or in the muscularis mucosae and propria. In active Crohn's disease, $\alpha_1(I)$ procollagen gene transcript levels were markedly increased in lamina propria cells. The number of labelled cells was higher than in control tissues and correlated with the cellular density of the inflammatory infiltrate. Interestingly, in Crohn's disease, the relative increase of $\alpha_1(III)$ transcripts in relation to $\alpha_1(I)$ and $\alpha_2(V)$ transcripts was significantly greater in fibrotic areas or stenoses than in inflamed specimens.

Considering the importance of cytokines in the pathogenesis of fibrosis, we wanted to analyse the regulatory influence of cytokines on collagen synthesis, which is potentially involved in the development of intestinal fibrosis. TGF-β has been shown to stimulate the expression of collagen and fibronectin and to increase protein production[40]. Therefore, we used a cell culture model of lamina propria fibroblasts isolated from patients with chronic inflammatory bowel disease. In a dose-dependent manner, TGF-β_1 stimulated synthesis of total proteins, collagens and pro-collagen type III peptide (PIIIP) as a marker for type III collagen synthesis. Interestingly, the effects of TGF-β_1 on type III collagen synthesis by lamina propria fibroblasts isolated from strictures were different from those exerted on type III collagen synthesis by lamina propria fibroblasts isolated from merely inflamed specimens. In Crohn's disease, the effect of TGF-β_1 on PIIIP synthesis in fibroblasts from strictures was significantly higher than that on PIIIP synthesis in fibroblasts of inflamed specimens from the same patients (see Figure 3). Similar findings were reported by W. F. Doe[41]. He demonstrated that collagen production from freshly isolated fibroblasts in Crohn's disease was significantly greater than in normal fibroblasts from control patients. Exposure to TGF-α_1 or insulin growth factor (IGF-1) results in an increased total collagen production in Crohn's disease fibroblasts compared with normal fibroblasts. In this context, it should be stressed that the concentration of IGF-1 in whole-gut lavage is increased in patients with intestinal strictures compared with patients with inflammation or controls[42]. The mechanisms responsible for the disease-specific effects of cytokines and growth factors on collagen synthesis by human intestinal mesenchymal cells are not understood. One level of control may be achieved through differential expression of TGF-β receptor isoforms through which TGF-β_1 may mediate specific biological functions. Three receptor subtypes have been identified (for review, see Reference 43). Differential expression of receptor isoforms in normal and fibrotic tissues may account for differential TGF-β effects on matrix metabolism. In the mouse embryo, type II receptor expression is greater in undifferentiated mesenchyme than in more mature cells[44]. Preliminary data indicate that distribution of TGF-β receptor subtypes is different in specimens from patients with Crohn's disease

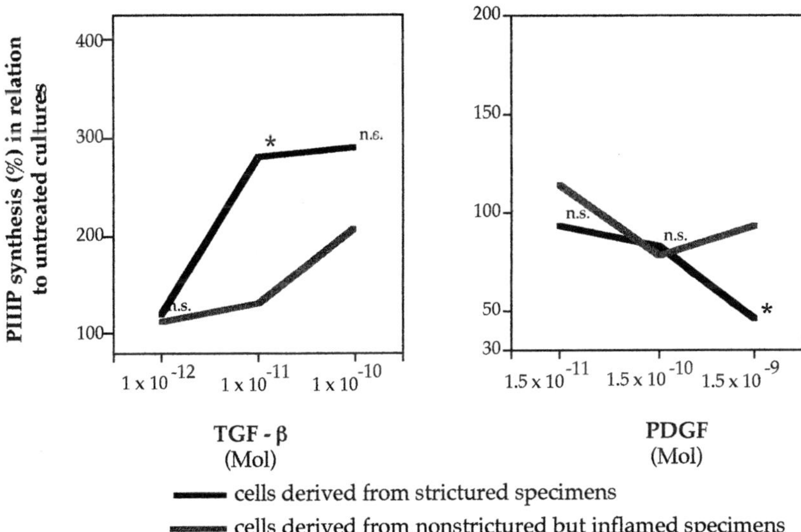

Figure 3 Effect of TGF-β_1 and PDGF on PIIIP synthesis by lamina propria fibroblasts derived from strictured and non-strictured but inflamed Crohn's disease specimens. Results are expressed as median of PIIIP synthesis. The amount of PIIIP (ng/μg DNA) in the cultures exposed to TGF-β_1 and PDGF is expressed relative to unstimulated controls (100%). n.s., non-significant differences at the 5% level; * $p \leq 0.05$

compared with controls. Using *in-situ* hybridization, Northern blot analysis and Western blotting, Martignoni and coworkers were able to demonstrate increased TGF-β type II receptor expression in Crohn's disease[45].

The concept that functionally distinct fibroblast subsets are responsible for the development of intestinal fibrosis is further supported by results of animal models of lung fibrosis. Molecular, genetic and immunohistological analysis demonstrated that pulmonary fibroblasts represent a mixture of cells which can be divided into morphologically and functionally different subsets. These subpopulations displayed differences in surface marker expression, response to and synthesis of cytokines and extracellular matrix protein production. In radiation-induced lung fibrosis, the percentage of so-called Thy-1$^+$ fibroblasts was increased[46]. Thy-1$^+$ fibroblasts constitutively produced more extracellular matrix protein than Thy-1$^-$ fibroblasts and more readily proliferated in response to cytokines IL-4, IL-1α and IL-6. Sempowski *et al.* described that IL-4 dramatically elevates the total amount of collagen production and the steady-state mRNA level of types I and III collagen in Thy-1$^+$ fibroblasts. By contrast, collagen production by Thy-1$^-$ fibroblasts was refractory to IL-4. IFN-γ, which is an antagonistic cytokine for IL-4, decreased collagen production by more than 50% in Thy-1$^+$ and Thy-1$^-$ fibroblasts[47]. Overall, these data further support the hypothesis that selective expansion of functionally distinct fibroblast subsets is important in the transition from a benign wound healing process to chronic fibrosis.

SUMMARY

Increasing data highlight the role of intestinal fibroblasts in IBD: their heterogeneity and their role in the pathogenesis of intestinal fibrosis in inflammatory bowel disease. It is tempting to speculate that disturbances in the relationships between different mesenchymal cell clones may contribute to the manifestations of intestinal diseases. Defective subepithelial myofibroblast organization may contribute to villous atrophy in an inflammatory bowel condition, such as coeliac disease. There are clear differences between mesenchymal cells in CD and UC, which may explain the different clinical manifestations. Over-representation of defined mesenchymal cell clones within the connective tissue may be a relevant contributory factor to fibrotic manifestations in Crohn's disease. Further studies are required to characterize the differences occurring in mesenchymal cells in terms of their response to cytokines in inflammatory bowel disease. The forthcoming challenge is to find specific markers in these fibroblasts to help understand the nature and treatment of these diseases.

References

1. Fiocchi C. Intestinal inflammation: a complex interplay of immune and nonimmune cell interactions. Am J Physiol. 1997;273:G769–75.
2. Young HE, Mancini ML, Wright RP *et al.* Mesenchymal stem cells reside within the connective tissues of many organs. Dev Dyn. 1995;202:137–44.
3. Schmitt-Gräff A, Desmouliere A, Gabbiani G. Heterogeneity of myofibroblast phenotypic features: an example of fibroblastic cell plasticity. Virchows Arch. 1994;425:3–24.
4. Berschneider HM, Powell DW. Fibroblasts modulate intestinal secretory responses to inflammatory mediators. J Clin Invest. 1992;89:484–9.

5. Mathan M, Hermos JA, Trier JS. Structural features of the epithelio-mesenchymal interface of rat duodenal mucosa during development. J Cell Biol. 1972;52:577–88.
6. Haffen K, Kedinger M, Simon-Assmann PM, Lacroix B. Mesenchyme-dependent differentiation of intestinal brush border enzymes in the gizzard endoderm of the chick embryo. In: Embryonic Differentiation: Part B: Cellular Aspects. New York: A. Liss; 1982:261–70.
7. Ishizuya OA, Mizuno T. Intestinal cytodifferentiation in vitro of chick stomach endoderm induced by the duodenal mesenchyme. J Embryol Exp Morphol. 1984;82:163–76.
8. Haffen K, Lacroix B, Kedinger M, Simon AP. Inductive properties of fibroblastic cell cultures derived from rat intestinal mucosa on epithelial differentiation. Differentiation. 1983;23:226–33.
9. Correa P. Chronic gastritis as a cancer precursor. Scand J Gastroenterol Suppl. 1984;104:131–6.
10. Stallmach A, Hahn U, Merker HJ, Hahn EG, Riecken EO. Differentiation of rat intestinal epithelial cells is induced by organotypic mesenchymal cells in vitro. Gut. 1989;30:959–70.
11. Fritsch C, Simon AP, Kedinger M, Evans GS. Cytokines modulate fibroblast phenotype and epithelial–stroma interactions in rat intestine. Gastroenterology. 1997;112:826–38.
12. Aufderheide E, Ekblom P. Tenascin during gut development: appearance in the mesenchyme, shift in molecular forms, and dependence on epithelial–mesenchymal interactions. J Cell Biol. 1988;107:71–9.
13. Riedl S, Kadmon M, Tandara A et al. Mucosal tenascin C content in inflammatory and neoplastic diseases of the large bowel. Dis Colon Rectum. 1998;41:86–92.
14. Bucala R, Ritchlin C, Winchester R, Cerami A. Constitutive production of inflammatory and mitogenic cytokines by rheumatoid synovial fibroblasts. J Exp Med. 1991;173:569–74.
15. Elias JA, Reynolds MM. Interleukin-1 and tumor necrosis factor synergistically stimulate lung fibroblast interleukin-1 alpha production. Am J Respir Cell Mol Biol. 1990;3:13–20.
16. Libby P, Ordovas JM, Birinyi LK, Auger KR, Dinarello CA. Inducible interleukin-1 gene expression in human vascular smooth muscle cells. J Clin Invest. 1986;78:1432–8.
17. Gruss HJ, Scott C, Rollins BJ, Brach MA, Herrmann F. Human fibroblasts express functional IL-2 receptors formed by the IL-2R alpha- and beta-chain subunits: association of IL-2 binding with secretion of the monocyte chemoattractant protein-1. J Immunol. 1996;157:851–7.
18. Krzesicki RF, Fleming WE, Winterrowed GE, Hatfield CA, Sanders ME, Chin JE. T lymphocyte adhesion to human synovial fibroblasts. Role of cytokines and the interaction between intercellular adhesion molecule 1 and CD11a/CD18. Arthritis Rheum. 1991;34:1245–53.
19. Piela TH, Korn JH. Lymphocyte–fibroblast adhesion induced by interferon-gamma. Cell Immunol. 1988;114:149–60.
20. Fibbe WE, Van DJ, Billiau A et al. Human fibroblasts produce granulocyte-CSF, macrophage-CSF, and granulocyte-macrophage-CSF following stimulation by interleukin-1 and poly(rI).poly(rC). Blood. 1988;72:860–6.
21. Leizer T, Cebon J, Layton JE, Hamilton JA. Cytokine regulation of colony-stimulating factor production in cultured human synovial fibroblasts: I. Induction of GM-CSF and G-CSF production by interleukin-1 and tumor necrosis factor. Blood. 1990;76:1989–96.
22. Rolfe MW, Kundel SL, Standiford TJ et al. Pulmonary fibroblast expression of interleukin-8: a model for alveolar macrophage-derived cytokine networking. Am J Respir Cell Mol Biol. 1991;5:493–501.
23. Hamilton JA, Waring PM, Filonzi EL. Induction of leukemia inhibitory factor in human synovial fibroblasts by IL-1 and tumor necrosis factor-alpha. J Immunol. 1993;150:1496–502.
24. van Damme J, Schaafsma MR, Fibbe WE, Falkenburg JH, Opdenakker G, Billiau A. Simultaneous production of interleukin 6, interferon-beta and colony-stimulating activity by fibroblasts for viral and bacterial infection. Eur J Immunol. 1989;19:163–8.
25. Xing Z, Jordana M, Braciak T, Ohtoshi T, Gauldie J. Lipopolysaccharide induces expression of granulocyte/macrophage colony-stimulating factor, interleukin-8, and interleukin-6 in human nasal, but not lung fibroblasts: evidence for heterogeneity within the respiratory tract. Am J Respir Cell Mol Biol. 1993;9:255–63.
26. Hogaboam CM, Snider DP, Collins SM. Activation of T lymphocytes by syngeneic murine intestinal smooth muscle cells. Gastroenterology. 1996;110:1456–66.
27. Khan I, Blennerhassett MG, Kataeva GV, Collins SM. Interleukin 1 beta induces the expression of interleukin 6 in rat intestinal smooth muscle cells. Gastroenterology. 1995;108:1720–8.
28. Pang G, Couch L, Batey R, Clancy R, Crippo A. GM-CSF, IL-1a, IL-1b, IL-6, IL-8, IL-10, ICAM-1 and VCAM-1 gene expression and cytokine production in human duodenal fibroblasts stimulated with lipopolysaccharide, IL-1α and TNF α. Clin Exp Immunol. 1994;96:437–43.

29. Strong SA, Pizarro TT, Klein JS, Cominelli F, Fiocchi C. Proinflammatory cytokines differentially modulate their own expression in human intestinal mucosal mesenchymal cells. Gastroenterology. 1998;114:1244–56.
30. Rogler G, Vogl D, Jehl S *et al.* Induction of cytokine synthesis in intestinal myofibroblasts by NFκB. German J Gastroenterol. 1998;36:668 (German abstract).
31. Hagoboam CM, Snider DP, Collins SM. Cytokine modulation of T-lymphocyte activation by intestinal smooth muscle cells. Gastroenterology. 1997;112:1986–95.
32. Scott S, Pandolfi F, Kurnick JT. Fibroblasts mediate T cell survival: a proposed mechanism for retention of primed T cells. J Exp Med. 1990;172:1873–6.
33. Falk MH, Meier T, Issels RD, Brielmeier M, Scheffer B, Bornkamm GW. Apoptosis in Burkitt lymphoma cells is prevented by promotion of cysteine uptake. Int J Cancer. 1998;75:620–5.
34. Ina K, Binion DG, West GA, Dobrea GM, Fiocchi C. Secretion of soluble factors and phagocytosis by intestinal fibroblasts regulate T-cell apoptosis. Gastroenterology. 1995;108:841 (abstract).
35. Ina K, Kusugami K, Fiocchi C. Enhanced interaction of intestinal fibroblasts with T-cells in inflammatory bowel disease (IBD). Gastroenterology. 1996;110:930 (abstract).
36. Graham MF, Diegelmann RF, Elson CO *et al.* Collagen content and types in the intestinal strictures of Crohn's disease. Gastroenterology. 1988;94:257–65.
37. Alexander AC, Irving MH. Accumulation and pepsin solubility of collagens in the bowel of patients with Crohn's disease. Dis Colon Rectum. 1990;33:956–62.
38. Stallmach A, Schuppan D, Lazar D, Riese H, Riecken E. Increased collagen type III synthesis by lamina propria fibroblasts from strictures in Crohn's disease. Gastroenterology. 1992;102:1920–9.
39. Matthes H, Herbst H, Schuppan D *et al.* Cellular localization of procollagen gene transcripts in inflammatory bowel diseases. Gastroenterology. 1992;102:431–42.
40. Ignotz RA, Massague J. Transforming growth factor-β stimulates the expression of fibronectin and collagen and their incorporation into the extracellular matrix. J Biol Chem. 1986;261:4337–45.
41. Doe WF. Are there other important cells? Characterization of intestinal fibroblasts in Crohn's disease. In: Andus T, Goebell H, Layer P, Scölmerich J, editors. Inflammatory Bowel Diseases – From Bench to Bedside. Dordrecht, Boston, London: Kluwer Academic Publishers; 1997:126–9.
42. Gosh S, Humphreys K, Papachrysostomou M, Ferguson A. Detection of insulin-like growth factor-1 and transforming growth factor-β in whole gut lavage fluid: a novel method of studying intestinal fibrosis. Eur J Gastroenterol Hepatol. 1997;9:505–8.
43. Roberts AB, Sporn MB, eds. The transforming growth factor-βs. Heidelberg: Springer-Verlag; 1990:419–72.
44. Lawler S, Candia AF, Ebner R *et al.* The murine type II TGF-β receptor has a coincident embryonic expression and binding preference for TGF-β1. Development. 1994;120:165–75.
45. Martignoni ME, Friess H, di Mola FF *et al.* TGFβ and its receptors: A key role in Crohn's disease. German J Gastroenterol. 1998;36:728 (German abstract).
46. Froncek MJ, Derdak S, Felch ME, Silvera MR, Watts HB, Phipps RP. Cellular and molecular characterization of Thy-1– and Thy-1+ murine lung fibroblasts. In: Phipps RP, ed. Pulmonary fibroblast heterogeneity. Boca Raton, FL: CRC Press; 1992: 135–98.
47. Sempowski GD, Derdak S, Phipps RP. Interleukin-4 and interferon-γ discordantly regulate collagen biosynthesis by functionally distinct lung fibroblast subsets. J Cell Physiol. 1996;167:290–6.

16
The role of extracellular matrix proteins in IBD

P. POZAROWSKI and A. GORSKI

EXTRACELLULAR MATRIX PROTEINS IN NORMAL CONDITIONS

Leukocytes are in constant movement through the whole human body. Naive B and T cells using specific 'homing' receptors migrate via high endothelial venules (HEV) into secondary lymphoid tissue such as Peyer's patches or peripheral lymph nodes. Memory lymphocytes and lymphoblasts possess tissue-restricted migration abilities to extralymphoid sites such as mucosal epithelium or skin. Neutrophils, monocytes and lymphocytes migrate into inflamed tissues in response to inflammatory stimulation[1]. During these migrations they not only pass through different microenvironments but also these local conditions, far from being inactive bystanders, also influence them. Furthermore, they have their functions in specific local conditions defined by extracellular matrix (ECM) proteins, the fluid in which they are immersed, and different factors secreted by surrounding cells at the site of destination (e.g. inflamed areas).

Structure of ECM

Extracellular matrix has an influence upon cell growth, differentiation, adhesion and migration in normal and pathological conditions[2]. The skeleton, or rather a skeletal complex network, of ECM is formed from proteins. The molecules that comprise the ECM consist of glycoproteins and complex carbohydrates known as glycosaminoglycans, usually covalently linked to core proteins to form proteoglycans[3]. These are structurally and functionally very heterogeneous. Thus, depending on the origin of tissues, the state of development of the organism and the macromolecular consistency of ECM may be quite different[4]. Fibronectin, collagens, elastin, laminin, thrombospondin, tenascin and entactin are among the most important ECM glycoproteins. Proteoglycans – much more abundant, heterogeneous and perhaps functionally the most versatile non-fibrillar component of ECM – consist mainly of perlecan, decorin, biglycal and fibromodulin[4]. The fibrous backbone of ECM is composed of fibrillar collagens (types I, II, III) and elastin, which are linked to the non-fibrillar collagens (type IV),[5] laminin and entactin. These are assembled into a complex network forming basement membrane, which is specialized ECM separating epithelial and endothelial cells from the underlying tissues[3,4]. All these proteins are immersed in the hydrated carbohydrate gel consisting mainly of hyaluronic acid (HA, also hyaluronate or hyaluronan)[3]. It is worth mentioning that these ECM components are produced not only by fibroblast, or other tissue cells, but migatory mono-nuclear cells themselves (macrophages and T cells) are able to secrete at least some of them (i.e. fibronectin)[3,6]. Moreover, they can realize a wide array of cytokines, chemokines and matrix-degrading enzymes into the inflammatory milieu, all of which can have an influence upon the rapidly changing situation[7].

Immunomodulatory role of ECM

Depending on ECM, cellular responses may range from swift and selective (e.g. adhesion and chemotaxis) to slow and prolonged (e.g. cell proliferation and dif-ferentiation)[4]. T cell stimulation through the complex of T cell antigen receptor and CD3 in the absence of other signals is insufficient for their full activation, and could even induce T cell anergy. Therefore, other additionally costimulatory signals are obligatory for their effective action. Such signals could be provided by various interactions between T cells and antigen-presenting cells, e.g. CD2/LFA-3, or CD28/CD80. Recent data show that ECM proteins can strongly costimulate T cells; moreover, costimulation takes place in the absence of antigen-presenting cells[6]. ECM proteins also play a protective role, not only for lymphocytes but also for epithelia and endothelial cells. Adherent cells are pro-tected from apoptosis by interactions with ECM proteins. Normally they undergo apoptosis when they are detached from ECM proteins; this pheno-menon is termed anoikis[8].

ECM receptors on cells

ECM proteins also play a key role in cell movement through the various tissues. Cell adhesion to ECM proteins not only helps in transmigration through the endothelial layer, but is also necessary for the migration of other tissues under normal and pathological conditions. The mechanism of this process has not yet been established. Probably it is not a simple cell migration on ECM proteins using specific receptors for these proteins. Rather – according to other hypo-theses, the cells utilize $\alpha v\beta 3$ integrins to bind endogenously produced fibro-nectin (found on T cells[9,10]), which binds to underlying ECM proteins such as collagens. The processes of attachment or detachment are produced by release of adherent or non-adherent isomers of some ECM proteins (e.g. thrombospondin), their binding to CD36 and $\alpha v\beta 3$ integrins forming active complexes associated with actin fibres. Such events take place locally on the cell surfaces – mostly attachment on the cell leading edges and mostly detachment on other parts of cells[11].

Cell interactions with ECM proteins are produced by two kinds of receptors – integrins and less-characterized surface-associated proteoglycans. The integrins are a supergene family of α and β subunits that together form α–β heterodimeric associations on the cell surfaces. Currently more than 15 α subunits and at least eight β chains have been characterized, but permutations are restricted, and only about 20 α–β receptor combinations have been identified. The most important integrins involved in T cell interactions with ECM proteins are $\beta1$ (VLA – very late antigen) integrins. They consist of a common $\beta1$ subunit connected to various α units (from $\alpha1$ to $\alpha8$)[11,12]. Integrin interactions with ECM proteins are complicated – one integrin can interact with more than one protein (e.g. VLA-1 with collagen I and IV). The opposite situation can also take place – for example fibronectin is recognized by VLA-4 and VLA-5. Moreover, the signals of T cell ECM protein adhesion and costimulation can be provided by completely different receptors (e.g. T cell adhesion to collagen IV: VLA-1, VLA-2 and CD26; costimulation: VLA-3 and CD26) (see Table 1). T cell adhesion to ECM protein is regulated in two different ways. First, VLA binding activity of the T cell is rapidly and strongly augmented by cell activation without a change in the level of their expression (qualitative changes). Secondly, memory cells express three to four times more VLA-4, 5 and 6 than do naive cells (quantitative changes)[3,13]. Integrins can transduce information from the outside into the inside of cells, and they also signal back from the inside out[14] (e.g. post-activatory qualitative and quantitative changes). Although the ligand binding by these integrins involves interactions between α and β subunits, the intracellular signal seems to be transduced mainly by the cytoplasmic domain of β chain interactions with two major cytoskeletal proteins – talin and α-actin[4]. The process of organizing the cytoskeleton, activation of the Na^+/H^+ antiporter, changes in cytoplasmic Ca^{2+} concentration and activation of pp^{125} focal adhesion kinase (pp^{125FAK}) are the most established intracellular events mediated by integrins[14]. Moreover, some surface molecules can modulate signal transduction via integrins (CD4 in T cells)[15]. All

Table 1 Receptors involved in T cell interactions with ECM proteins

ECM proteins	Adhesion mediating receptors	Costimulation mediating receptors
Collagen I	VLA-1 VLA-2	VLA-3 CD26
Collagen IV	VLA-1 VLA-2 CD26	VLA-3 CD26
Fibronectin	VLA-4 VLA-5 CD26	VLA-5 VLA-4
Laminin	VLA-6	VLA-6
Thrombospondin	VLA-4 VLA-5 $\alpha v \beta 3$	–
Elastin	67 kDa EBP VLA-3	VLA-3
Tenastin	VLA-4	

VLA, very late antigen; EBP, elastin binding protein; –, data not available.

these events can finally lead to induction of several genes (e.g. interleukin 1 (IL-1), IL-2, IL-4, or tumour necrosis factor alpha (TNF-α) in T cells or other cells)[6].

ECM IN IBD

Although much scientific study has taken place recently, the pathogenesis of inflammatory bowel disease (IBD) is still unknown. We cannot even say clearly whether ulcerative colitis (UC) and Crohn's disease (CD) are discrete entities or different expressions of the same disease[16], but the immunological influence on the pathogenesis of IBD is a fact.

ECM interactions with cytokines

Many IBD reports concern the role of cytokines in the pathogenesis of IBD, but their interactions with ECM have been largely ignored. It is now clear that ECM not only serve as the functional storage of cytokines, but can also restrict or modulate cytokine activities at target sites[7]. The best examples of these relations are interactions between the proactivatory cytokine TNF-α (the levels of which are increased in IBD patients[17]), and laminin and fibronectin. TNF-α not only binds avidly to laminin and fibronectin, and is stored in complexes formed with these proteins, but they can also regulate the bioavailability and activity of TNF-α[7,18]. Moreover, some cytokines (e.g. basic fibroblast growth factor) can stimulate cells only in binding with heparan sulphate proteoglycans[4]. Migratory cells (monocytes/macrophages, neutrophils and especially T cells) can produce and release heparanase (endo-β-D-glucuronidase), which cleaves heparan sulphate molecules of the ECM, releasing various cytokines and growth factors bound to them and facilitating cell movement and migration through extravascular tissues. Furthermore, heparanase activities are regulated by local pH. Heparanase is enzymatically quiescent at the physiological pH of 7.2 (although it can still be stored in ECM), but is active at relatively acidic pH values (6.4–6.8)[7]. Such conditions can be present locally in the gut of IBD patients. Furthermore, it is not only cytokines which can interact with ECM, migratory cells and heparanase, but chemokines also can react. RANTES and macrophage inflammation protein 1β (MP-1β) have been most studied[7,19]. Some reports show that they are involved in the pathogenesis of IBD[20].

Alterations in ECM receptors

Lymphocytes and other cells interact with ECM proteins with the help of their receptors. Although peripheral blood lymphocyte (PBL) subsets of patients with IBD do not differ from healthy controls (they are only more activated)[21], there are significant alterations in IBD and normal intestinal lymphocyte integrin pattern. UC T cells express significantly more $\alpha2$, $\alpha6$ and less $\beta7$ and $\alpha4$ integrins, but B cells have significantly less $\alpha4$ integrins and more $\alpha2$, $\alpha3$, $\alpha5$ and $\alpha6$ integrins. On the other hand CD T lymphocytes show an increase of $\alpha6$ integrins and a decrease of $\beta7$ integrins. CD B cells have fewer $\beta7$ and $\alpha4$ integrins and more $\alpha2$ and $\alpha5$ integrins[22]. These findings are supported by observations that VLA-4 is expressed on most lymphocytes of lymph follicles in IBD[23]. All these changes in expression of ECM receptors have an influence on the abilities of lamina propria lymphocyte to adhere and to be constimulated by ECM proteins. The most interesting finding is the decreased number of $\alpha 4\beta 7$ molecules. This integrin is responsible for lymphocyte gut homing via their ligation not only with mucosal addressin cell adhesion molecule-1 (MAdCAM-1), but also VCAM-1 and fibronectin. The $\alpha 4\beta 7$ integrin percentage reduction observed here is relative, and is probably caused by a greater than normal influx of non-specific gut lymphocytes forcing by inflammatory factors. Moreover, $\alpha 4\beta 7$ integrin also seems to increase the CD3-dependent activation of gut lymphocytes[24].

The importance of integrins in the pathogenesis of bowel inflammations is proved in animal studies, in which the use of the monoclonal antibodies anti-$\alpha 4$ integrins (blocking VLA-4 and $\alpha 4\beta 7$), anti-$\beta 7$ integrins and anti-MAdCAM-1 was effective in animal treatment[25,26].

Lymphocyte interactions with ECM

In our own research we have examined peripheral blood T cell adhesion to ECM proteins (fibronectin, elastin and collagen IV) and also their (fibronectin, elastin, collagen I and collagen IV) costimulatory abilities in UC patients. We have found significantly greater T cell adhesion to fibronectin and collagen IV. Generally, these changes are stronger in acutely ill patients than in chronic patients. Our findings suggest not only the importance of typical ECM protein (e.g. fibronectin), but also, what is more relevant, the importance of basement membrane proteins (i.e. collagen IV) in the pathogenesis of UC. The question arises whether UC is a new example of vasculitis. We cannot answer this clearly (Pozarowski, unpublished), but some reports showing the importance of lymphocyte (or other cells)–endothelial interactions support this hypothesis[27–31] (for review also see refs 32–34). The results from studies by Ito and co-workers are similar to some of our results; they indirectly proved the involvement of integrin–fibronectin interactions in the pathogenesis of UC[35]. The local importance of fibronectin emphasizes its increased deposition in the rectum[36], in contrast to the decrease in its serum level in UC patients[37]. Remodelling of ECM components is also present in CD. Long-lasting inflammation is accompanied by the deposition of fibrotic tissue containing excessive amounts of collagen types I, III and V. Moreover, collagen I degradation is increased not only in active CD, but also in patients entering clinical remission[38]. This could suggest continuous character of ECM changes in the gut of a patient suffering from CD, even during remissions.

Much has been directed towards detecting a bacterial agent responsible for the appearance of IBD. Although local tolerance to autologous intestinal flora is broken in inflamed IBD intestine[39], the pathogenic role of any specific bacteria has not yet been proved. The possibility that *Yersinia enterocolitica* is involved in the pathogenesis of IBD cannot be excluded[40]. *Yersinia* invasin protein has an influence on T lymphocyte interactions with ECM. It is not only a $\beta 1$-integrin ligand, but it also can induce costimulation, migration on fibronectin and collagen IV, and pseudopodia formation of T lymphocytes[41]. Moreover, other bacterial proteins can also influence the local immunity of patients suffering from IBD.

CONCLUSIONS

Our knowledge concerning the role of ECM in IBD pathogenesis is insufficient, but it seems that ECM, similar to its influence on the pathogenesis of other disorders[6], plays an important role in IBD patients. This chapter has described how changes in ECM protein composition, their receptors, interactions with cells, chemokines and cytokines have an influence on incorrect local immunological response. It is to be hoped that more intensive research on this topic will be carried out in the future. Studies on anti-integrin monoclonal antibody treatment abilities and the influence of ECM on apoptosis (not only on lymphocytes, but also on gut epithelial cells) are most interesting topics.

Acknowledgements

Many references had to be deleted to shorten this chapter, and we apologize to authors and readers for work that could not be cited. Some of the work reported in this chapter was supported by the Committee for Research (KBN) grants (4P05B04412 and 4P05B04709).

References

1. Hogg N, Berlin C. Structure and function of adhesion receptors in leukocyte trafficking. Immunol Today. 1995;16:327–30.
2. Guarino M, Christensen L. Immunohistochemical analysis of extracellular matrix components in synovial sarcoma. J Pathol. 1994;172:279–86.
3. Shimizu Y, Shaw S. Lymphocyte interactions with extracellular matrix. FASEB J. 1991;5:2292–9.
4. Raghow R. The role of extracellular matrix in postinflammatory wound healing and fibrosis. FASEB J. 1994;8:823–31.
5. Kuhn K. Basement membrane (type IV) collagen. Matrix Biol. 1994;14:439–45.
6. Gorski A, Kupiec-Weglinski JW. Extracellular matrix proteins, regulators of T-cell functions in healthy and diseased individuals. Clin Diagn Lab Immunol. 1995;2:646–51.
7. Gilat D, Cahalon L, Hershkoviz R, Lider O. Interplay of T cells and cytokines in the context of enzymatically modified extracellular matrix. Immunol Today. 1996;17:16–20.
8. Ruoslahti E, Reed JC. Anchorage dependence, integrins and apoptosis. Cell. 1994;77:477–8.
9. Hauzenberger D, Sundqvist KG. Fibronectin at the lymphocyte surface. Evidence for activation-dependent binding to VLA4 and VLA5 integrins. Scand J Immunol. 1993;37:87–95.
10. Pallis M, Robins RA, Powell RJ. Peripheral blood lymphocyte binding to a soluble FITZ–fibronectin conjugate. Cytometry. 1997;28:157–64.
11. Tooney PA, Agrez MV, Burns GF. The re-examination of the molecular basis of cell movement. Immunol Cell Biol. 1993;71:131–9.
12. Ruoslahti E. Integrins. J Clin Invest. 1991;87:1–5.
13. Shimizu Y, van Seventer GA, Horgan KJ, Shaw S. Regulated expression and binding of three VLA (β1) integrin receptors on T cells. Nature. 1990;345:250–3.
14. Rosales C, Juliano RL. Signal transduction by cell adhesion receptors in leukocytes. J Leukocyte Biol. 1995;57:189–98.
15. Hershkoviz R, Miron S, Cohen IR *et al.* T lymphocyte adhesion to fibronectin and laminin components of extracellular matrix is regulated by the CD4 molecule. Eur J Immunol. 1992;22:7–13.
16. Shanahan F. Pathogenesis of ulcerative colitis. Lancet. 1993;342:407–11.
17. Jewell DP. Immunology of inflammatory bowel disease – an update. J Gastroenterol. 1995;30(Suppl. VIII):78–82.
18. Alon R, Cahalon L, Hershkoviz R. TNF-α binds to the N-terminal domain of fibronectin and augments the β1-integrin-mediated adhesion of CD4+ T lymphocytes to the glycoprotein. J Immunol. 1994;152:1304–13.
19. Gilat D, Hershkoviz R, Mekori YA *et al.* Regulation of adhesion of CD4+ T lymphocytes to intact or heparinase-treated subendothelial extracellular matrix by diffusible or anchored RANTES and MIP-1β. J Immunol. 1994;153:4899–906.

20. Grimm MC, Doe WF. Chemokines in inflammatory bowel disease mucosa: expression of RANTES, macrophage inflammatory protein (MIP)-1α, MIP-1β, and γ-interferon-inducible protein-10 by macrophages, lymphocytes, endothelial cells and granulomas. Inflamm Bowel Dis. 1996;2:88–96.
21. MacDermott RP. Alterations in the mucosal immune system in ulcerative colitis and Crohn's disease. Med Clin N Am. 1994;78:1207–30.
22. Yacyshyn BR, Lazarovits A, Tsai V, Matejko K. Crohn's disease, ulcerative colitis, and normal intestinal lymphocytes express integrins in dissimilar patterns. Gastroenterology. 1994;107:1364–71.
23. Pedersen G, Brynskov J, Nielsen OH, Bendtzen K. Adhesion molecules in inflammatory and neoplastic intestinal diseases. Dig Dis. 1995;13:322–36.
24. Sarnacki S, Begue B, Buc H et al. Enhancement of CD3-induced activation of human intestinal intraepithelial lymphocytes by stimulation of the β7-containing integrin defined by HML-1 monoclonal antibody. Eur J Immunol. 1992;22:2887–92.
25. Podolski D, Lobb R, King N et al. Attenuation of colitis in the cotton-top tamarin by anti-α4 integrin monoclonal antibody. J Clin Invest. 1993;92:372–80.
26. Picarella D, Hurlbut P, Rottman J et al. Monoclonal antibodies specific for β7 integrin and mucosal addressin cell adhesion molecule-1 (MAdCAN-1) reduce inflammation in the colon of *scid* mice reconstituted with CD45RB[high] CD4+ T cells. J Immunol. 1997;158:2099–106.
27. Schurmann GM, Bishop AE, Facer P et al. Increased expression of cell adhesion molecules P-selectin in active inflammatory bowel disease. Gut. 1995;36:411–18.
28. Nielsen OH, Brynskov J, Vainer B. Increased mucosal concentration of soluble intercellular adhesion molecule-1 (sICAM-1), sE-selectin, and interleukin-8 in active ulcerative colitis. Dig Dis Sci. 1996;41:1780–5.
29. Kirman I, Nielsen OH. LFA-1 subunit expression in ulcerative colitis patients. Dig Dis Sci. 1996;41:670–6.
30. Malizia G, Calabrese A, Cottone M et al. Expression of leukocyte adhesion molecules by mucosal mononuclear phagocytes in inflammatory bowel disease. Gastroenterology. 1991;100:150–9.
31. Jones SC, Banks RE, Haider A et al. Adhesion molecules in inflammatory bowel disease. Gut. 1995;36:724–30.
32. Shimizu Y, Newman W, Tanaka Y, Shaw S. Lymphocyte interactions with endothelial cells. Immunol Today. 1992;13:106–12.
33. Carlos TM, Harlan JM. Leukocyte–endothelial adhesion molecules. Blood. 1994;84:2068–101.
34. Adams DH, Shaw S. Leucocyte–endothelial interactions and regulation of leucocyte migration. Lancet. 1994;343:831–6.
35. Ito M, Hirata S, Arai S, Takahshi T. T cell adherence and mucosal injury in ulcerative colitis: involvement of integrin–fibronectin interaction *in situ*. J Gastroenterol. 1995;30(Suppl. VIII):70–2.
36. Scott DL, Morris CJ, Blacke AE et al. Distribution of fibronectin in the rectal mucosa. J Clin Pathol. 1981;34:749–58.
37. Stadnicki A, Hrycek A, Stasiura H, Jacek Hartleb. Plasma fibronectin and some humoral factors in ulcerative colitis patients. Arch Gastroenterohepatol. 1994;13:79–82.
38. Kjeldsen J, Schaffalitzky de Muckadell OB, Junker P. Seromarkers of collagen I and III metabolism in active Crohn's disease. Relation to disease activity and response to therapy. Gut. 1995;37:805–10.
39. Duchmann R, Kaiser I, Hermann E et al. Tolerance exists towards resident intestinal flora but is broken in active inflammatory bowel disease (IBD). Clin Exp Immunol. 1995;102:448–55.
40. Thayer WR, Chitnavis V. The case for an infectious etiology. Med Clin N Am. 1994;78:1233–47.
41. Arencibia I, Suarez NC, Wolf-Watz H, Sunqvist K. *Yersinia* Invasin, a bacterial β1-integrin ligand, is a potent inducer of lymphocyte motility and migration to collagen type IV and fibronectin. J Immunol. 1997;159:1853–9.

17
Heat shock proteins in IBD

D. LUDWIG, M. STAHL and E. F. STANGE

INTRODUCTION

Heat shock proteins (Hsp) are highly conserved intracellular proteins, present constitutively in most mammalian and also procaryotic cells[1–3]. Hsp synthesis is induced by a variety of stimuli including heat, ischaemia/reperfusion, inflammation and microbial infection[3–5]. Heat shock proteins – also called stress proteins – are classified by their molecular weight[6] and especially the proteins of the 60 and 70 kDa family are known to play an important role in maintaining cellular homeostasis by interacting with the intracellular transport and folding of proteins[3]. Moreover these proteins are thought to participate directly in antigen presentation of proteins and may act as autoantigens[7,8]. Autoantibodies and reactive T cells against different Hsp have been found in various diseases including inflammatory bowel disease (IBD)[9–11] and may be caused by molecular mimicry due to the high-grade homology between human and microbial, especially mycobacterial, Hsp[12–14]. There is some information about the Hsp-60 response at the site of inflammation in IBD[15,16], but few data are available concerning the 27, 70 and 90 kDa Hsp.

Hsp27

The 27 kDa protein of the group of small Hsp is encoded by a single gene located on chromosome 7[17]. This protein is the most highly induced when cells are exposed to heat shock, or after treatment with steroid hormones. Low levels are found in most mammalian cells, especially in nerval tissue, smooth muscle and skeletal muscle[18].

In the human colon the protein is expressed moderately in epithelial cells and some mononuclear cells of the lamina propria. The most important immunoreactivity is observed in smooth muscle cells, endothelial cells and nervous tissue cells (Figure 1), even enhanced in IBD. The cellular localization of Hsp27 in unstressed cells is generally perinuclear, while a redistribution to the nucleus is observed during heat shock or following incubation with some cytokines. This suggests that Hsp27 protects against and/or repairs cellular damage.

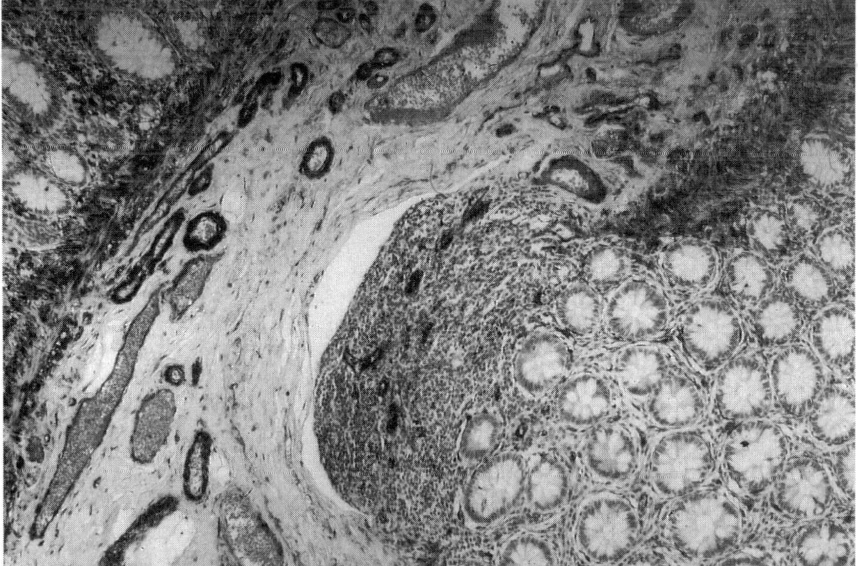

Figure 1   Distribution pattern of Hsp27 in the colonic mucosa (tissue resection specimen)

Additionally, this protein is essential in the signal transduction of actin micro-filaments[18]. A specific role of Hsp27 in IBD remains to be established.

Hsp60

Most reports have focused on the 60 kDa protein, which shows a high grade of homology between mycobacteria, other microorganisms and human cells. Molecular mimicry could be the basis for a possible link between the immune response to infection and autoimmunity[19]. Support for this hypothesis has been furnished by several reports: (a) exposure of monocytic cells to mycobacterial Hsp60 stimulates the release of tumour necrosis factor alpha (TNF-α) and inter-leukin 1 beta (IL-1β), even in the absence of sensitized T cells[20], (b) interferon gamma (IFN-γ) and TNF-α induce increased expression of Hsp60 in mono-cytic cell lines[21], (c) T cells specific for epitopes in self-Hsp60 are activated during a sterile inflammation, without previous exposure to exogenous Hsp[22], (d) the synthesis of Hsp60 is increased in intestinal epithelium in ulcerative colitis[15], and (e) Hsp60 is strongly expressed by B7-positive antigen-presenting cells in the mucosa of patients with IBD[16]. The latter finding is of particular interest since B7, a member of the immunoglobulin superfamily expressed on professional antigen-presenting cells[23], has an essential role in T cell activation. Abnormal T cell reactivity is a common finding, especially in Crohn's disease[12]. Hsp60 as cross reactive and immunodominant antigen may thereby enhance the state of T cell activation and be responsible for the persistence of increased immune reactivity[16].

Hsp70

The most highly inducible Hsp belong to the Hsp70 family, which includes both the constitutive protein (Hsp70c) essential for cellular function, and the inducible form (Hsp70i) which increases in response to environmental stress[6]. In stressed cells Hsp70 localizes to, and strongly associates with, the nucleus to protect intracellular proteins from denaturation resulting in cellular dysfunction. Other functional properties include the prevention of misfolding or aggregation of proteins, thus maintaining cellular integrity. This so-called function as 'molecular chaperone' includes differential binding capabilities of the Hsp60 and Hsp70 system, suggesting a function in a sequential manner[24]. An immunological role including intracellular antigen processing and surface expression of these antigens has been suggested as for Hsp60. A strong Hsp70 immunoreactivity has been found in thyroid follicles of patients with autoimmune thyroiditis, markedly reduced in patients treated with antithyroid drugs and absent in multinodular goitre and in normal thyroid tissue[25]. Moreover, the observed cell surface expression of the 72 kDa protein in retro-ocular fibroblasts of patients with Graves' ophthalmopathy, absent in cells of healthy controls, further supports an important role in the immune process[26]. Elevated antibody levels directed against mycobacterial and human Hsp72 in Crohn's disease (CD) but not in ulcerative colitis (UC), suggest differences in the pathogenesis of the two diseases[27].

The mucosal content of Hsp70, determined in biopsy specimens by semiquantitative immunoblot, is increased in patients with CD and UC in non-inflamed and inflamed mucosal areas, but also infectious colitis. Preliminary findings of semiquantitative polymerase chain reaction (PCR) revealed no differences in Hsp synthesis between diseased and healthy mucosa (Fellermann *et al.*, personal communication). The constitutive Hsp70 (Hsp70c), assessed by immunohistochemistry in tissue resection specimens, is moderately expressed in normal epithelial cells and some mononuclear cells in the lamina propria. The staining pattern for Hsp70c appears diffusely cytoplasmic, but granular for the inducible form (Hsp70i). The latter finding may be expression of aggregation or increased synthesis of proteins. In CD and UC the intensity of staining for Hsp70c is enhanced, and the relative number of positively stained mucosal mononuclear cells is increased. Induction of Hsp70 in these cells is only marginal, but not reduced compared to controls. Mucosal Hsp70 antibodies have been found in the majority of patients, but also in controls. Interestingly, these antibodies were exclusively of isotypes A or M, independent of the degree of mucosal inflammation. The absence of complement-binding IgG antibodies argues against a major pathogenetic role of these immunoglobulins in IBD.

Hsp90

Only few reports have dealt with Hsp90 in human diseases. This protein is also stress-inducible, and associates with numerous cytosolic and nuclear proteins involved in cell signalling. Most interestingly, Hsp90 induce reversible changes in the conformation of the glucocorticoid receptor, potentiating signalling activity[28]. The detection of IgG autoantibodies directed against Hsp90 in sera of patients with systemic lupus erythematosus (SLE), absent or at low levels in controls, points towards a possible role in autoimmune disorders[10,29]. The protective role of this protein has been shown in animal models[30]. In our studies there was no tendency towards increased expression in IBD tissue resection specimens. The cellular expression pattern has been found to be different, compared to other Hsp, since nerve cells or ganglions react intensely, even at higher dilutions. The protein is further detected in epithelial cells, mononuclear cells, granulocytes and giant cells, but also cells of small vessels (Figures 2 and 3). Mononuclear cells reacting are mainly macrophages (CD68+) or T lymphocytes (OPD4+), but not B lymphocytes (CD20+). A potential protective or immunogenic function of Hsp90 in IBD seems unlikely[31].

CONCLUSION

Heat shock proteins are constitutively expressed in the normal and diseased colonic mucosa. There are characteristic differences in cell populations positive for one or the other Hsp. The enhanced expression mainly of Hsp60 and 70 may reflect non-specific immune activation by inflammatory mediators or enhanced reactivity against luminal bacterial antigens. A relative deficiency of Hsp synthesis as the basis of mucosal inflammation seems unlikely, since the capacity of induction of these proteins was not found to be reduced. The similar prevalence and the absence of IgG isotype of mucosal Hsp70 antibodies in controls and

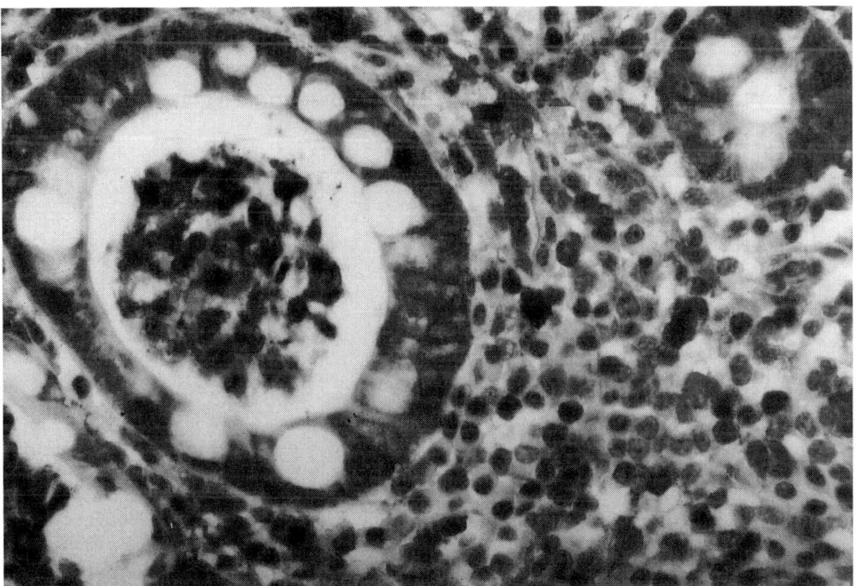

Figure 2 Localization of Hsp90 immunofluorescence in ulcerative colitis specimen. Staining of epithelial cells and some granulocytes and lamina propria mononuclear cells (original magnification ×250).

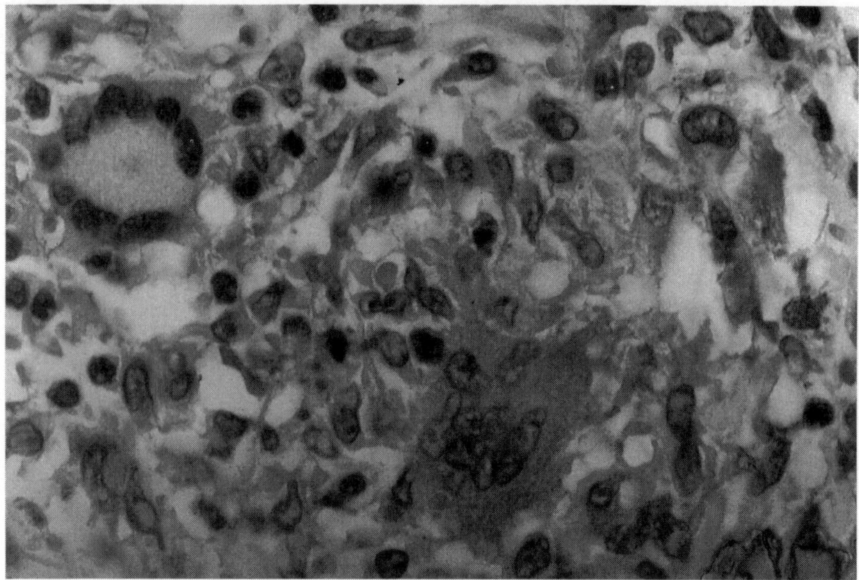

Figure 3 Immunohistochemical localization of Hsp90 in a giant cell in Crohn's disease (original magnification ×625).

IBD patients support the concept that mucosal antibodies in general represent an epiphenomenon of inflammation. A local protective or immunomodulatory function of Hsp70 is possible, whereas a humoral autoimmune response as pathogenetic event seems unlikely.

With increasing evidence of a major role of Hsp in mediating drug effects such as salicylates[32,33] and corticosteroids[34], further research in this area is awaited with interest.

References

1. Lindquist S, Craig EA. The heat-shock proteins. Annu Rev Genet. 1988;22:631–7.
2. Ang D, Liberek K, Showyra D, Zyclicz M, Georgopoulos C. Biological role and regulation of the universally conserved heat shock proteins. J Biol Chem. 1991;266:24233–6.
3. Kaufmann SHE. Heat shock proteins and the immune response. Immunol Today. 1990;11:129–36.
4. Welch WJ. How cells respond to stress. Sci Am. 1993;268:56–64.
5. Musch MW, Ciancio MJ, Sarge K, Chang EB. Induction of heat shock protein 70 protects intestinal epithelial cells from oxidant and thermal injury. Am J Physiol. 1996;270:C429–36.
6. Morimoto RI, Tissieres A, Georgopoulos C. Progress and perspectives of the biology of heat shock proteins and molecular chaperones. In: Morimoto RI, Tissieres A, Georgopoulos C, editors. The Biology of Heat Shock Proteins and Molecular Chaperones. New York: Cold Spring Harbor Laboratory Press; 1994:335–73.
7. Georgopoulos C, Welch WJ. Role of major heat shock proteins as molecular chaperones. Annu Rev Cell Biol. 1993;9:601–43.
8. Domanico SZ, DeNagel WE, Dahlseid JN, Green JM, Pierce SK. Cloning of the gene encoding peptide-binding protein 74 shows that it is a new member of the heat shock protein 70 family. Mol Cell Biol. 1993;13:3598–610.

9. De Graeff-Meeder ER, Voorhorst M, van Eden W *et al.* Antibodies to the mycobacteria 65-kd heat-shock protein are reactive with synovial tissue of adjuvant arthritic rats and patients with rheumatoid arthritis and osteoarthritis. Am J Pathol. 1990;137:1013–17.

10. Minota S, Koyasu S, Yahara I, Winfield J. Autoantibodies to the heat-shock protein hsp90 in systemic lupus erythematosus. J Clin Invest. 1988;81:106–9.

11. Elsaghier A, Prantera C, Bothamley G, Wilkins E, Jindal S, Ivanyi J. Disease association of antibodies to human and mycobacterial hsp70 and hsp60 stress proteins. Clin Exp Immunol. 1992;89:305–9.

12. Pirzer U, Schönhaar A, Fleischer B, Hermann E, Meyer zum Büschenfelde K-H. Reactivity of infiltrating T lymphocytes with microbial antigens in Crohn's disease. Lancet. 1991; 338:1238–9.

13. Sanderson JD, Moss MT, Tizard MLV, Hermann-Taylor J. *Mycobacterium paratuberculosis* DNA in Crohn's disease tissue. Gut. 1992;33:890–6.

14. Stainsby KJ, Lowes JR, Allan RN, Ibbotson JP. Antibodies to *Mycobacterium paratuberculosis* and nine species of environmental mycobacteria in Crohn's disease and control subjects. Gut. 1993;34:371–4.

15. Winrow VR, Mojdehi GM, Ryder SD, Rhodes JM, Blake DR, Rampton DS. Stress proteins in the colorectal mucosa: enhanced expression in ulcerative colitis. Dig Dis Sci. 1993;38:1994–2000.

16. Peetermans WE, D'Haens GR, Ceuppens JL, Rutgeerts P, Geboes K. Mucosal expression by B7-positive cells of the 60-kilodalton heat-shock protein in inflammatory bowel disease. Gastroenterology. 1995;108:75–82.

17. Hickey E, Brandon SE, Potter R, Stein G, Stein J, Weber LA. Sequence and organization of genes encoding the human 27kDa heat shock protein. Nucl Acids Res. 1986;14:4127–44.

18. Arrigo A-P, Landry J. Expression and function of the low-molecular-weight heat shock proteins. In: Morimoto RI, Tissieres A, Georgopoulos C, editors. The Biology of Heat Shock Proteins and Molecular Chaperones. New York: Cold Spring Harbor Laboratory Press; 1994:335–73.

19. Lamb JR, Bal V, Mendez-Samperio P *et al.* Stress proteins may provide a link between the immune reponse to infection and autoimmunity. Int Immunol. 1989;1:191–6.

20. Friedland JS, Shattock R, Remick DG, Griffin GE. Mycobacterial 65-kD heat shock protein induces release of proinflammatory cytokines from human monocytic cells. Clin Exp Immunol. 1993;91:58–62.

21. Ferm MT, Söderström K, Jindal S *et al.* Induction of human Hsp60 expression in monocytic cell lines. Int Immunol. 1992;4:305–11.

22. Anderton SM, van der Zee R, Goodacre JA. Inflammation activates self Hsp60-specific T-cells. Eur J Immunol. 1993;23:33–8.

23. Vandenberghe P, Delabie J, de Boer M, De Wolf-Peeters C, Ceuppens JL. *In situ* expression of B7/BB1 on antigen presenting cells and activated B cells: an immunohistochemical study. Int Immunol. 1993;5:317–21.

24. Frydman J, Hartl F-U. Molecular chaperone functions of Hsp70 and Hsp60 in protein folding. In: Morimoto RI, Tissieres A, Georgopoulos C, editors. The Biology of Heat Shock Proteins and Molecular Chaperones. New York: Cold Spring Harbor Laboratory Press; 1994:251–83.

25. Heufelder AE, Goellner JR, Wenzel BE, Bahn RS. Immunohistochemical detection and localization of a 72-kilodalton heat shock protein in autoimmune thyroid disease. J Clin Endocrinol Metab. 1992;74:724–31.

26. Heufelder AE, Wenzel BE, Gorman CA, Bahn RS. Detection, cellular localization, and modulation of heat shock proteins in cultured fibroblasts from patients with extrathyroidal manifestations of Graves' disease. J Clin Endocrinol Metab. 1991;73:2483–9.

27. Elsaghier A, Prantera C, Moreno C, Ivanyi J. Antibodies to *Mycobacterium paratuberculosis* specific protein antigens in Crohn's disease. Clin Exp Immunol. 1992;90:503–8.

28. Bohen BP, Yamamoto KR. Modulation of steroid receptor signal transduction by heat shock proteins. In: Morimoto RI, Tissieres A, Georgopoulos C, editors. The Biology of Heat Shock Proteins and Molecular Chaperones. New York: Cold Spring Harbor Laboratory Press; 1994:313–34.

29. Norton PM, Isenberg DA, Latchmann DS. Elevated levels of the 90 kd heat shock protein in a proportion of SLE patients with active disease. Mol Cell Biochem. 1988;130:49–55.

30. Zhao Y, Chacko S, Levin RM. Expression of stress proteins (Hsp 70 and Hsp 90) in the urinary bladder subjected to partial outlet obstruction. Mol Cell Endocrinol. 1993;98:49–54.

31. Stahl M, Ludwig D, Fellermann K, Stange EF. Intestinal expression of human heat shock protein 90 in patients with Crohn's disease and ulcerative colitis. Dig Dis Sci. 1998;43:1079–87.

32. Jurivich DA, Sistonen L, Kroes RA, Morimoto RI. Effect of sodium salicylate on the human heat shock response. Science. 1992;255:1243–5.
33. Burress GC, Musch MW, Jurivich DA, Welk J, Chang EB. Effects of mesalamine on the hsp72 stress response in rat IEC-18 intestinal epithelial cells. Gastroenterology. 1997;113:1474–9.
34. Pratt WB. The role of heat shock proteins in regulating the function, folding and trafficking of the glucocorticoid receptor. J Biol Chem. 1993;268:21455–8.

18
Regulation and function of eosinophils and mast cells: implications for the gastrointestinal tract

S. C. BISCHOFF and M. P. MANNS

INTRODUCTION

Eosinophils and mast cells are inflammatory effector cells, which often occur in parallel at sites of tissue inflammation. The crucial role of both cell types in mediating allergic inflammation is well documented. Apart from allergic reactions, a number of other diseases such as non-allergic inflammatory disease, parasitosis and tissue fibrosis, which are often located in the gastrointestinal tract, have been associated with mast cell and eosinophil accumulation and activation. Both cell types are found constitutively in normal human gut. Their number may be elevated in the course of intestinal inflammation. However, their precise role in gastrointestinal physiology and pathology remains to be elucidated. In the present chapter, our current knowledge on the regulation and function of human eosinophils and mast cells is summarized.

EFFECTOR FUNCTIONS OF HUMAN EOSINOPHILS

Upon activation, eosinophils release cationic proteins, such as eosinophil cationic protein (ECP), eosinophil-derived neurotoxin (EDN) and major basic protein (MBP). Moreover, eosinophils have cytotoxic potency by releasing eosinophil peroxidase (EPO) and oxygen free radicals. Apart from these pre-formed mediators, *de-novo*-synthesized mediators, such as prostaglandins (PGF$_2$), thromboxane (TxA$_2$) and platelet-activating factor (PAF), are released by activated eosinophils. Most recently it was shown that eosinophils are capable of producing cytokines, such as transforming growth factor-β (TGF-β) and interleukins[1-5]. The effector functions of eosinophils are summarized in Figure 1.

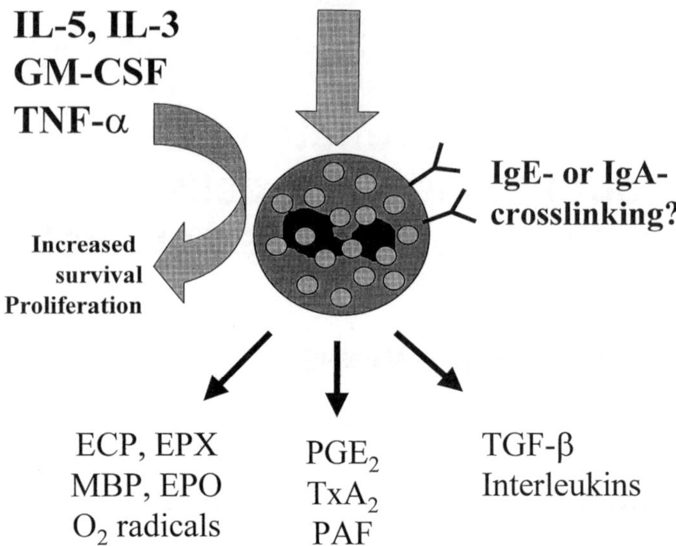

Figure 1 Regulation of human eosinophil effector functions. For details and abbreviations: see text

EFFECTOR FUNCTIONS OF HUMAN MAST CELLS

Mast cells exert their biological activities by releasing preformed mediators stored in cytoplasmatic granules (e.g. histamine, proteases) and *de-novo*-synthesized mediators (prostaglandins, leukotrienes) upon activation[5–12]. Similar to the findings in eosinophils, mast cells act not only as proinflammatory effector cells but also as immunoregulatory cells which may produce cytokines such as tumour necrosis factor-α (TNF-α) and possibly interleukins (Figure 2). However, most of these data are derived from animal studies, the results of which cannot be readily transferred to the human system[11]. However, we and others can confirm that human mucosal mast cells are capable of producing TNF-α and, upon activation, IL-5[8,9] (and our own unpublished results). In some individuals, mast cells may also produce small amounts of IL-4[8,9].

CYTOKINE PRODUCTION BY HUMAN EOSINOPHILS AND MAST CELLS

The fact that mast cells and eosinophils are capable of generating and releasing a number of immunoregulatory cytokines, such as TNF-α (mast cells), TGF-β (eosinophils), IL-4 (mast cells), IL-5 (eosinophils and mast cells) and IL-16

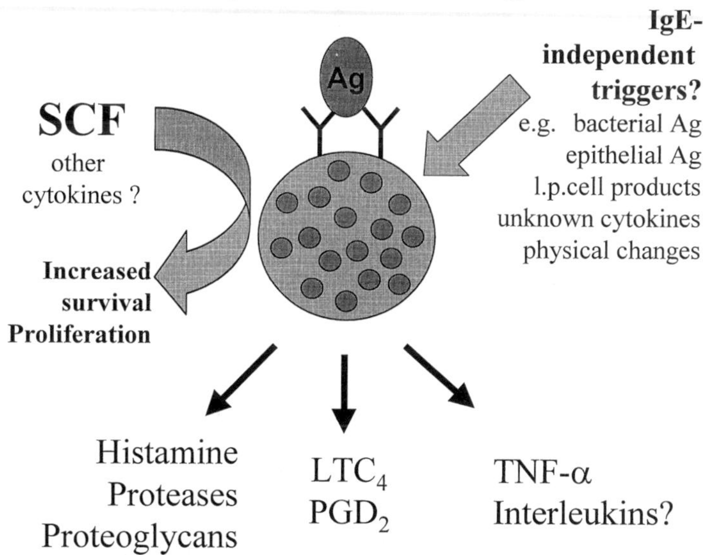

Figure 2   Regulation of human mast cell effector functions. For details and abbreviations: see text

(mast cells), strongly suggests that both cell types may act not only as pro-inflammatory cells but also as immunoregulatory components, which may have implications for their pathophysiological function in the gut (Figure 3). The role of mast cells and eosinophils as inflammatory effector cells in allergic reactions, but also in other chronic inflammatory diseases, such as Crohn's disease, ulcerative colitis, coeliac disease and eosinophilic gastroenteritis is well established[2,5,7,10,13–18]. However, the recent finding of cytokine production by these cell types may indicate that they also exert 'physiological' functions, such as immunoregulation, regulation of cell proliferation, maturation and function, as well as induction of immunological tolerance in the gut[1,3,9,11]. Eosinophils were suggested to be of particular importance in host defence against parasitic infections, namely worm infections, which are still relevant infectious diseases in underdeveloped countries[2,4]. The physiological functions of mast cells are less defined. Recent experiments performed in animals suggest that mast cells may be of importance for host defence against bacterial infection. In a mouse model of bacterial peritonitis, mast cells proved to be crucial for survival. The authors could show that this mast cell-dependent benefit was mostly due to TNF-α which is produced in significant quantities in the course of sepsis[11]. These animal data were confirmed by recently performed human studies showing that treatment with anti-TNF-α antibodies has no benefit in patients with bacterial sepsis. Apart from their function during bacterial infections, mast cells have been suggested to be involved in processes such as wound healing, tissue

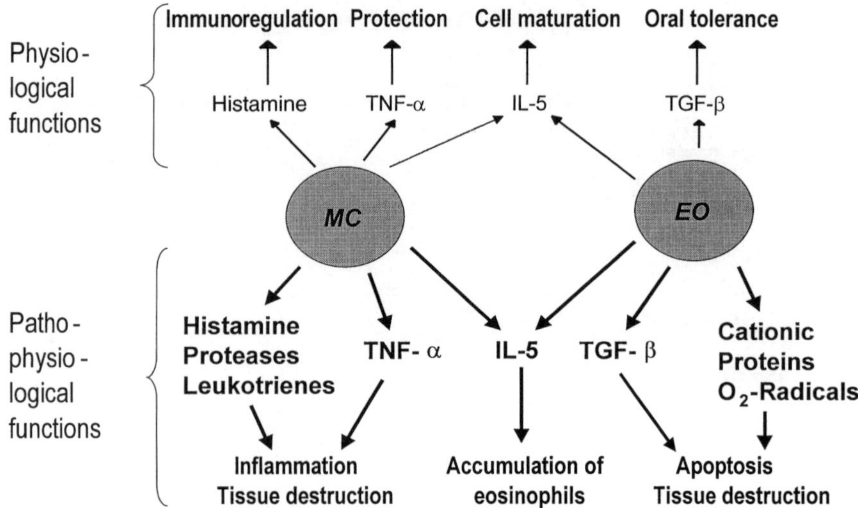

Figure 3 Hypothetical physiological and pathophysiological functions of human mast cells and eosinophils. For details and abbreviations: see text

fibrosis and tissue remodelling (through TGF-β and basic fibroblast growth factor, bFGF), regulation of epithelium and endothelium (histamine and leukotrienes) and eosinophil and basophil recruitment (IL-5)[5,7,9]. The possible physiological mast cell functions at the gastrointestinal barrier are summarized in Figure 4.

REGULATION OF EOSINOPHIL AND MAST CELL FUNCTIONS

During recent years, we have developed methods for mast cell and eosinophil isolation from human intestinal tissue (surgical specimens) allowing functional studies on the regulation of these cell types[19,20]. Using these methods, we could show that stem cell factor (SCF), the *c-kit* ligand, is a unique regulator of human mast cell function. It enhances mediator release in response to IgE-crosslinking, which is still the most potent triggering event. IgE-independent triggers (e.g. C5a or substance P) have been described for human skin mast cells but not for human mucosal mast cells[6,10,19,20]. Furthermore, we can define a particular set of lymphokines (IL-3, IL-5 and GM-SCF) which profoundly modulates human eosinophil function[21]. Finally, we can define several new agonists triggering eosinophils for mediator release (e.g. the anaphylatoxins C3a and C5a, eotaxin and other members of the CC-chemokine family, the bacterial product fMLP and PAF). It is tempting to speculate that such agonists play a crucial role in regulating human mast cell and eosinophil function. However, the clinical relevance of each of these mediators has to be defined in future studies.

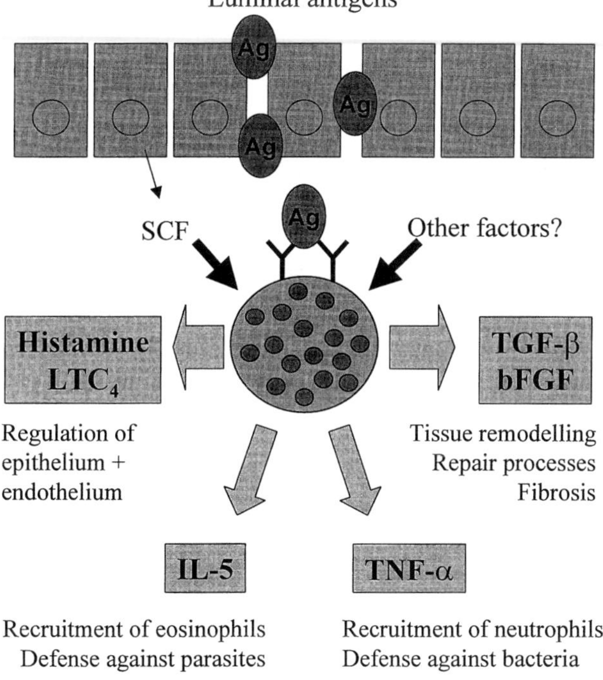

Figure 4 Immunoregulatory role of mast cells at the gastrointestinal barrier. For details and abbreviations: see text

CLINICAL IMPLICATIONS

The mechanisms of the mucosa-associated lymphoid system (MALT) are not yet fully understood. However, several studies indicate that a number of gastrointestinal diseases, including hypersensitivity reactions and inflammatory bowel disease, are based on alterations of the gut immune system, namely on the loss of immune tolerance[22–24]. Whereas lymphocytes and other cellular components of the gastrointestinal immune system have been characterized in detail in many studies, other cells, such as eosinophils and mast cells, which we found constitutively in the human gastrointestinal mucosa, have been studied rarely. Therefore, the clinical significance of these cell types in the gut is largely unclear. Eosinophils can be monitored by histological and immunohistological means, but also by measuring eosinophil-derived mediators, such as EDN or ECP, in serum and stool samples[13,18,25]. We were able to show that the faecal EDN levels are substantially elevated in patients with inflammatory bowel disease as well as in patients suffering from abdominal symptoms related to food allergy (Figure 5)[13]. Monitoring mast cell activation or accumulation in the intestinal tract is more complicated because mast cells cannot be readily detected in routine biopsy specimens since their staining properties are lost after formalin fixation[26]. Moreover,

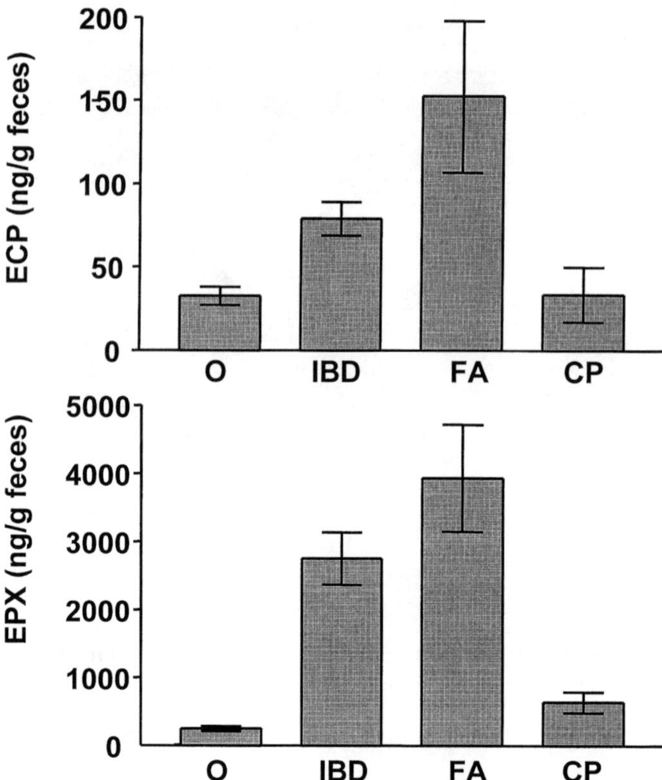

Figure 5 Eosinophil activation markers in stool samples. ECP, eosinophil cationic protein; EPX, eosinophil protein X (= eosinophil-derived neurotoxin); O, healthy control individuals; IBD, inflammatory bowel disease; FA, food allergy; CP, control patients with other gastrointestinal diseases. Data (mean ± SD) from Reference 13

mast cell mediators are either not stable enough or not sufficiently concentrated for measurement in stool samples[13].

Our data confirm previous studies suggesting that eosinophils are involved in a number of gastrointestinal diseases, including gastrointestinal allergy[14,27], inflammatory bowel disease[13,15,18,25,28] and eosinophilic enteritis[2–4]. Mast cells have been implicated in the same kind of diseases[1,5,10,14,17,28,29]. A number of studies indicate that mast cells and eosinophils are involved in allergic inflammation of the gut[1,7,14,27]. However, according to some recent findings, it is tempting to speculate that the mechanism of allergic inflammation, which is characterized by an infiltration and activation of mast cells, basophils, eosinophils and lymphocytes of the Th-2 type (Figure 6), may be of relevance also for other forms of chronic intestinal inflammation, such as ulcerative colitis[10,29,30], Crohn's disease[15,17,30], coeliac disease[16], eosinophil gastroenteritis, idiopathic diarrhoea[31], and possibly also for irritable bowel syndrome[32,33]. Therefore, allergic reactions should be considered in the differential diagnosis of such bowel diseases (Figure 7). On the other hand, the functions of mast cells and eosinophils may not be restricted to allergic reactions, as shown recently in the above-mentioned studies on the roles of mast cells and TNF-α in bacterial peritonitis[11], and the importance of eosinophils in intestinal parasitosis[2,4].

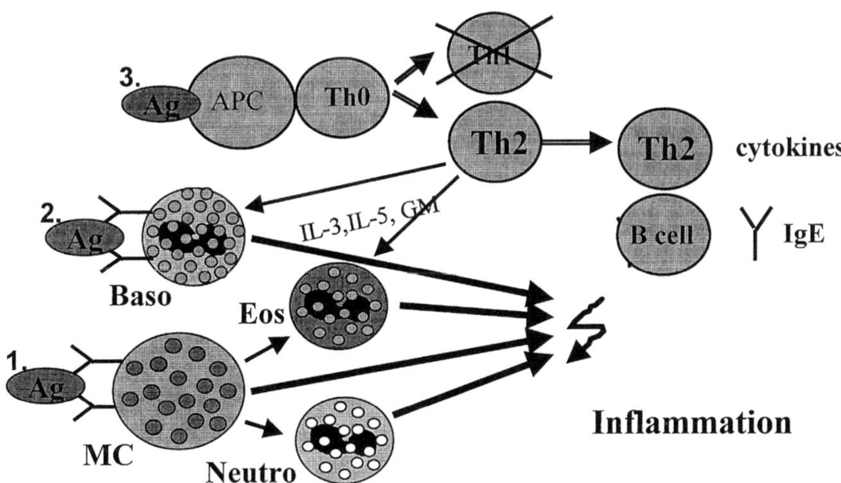

Figure 6 Pathogenesis of allergic inflammation – current concepts. For details and abbreviations: see text

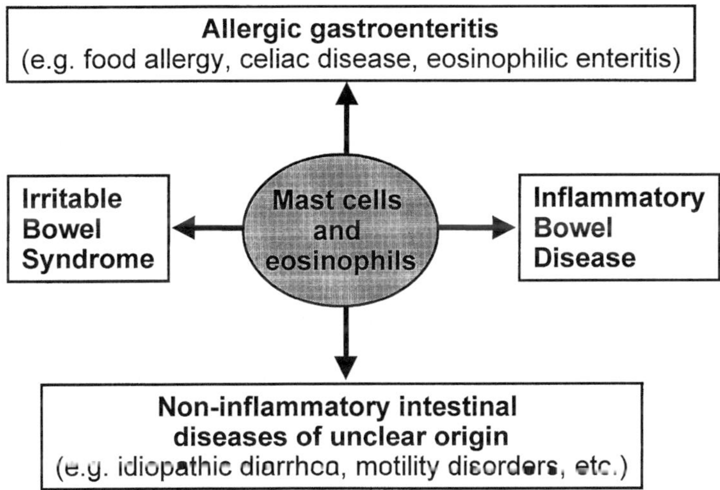

Figure 7 Gastrointestinal diseases associated with mast cells and eosinophils

References

1. Bischoff SC. Mucosal allergy: role of mast cells and eosinophil granulocytes in the gut. Baillieres Clin Gastroenterol. 1996;10:443–59.
2. Futura GT, Ackerman SJ, Wershil BK. The role of eosinophils in gastrointestinal disease. Curr Opin Gastroenterol. 1995;11:541–7.
3. Levy AM, Kita K. The eosinophil in gut inflammation: Effector or director? Gastroenterology. 1996;110:952–4.
4. Weller PF. The immunobiology of eosinophils. N Engl J Med. 1991;324:1110–18.
5. Wershil BK, Galli SJ. Gastrointestinal mast cells. New approaches for analyzing their function in vivo. Gastroenterol Clin N Am. 1991;20:613–27.
6. Befus AD, Dyck N, Goodacre R, Bienenstock J. Mast cells from the human intestinal lamina propria. Isolation, histochemical subtypes, and functional characterization. J Immunol. 1987;138:2604–10.
7. Bischoff SC, Wedemeyer J, Wagner S, Meier PN, Manns MP. Human mast cells and basophils: new concepts and their relevance for the gastrointestinal tract. Z Gastroenterol. 1994;32:64–70.
8. Bradding P, Okayama Y, Howarth PH, Church MK, Holgate ST. Heterogeneity of human mast cells based on cytokine content. J Immunol. 1995;155:297–307.
9. Church MK, Levi-Schaffer F. The human mast cell. J Allergy Clin Immunol. 1997;99:155–60.
10. Fox CC, Lazenby AJ, Moore WC, Yardley JH, Bayless TM, Lichtenstein LM. Enhancement of human intestinal mast cell mediator release in active ulcerative colitis. Gastroenterology. 1990;99:119–24.
11. Galli SJ, Wershil BK. The two faces of the mast cell. Nature. 1996;381:21–2.
12. Ishizaka T, Mitsui H, Yanagida M, Miura T, Dvorak AM. Development of human mast cells from their progenitors. Curr Opin Immunol. 1993;5:937–43.
13. Bischoff SC, Grabowsky J, Manns MP. Quantification of inflammatory mediators in stool samples of patients with inflammatory bowel disorders and controls. Dig Dis Sci. 1997;42:394–403.
14. Crowe SE, Perdue MH. Gastrointestinal food hypersensitivity: basic mechanisms of pathophysiology. Gastroenterology. 1992;103:1075–95.
15. Desreumaux P, Brandt E, Gambiez L et al. Distinct cytokine patterns in early and chronic ileal lesions of Crohn's disease. Gastroenterology. 1997;113:118–26.
16. Hed J. Coeliac disease: a food allergy? Monogr Allergy. 1996;32:204–10.
17. Knutson L, Ahrenstedt Ö, Odling B, Hällgren R. The jejunal secretion of histamine is increased in active Crohn's disease. Gastroenterology. 1990;98:849–54.
18. Levy AM, Gleich GJ, Sandborn WJ, Tremaine WJ, Steiner ML, Phillips SF. Increased eosinophil granule proteins in gut lavage fluid from patients with inflammatory bowel disease. Mayo Clin Proc. 1997;72:117–23.
19. Bischoff SC, Dahinden CA. C-kit ligand: a unique potentiator of mediator release by human mast cells. J Exp Med. 1992;175:237–44.
20. Bischoff SC, Schwengberg S, Raab R, Manns MP. Functional properties of human intestinal mast cells cultured in a new culture system. Enhancement of IgE receptor-dependent mediator release and response to stem cell factor. J Immunol. 1997;159:5560–7.
21. Takafuji S, Bischoff SC, de Weck AL, Dahinden CA. IL-3 and IL-5 prime normal human eosinophils to produce leukotriene C4 in response to soluble agonists. J Immunol. 1991;147:3855–61.
22. Brandtzaeg P. History of oral tolerance and mucosal immunity. Ann NY Acad Sci. 1996;778:1–27.
23. Romagnani S. Th1 and Th2 in human diseases. Clin Immunol Immunopathol. 1996;80:225–35.
24. Schreiber S, Raedler A, Stenson WF, Mac Dermott RP. The role of the mucosal immune system in inflammatory bowel disease. Gastroenterol Clin N Am. 1992;21:451–502.
25. Makiyama K, Kanzaki S, Yamasaki K, Zea-Iriarte W, Tsuji Y. Activation of eosinophils in the pathophysiology of ulcerative colitis. J Gastroenterol. 1995;30:64–90.
26. Strobel S, Miller HRP, Ferguson A. Human intestinal mucosal mast cells: evaluation of fixation and staining techniques. J Clin Pathol. 1981;34:851–8.
27. Bischoff SC, Mayer J, Wedemeyer J et al. Colonoscopic allergen provocation (COLAP): a new diagnostic approach for gastrointestinal food allergy. Gut. 1997;40:745–53.
28. Bischoff SC, Wedemeyer J, Herrmann A et al. Quantitative assessment of intestinal eosinophils and mast cells in inflammatory bowel disease. Histopathology. 1996;28:1–13.

29. King T, Biddle W, Bhatia P, Moore J, Miner PB. Colonic mucosal mast cell distribution at line demarcation of active ulcerative colitis. Dig Dis Sci. 1992;37:490–5.
30. Ballegaard M, Bjergstrom A, Bronndum S, Hylander E, Jensen L. Self-reported food intolerance in chronic inflammatory bowel disease. Scand J Gastroenterol. 1997;32:569–71.
31. Crowe SE, Luthra GK, Perdue MH. Mast cell mediated ion transport in intestine from patients with and without inflammatory bowel disease. Gut. 1997;41:785–92.
32. Jones VA, McLaughlan P, Shorthouse M, Workman E, Hunter JO. Food intolerance: a major factor in the pathogenesis of irritable bowel syndrome. Lancet. 1982;2:1115–17.
33. Zwetchkenbaum JF, Burakoff R. Food allergy and the irritable bowel syndrome. Am J Gastroenterol. 1988;83:901–4.

Section V
Epithelial Barrier in IBD

19
Role of epithelial cells in IBD

R. S. BLUMBERG

INTRODUCTION

The epithelial layer of the intestine, above the basal membrane (BM), consists predominantly of two cell types: intestinal epithelial cells (IEC) and intestinal intraepithelial lymphocytes (iIEL). It is thus appropriate in considering IEL biology relative to inflammatory bowel disease (IBD) to consider these cells as a functional unit (Figure 1). These two cell types are separated from the underlying lamina propria by the basal lamina, and probably function together in a variety of immune functions that regulate the integrity of mucosal barrier function and responses to luminal antigen.

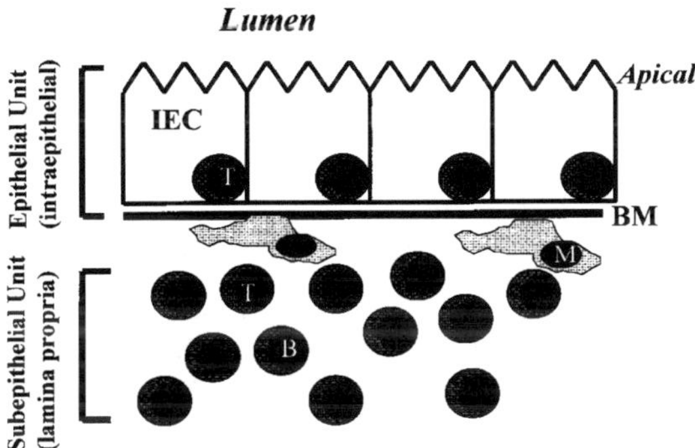

Figure 1 Structure of the epithelial unit: The normal human intestine has two anatomically and functionally distinct compartments that are separated from each other by the basement membrane (BM). Above the BM is the epithelial unit which consists of two cell types: the intestinal epithelial cell (IEC) and intraepithelial lymphocyte (iIEL), which is a unique T lymphocyte. Below the BM is the subepithelial unit, or lamina propria, which consists of a variety of cellular elements including macrophages (M), T lymphocytes (T), and B lymphocytes (B). Whereas the T cells in the lamina propria are memory cells involved in the production of cytokines, the B lymphocytes are skewed towards differentiation as IgA blasts for the production of dimeric IgA

iIEL are T lymphocytes with many characteristics distinguishing them from lamina propria T lymphocytes and peripheral blood T lymphocytes[1]. T lymphocytes recognize processed nominal antigens derived from the degradation of larger molecules in the context of a major histocompatibility complex (MHC) antigen on the cell surface of an antigen-presenting cell such as an IEC. The structure on the cell surface of the T cell responsible for this antigen recognition in the context of MHC is the T cell receptor (TCR) which, in the majority of cells, consists of a heterodimeric glycoprotein, $\alpha\beta$. A second type of TCR, the $\gamma\delta$-TCR, can also adorn T cells. Each T cell expresses a particular $\alpha\beta$ TCR in a clonal fashion. Since the TCR must recognize a large number of potential antigen/MHC combinations, the repertoire of TCR is potentially enormous ($\sim 10^{16}$). T cells are divided into two broad types: CD8+ T cells which recognize antigen in the context of MHC class I due to CD8–MHC class I interactions, and CD4+ T cells which recognize antigen in the context of MHC class I due to CD4–MHC class II interactions.

In humans, iIEL are predominantly TCR $\alpha\beta$+; however, TCR $\gamma\delta$+ cells are enriched compared to peripheral blood, although they still represent the minority. In the small bowel the vast majority of iIEL are CD8+ (Figure 2). In the large bowel, however, up to two-thirds of the TCR $\alpha\beta$+ cells may be either CD4+ or express the double negative phenotype (CD4– CD8–). iIEL are oligoclonal in that they express only a limited number of different TCR despite the abundance of different antigens present in the intestinal lumen[1–3]. iIEL remain in direct contact

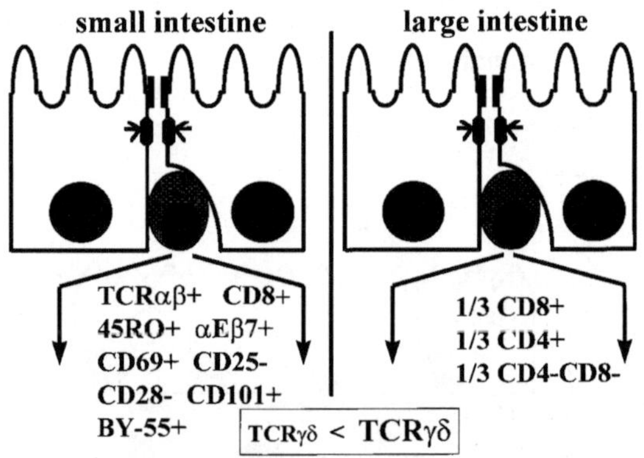

Figure 2 The intraepithelial lymphocyte: Intraepithelial lymphocytes (iIEL) are a unique group of T cells that reside along the basolateral surface of the IEC. The phenotype of these cells differs between the small intestine and large intestine. In the small intestine these cells are relatively homogeneous in that 95% of these cells are TCR-$\alpha\beta$+, CD8+, CD45RO+ (memory marker), αEβ7+ (ligand for E-cadherin on IEC), CD69+ (early T-cell activation antigen), CD25– (IL-2 receptor), CD28– (major co-stimulatory molecule that binds ligands on APC, such as CD80 and CD86), CD101+ (potential co-stimulatory molecule on iIEL), and BY-55+ (a novel, killer inhibitory receptor-like molecule). In the large intestine the vast majority of the iIEL are again TCR-$\alpha\beta$+. However, in the large intestine approximately one-third of iIEL are CD8+, one-third CD4+ and one-third double negative. Although TCR-$\gamma\delta$ iIEL are enriched in the epithelium, especially in the colon, they represent a minority of the lymphocytes. iIEL, both TCR-$\alpha\beta$+ and $\gamma\delta$+, express a limited number of TCR (i.e. oligoclonal). These phenotypic characteristics suggest that iIEL represent a memory population of lymphocytes that localize to the basolateral surface of the epithelium for the purposes of recognition of a limited number of antigens in the context of a MHC class I-like molecule

with the basolateral portion of the IEC and probably do not recirculate consistent with a role in local immunosurveillance of the epithelial cell surfaces (see below).

A major unifying hypothesis for IBD pathogenesis is that IBD represents a dysregulated mucosal immune response to antigens in a genetically susceptible host that is subject to modification by a variety of environmental factors. This subsequently leads to chronic inflammation, tissue injury and clinical symptoms. At the centre of this hypothesis is antigen. In IBD it continues to remain controversial as to whether the dysregulated response observed in this disease represents an appropriate response to a foreign antigen (i.e. an infection) or an inappropriate response to an innocuous antigen (i.e. normal intestinal flora or autoantigen). Nonetheless, it is clear that some component of the luminal milieu is the focus of the mucosal immune response. As such, the epithelial unit, as the first cellular elements to come in contact with luminal events, must be a major consideration in understanding IBD pathophysiology. Similarly, antigen and the immune response to antigen must also be considered as a central focus.

The immune response fundamentally functions in the recognition of foreign antigen. Confronted with antigen that is perceived as foreign, the first series of immune responses that are initiated are those related to the innate immune system. The innate immune responses is a 'hard-wired' system that is mobilized immediately and consists of soluble (e.g. complement, kinin system) and cellular (e.g. neutrophils and natural killer cells) elements. The second and more enduring events associated with the immune response are those related to cognate (or antigen-specific) immune events. This response is often called adaptive or acquired immunity, which has three phases (initiation, recruitment and amplification). The adaptive response is initiated by recognition of antigen presented by an antigen-presenting cell (APC) to a T cell which subsequently leads to activation of both cell types as manifest by the secretion of cytokines and new membrane receptors. This is associated with recruitment of new cell types including those associated with the innate immune response, which amplify the immune response through the secretion of additional soluble mediators (e.g. cytokines, chemokines, inflammatory mediators). The adaptive immune response is characterized by memory and down-regulation unless antigen is not removed and/or dysregulation occurs. Needless to say, the epithelial unit, as a novel APC–T cell pair, may function in innate and adaptive responses to antigen which contribute significantly to IBD pathogenesis.

IEC form a continuous monolayer, that separates the outside world from the human body. Some IEC, M cells, are specialized to express a unique microvillus fold structure for the purposes of sampling antigen, especially particulate antigen. However, the vast majority of iIEL represent the absorptive enterocyte which has four main groups of functions relevant to IBD pathogenesis. These are their barrier, transport, immunosurveillance and immunoregulation functions as discussed in more detail below (Figure 3).

BARRIER FUNCTION

The barrier formed by the IEC consists of the cells themselves, of the tight junctions sealing the spaces between the cells (tight junction and desmosomes) and

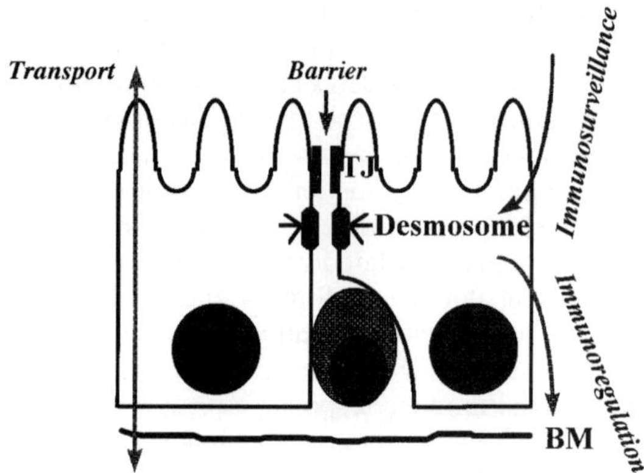

Figure 3 Functions of the epithelial unit: The epithelial unit has four major functions: transport function, barrier function, immunoregulation function and immunosurveillance function. TJ, tight junction; BM, basement membrane

of the mucus and soluble molecules (intestinal trefoil factor, complement and cryptins) secreted by them (Figure 4)[4]. This provides a passive means to exclude most macromolecules, including bacteria and antigens, from entering the body (no leak in) and at the same time minimizing fluid and electrolyte loss into the intestinal lumen (no leak out). The epithelium is also actively involved in maintaining homeostasis by virtue of regulation of fluid and electrolyte absorption and absorption of nutrients. This barrier function is regulated by complex interactions with the endocrine and the nervous system as well as by local, immunologically active cells and by locally secreted mediators that function in a paracrine manner[5,6]. For example human IEC growth[7] and barrier function[8] can be modulated by mucosa-derived lymphocytes through interleukin 4 (IL-4) and interferon-γ (IFN-γ) secreted by lymphocytes[9].

The intestine is exposed to a variety of foreign antigens, particularly microorganisms such as bacteria and their products, particularly in the colon, and

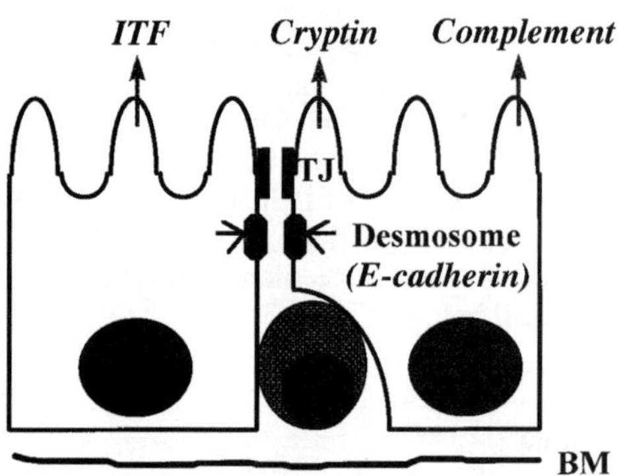

Figure 4 Role of epithelial unit in barrier function: For an explanation of this figure, see the text. The approximate locations of the tight junction (TJ) and desmosome are indicated

food-derived antigens. Therefore, the intestine has to be considered as an external body surface. One way to prevent these antigens from entering the body is to form a non-specific barrier. In the intestine this barrier consists of the IEC monolayer[4], sealed by tight junctions, and of the mucus secreted by IEC, with the main components, mucin glycoproteins, being well characterized[10]. This barrier function can be modulated by T cells and cytokines as briefly mentioned above[8,9]. Direct disruption of this barrier by inhibiting desmosome function through disruption of E-cadherin, for example, leads to an IBD-like illness in mice[11]. A non-specific defence mechanism consists of secreted intestinal trefoil factor (ITF), one of the three known mammalian trefoil peptides[12]. ITF is secreted into the mucus by IEC and is relatively resistant against protease digestion, probably due to its compact structure with three disulphide bonds. In *in-vitro* model systems ITF increases the migration of IEC towards a lesion, implicating an important role in wound healing. Furthermore, in animal models and in monolayers of IEC lines, ITF has a preventive protective effect against injury due to pharmacological challenges (ethanol, indomethacin) and exposure to *Clostridium difficile* toxin A. In addition, an IBD-like process can develop in mice deficient in ITF[13]. It is likely, therefore, that ITF plays a role in maintaining intestinal mucosal integrity by providing innate resistance to mucosal injury.

IEC also secrete soluble components of the innate immune response that potentially may directly neutralize and/or inactivate microorganisms and their noxious products and must be considered a part of the barrier function of IEL. These include complement components and cryptdins. Caco2, a human IEC cancer cell line, for example, secretes complement components, including C3, C4 and factor B[14]. Furthermore, complement secretion can be up-regulated in this model system by IL-1α, IL-6, tumour necrosis factor-α (TNF-α) and INF-γ. Paneth cells in the small intestine, a subtype of IEC, secrete at least two different cryptdins, a group of defensins that are antimicrobial[15–17].

TRANSPORT FUNCTIONS

The transport function of IEC in the context of mucosal immune function is related to the manner in which the IEC directly and indirectly transports luminal antigen. Athough less well characterized than that associated with the specialized M cell, there is a great deal of evidence in support of a direct role of the IEC in antigen transport. Three types of direct antigen transport by the IEC have been suggested: a cellular pathway which embodies the concept of antigen uptake, processing and presentation of antigen from the lumen to local T cells (see below in discussion on immunosurveillance)[18], the paracellular pathway which reflects the uptake of antigen through tight junctions and a transcellular pathway which directs luminal antigen directly across the IEC into the lamina propria unperturbed. The transcellular pathway is, in part, antigen-non-specific, which relates to fluid-phase endocytosis[19]. In addition, the transcellular pathway reflects a transcytotic pathway which may be antigen-specific by virtue of antigen binding to antibody (either IgA, IgM or IgG) which binds to antibody receptors involved in transcytosis (Figure 5). These include the polymeric immunoglobulin receptor (pIgR) and neonatal Fc receptor for IgG (FcRn). The

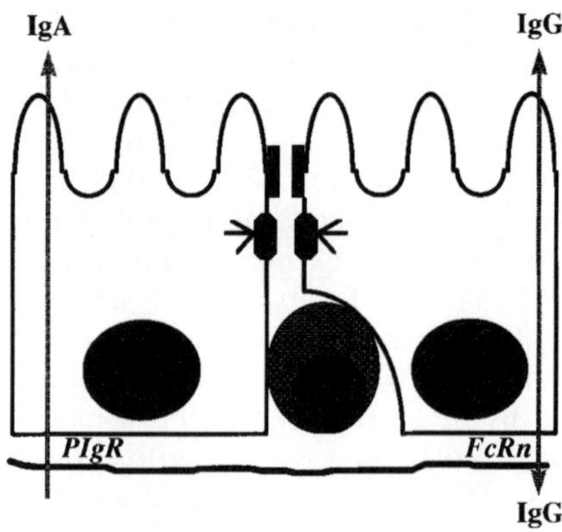

Figure 5 Transport functions of the epithelial unit: In addition to non-specific fluid-phase transport of antigens across the epithelial cell, two receptor-specific pathways exist in the epithelial cell related to the polymeric Ig receptor (PIgR) involved in the unidirectional transport of IgA from the basolateral to apical cell surface of the epithelium and processes related to the neonatal Fc receptor (FcRn) which is an MHC class I-like molecule involved in the bi-directional transport of IgG across the epithelial cell

transport of polymeric IgA and IgM represents a specific line of defence and means of antigen transport which is an end-product of the specific (or adaptive) immune response. The primary secretory immunoglobulin in the intestine is IgA. IgA is present as a monomer in the peripheral blood but predominantly as a homodimer in the intestine and intestinal lumen. IgA is synthesized by plasma cells within the lamina propria, below the epithelial layer. IEC express receptors for polymeric IgA (pIgR) on their basolateral surface which facilitate the uptake and transcellular transport of dimeric IgA (dIgA) to the apical surface of the IEC. A portion of the PIgR includes the secretory component which becomes associated with the apically secreted dIgA through a proteolytic cleavage event. The secreted product is known as secretory IgA[20,21]. Cytokines that up-regulate the receptor for polymeric IgA and its mRNA *in vitro* are INF-γ, TNF-α, IL-4[22,23] and, at least in rat epithelial cells, transforming growth factor-β (TGF-β)[24]. This receptor is also up-regulated in *in-vitro* cell culture systems by butyrate[25], a bacterial product. *In vivo* there is strong expression of this receptor in inflammatory conditions of the gut[26]. PIgR transport of polymeric IgA and Ig is unidirectional (basolateral or abluminal to apical or luminal).

Adult human IEC express a Fc receptor for monomeric IgG: the MHC class I-like neonatal Fc receptor (FcRn). The FcRn is considered an MHC class Ib molecule. Such molecules are classified as either gene products which are encoded within the classical MHC class I locus (HLA-A, B, C) on chromosome 6 and include HLA-E, F, G. H (*Hfe* gene associated with haemochromatosis) and the MHC class I chain-related gene A (MICA; see below) or gene products which are encoded outside the MHC class locus and include FcRn, the zinc-α2-glycoprotein, the MR1 gene, CD1 (see below) and an activated protein-C receptor[27] (Figure 6). These MHC class Ib molecules characteristically have MHC class I-like exon–intron structure, a functional relationship with β2m with some exceptions[27], a restricted cellular and tissue distribution unlike the ubiquitously expressed class-

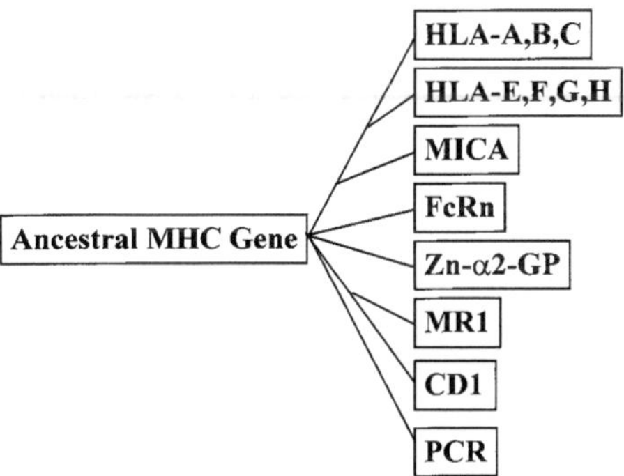

Figure 6 Summary of MHC-related molecules: The classical MHC class I molecules consist of the HLA-A, B and C genes encoded on chromosome 6 within the MHC locus. The human host also contains a large number of MHC class I-related genes[27]. These genes, often called MHC class Ib genes, consist of two types: those that are linked to the MHC locus on chromosome 6 (HLA-E, F, G, H and the MHC class I chain-related gene A [MICA]) and those that are encoded outside the MHC locus. These latter include the neonatal Fc receptor for IgG transport (FcRn), a circulating serum protein of unknown function called the zinc-α2-glycoprotein, the MR1 gene, the CD1 gene family (CD1-A, B, C, D and E) and activated protein C receptor expressed by endothelium (PCR)

ical class I (HLA-A, B, C), limited allelism (or non-polymorphic) and have distinct immunological functions through binding specific, evolutionarily conserved, ligands.

The FcRn was previously believed to be expressed in the intestine only during neonatal life, but has recently been shown to be expressed in adult life[28], including adult human IEC[29]. The receptor is functionally intact, binds human IgG at pH 6 but not at pH 8 and is responsible for the bidirectional transport of IgG across model IEC monolayers (ref. 30, and unpublished data). The same molecule is considered important in transporting maternal IgG in the newborn through the intestinal epithelial layer and, as a corollary, *in utero* through the placental layers. In adults it is possible that these Fc receptors could play a role in sampling immune complexes composed of IgG and foreign antigens, and transferring them into the lamina propria where they could be taken up and further processed by professional APC such as macrophages within the lamina propria. The relevance of this to IBD is unknown, but it is clear that IgG levels are markedly up-regulated[31].

IMMUNOREGULATORY FUNCTIONS IN INNATE AND ACQUIRED IMMUNITY

Although the biological function of the IEC–iIEL unit is presently unknown, it is likely that these cells participate together in regulating mucosal integrity, epithelial cell growth and renewal and, possibly, regulation of immune responses including those related to the development of local suppression of responses to luminal antigen. Moreover, a unique group of macromolecular interactions may be involved in these processes (Figure 7). IEC express E-cadherin that may

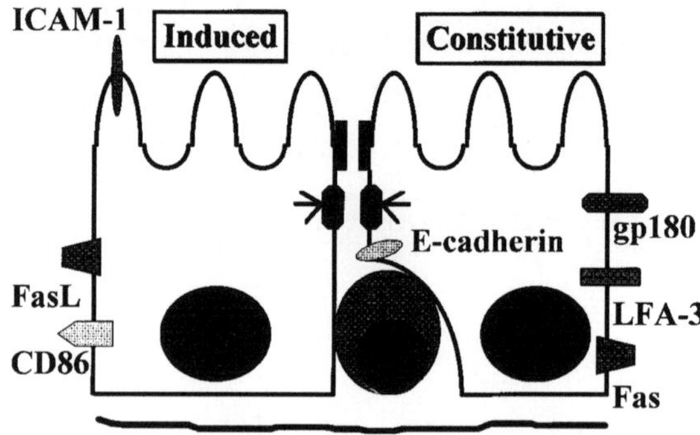

Figure 7 Immunoregulatory functions of IEC related to potential T-cell interactions: Molecules potentially involved in immunoregulatory functions are indicated as either those that are constitutively expressed by the IEC or those whose expression is induced

be involved, together with the integrin $\alpha E\beta 7$[32] to localize iIEL to the basolateral surface of the intestinal epithelium[33]. Intestinal epithelial cancer cell lines also bind iIEL via an $\alpha E\beta 7$-dependent mechanism as defined by the inhibition of this binding by the antibody HML-1, which recognizes $\alpha E\beta 7$[34]. E-cadherin–$\alpha E\beta 7$ interactions probably provide not only important adhesive functions for IEC–iIEL interactions but also probably provide important regulatory intracellular signals. $\alpha E\beta 7$ ligation on iIEL can modulate anti-CD3-mediated signals[35]. Moreover, E-cadherin ligation by $\alpha E\beta 7$ on iIEL may theoretically modulate epithelial cell growth[36] since E-cadherin binds catenins which also internet with products of the APC gene, a tumour suppressor gene[37]. In some circumstances IEC can also express intercellular adhesion molecule-1 (ICAM-1) and lymphocyte function-associated antigen 3 (LFA-3; CD58)[38], which may play important functions in adhesion and activation of leukocytes, including T cells, to IEC. Interestingly, ICAM-1, an immunoglobulin supergene family member which functions as a ligand for the $\beta 2$-integrin, $\alpha\Lambda\beta 7$ (LFA-1), is regulated in IBD and restricted to the apical surface of the IEC when expressed[39]. This suggests that the IEC may actively segregate particular immune adhesion molecules to specific membrane domains of the cell, creating distinct subcellular functional compartments. This may function to restrict these molecules to a desirable location for leukocyte interactions.

IEC seem to preferentially stimulate proliferation of CD8+ T cells[40] (see below). All the evidence to date suggests that the stimulatory CD8+ T cell ligand is neither a classical MHC class I nor class II antigen despite expression of both on the IEC surface. It has been hypothesized that this may be related to a pathway that generates local immunosuppression, since these stimulated T cells exhibit suppressor activity[41]. The stimulatory signal appears to consist of a 180 kDa glycoprotein (gp 180), perhaps in association with CD1d (see below). gp180 is a CD66e-like molecule which is expressed on normal IEC, binds CD8 and activates the CD8-associated tyrosine kinase p56lck[42,43]. gp180 is down-regulated in IBD, suggesting that diminished activation of CD8+ lymphocytes may occur under this circumstance[44].

The Fas (CD95) and Fas-ligand (FasL; CD95L) system is of particular potential relevance to IBD. Ligation of Fas by FasL, usually expressed by an activated T cell, leads to death by apoptosis of the Fas-bearing target such as an IEC[45]. Recent evidence suggests that the Fas–FasL system may be activated in IBD resulting in IEC destruction and theoretically further compromise of the epithelial barrier[46]. On the other hand, IEC cancers, such as occur in IBD, may be associated with FasL expression by the IEC, leading to a Fas counterattack on the lymphocyte[47].

Full activation of a T cell requires two signals: an antigen-specific (cognate) signal delivered to the TCR by the MHC molecule on the APC and a second antigen-independent (non-cognate) signal delivered by a co-stimulatory molecule on the APC. Major co-stimulatory molecules for T cells are the B7.1 (CD80) and B7.2 (CD86) molecules which bind to activate CD28 on the T cell. Although resting IEC are CD80/CD86 negative, studies with gastric epithelial cells suggest that inflammatory conditions can induce CD80/CD86[48]. Since most CD8+ iIEL are CD28–, this is most relevant to CD4+ iIEL which are most prominent in the colon. Whether this occurs in IBD is unknown.

It is also likely that IEC down-regulate the function of T cells. Supernatant from crude intestinal mucosa inhibits CD3-mediated proliferation of T lymphocytes *in vitro*[49–51]. It has also been shown that a soluble, inhibitory factor is produced by various intestinal epithelial cell lines such as HT29[52,53], T84 and Caco2, but not by a non-epithelial cell line, HL-60[54]. This factor only inhibits CD3-mediated proliferation of T lymphocytes, whereas the response to CD2-mediated signals is preserved[54]. In rats, a factor derived from epithelial cells that inhibits proliferation of T cells after concanavalin A stimulation has been described[55]. In summary, there are probably factor(s) produced by IEC that help minimize the response of T lymphocyte to antigen-mediated activation. Together with the tendency of IEC to stimulate CD8+ T cells, this may restrain local immune activation to the luminal antigenic milieu.

In addition to these soluble mediators described above, IEC are also capable of secreting cytokines[56] and, in turn, express cytokine receptors (Figure 8). Human IEC lines constitutively express IL-8 and TGF-β[57]. Best examined is the regulation of IL-8 production. IL-8 production by IEC lines is stimulated by various proinflammatory cytokines such as TNF-α, IL-1α and IFN-γ[58]. The effect of IFN-γ is further enhanced by co-stimulation with epidermal growth factor (EGF). The effect of bacterial lipopolysaccharide (LPS) on IL-8 production by IEC lines is cell line dependent. IL-8 production by Caco-2 cells and T84 cells seems not to be stimulated by LPS[57,59]. Other IEC lines, such as SW620 and to a lesser extent HT29, can be stimulated to secrete IL-8 by LPS[58]. mRNA for IL-8 is up-regulated within 90 min after bacterial infection of an IEC line (T84), a cervical epithelial cell line (HeLa) and a fibroblast cell line (WI-38)[59]. Infection of IEC lines with invasive bacteria, but not with non-invasive bacteria, up-regulates several other proinflammatory cytokines beside IL-8, including monocyte chemotactic protein 1, granulocyte macrophage colony stimulating factor (GM-CSF) and TNF-α[60,61]. The same four cytokines, as well as IL-6 and IL-7, were also found in freshly isolated human IEC[57,60] or by immunohistochemistry and *in-situ* hybridization of intestinal mucosa[62], making it likely that they are playing a role *in vivo*. IL-6 production by human

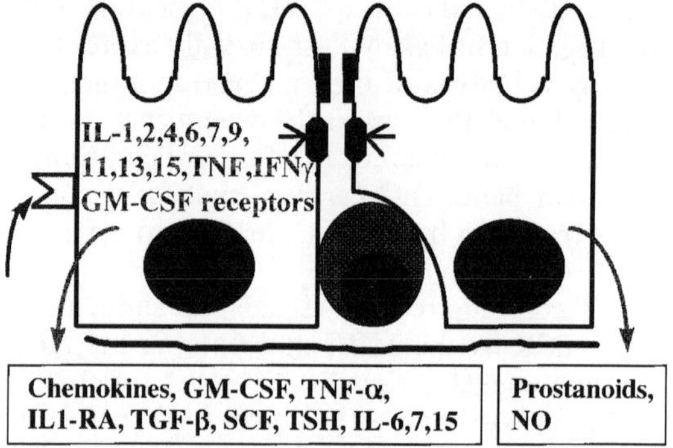

Figure 8 Immunoregulatory functions of IEC related to soluble mediators and their receptors: An ever-growing number of cytokines, growth factors and receptors for these molecules are being identified in IEC. TNF (tumour necrosis factor), IFN-γ (interferon-γ), GM-CSF (granulocyte macrophage-colony stimulating factor), IL-1-RA (IL-1-receptor antagonist), TGF-β (transforming growth factor-β), SCF (stem cell factor), TSH (thyroid-stimulating hormone), NO (nitrous oxide)

IEC is up-regulated by IL-1α[63]. Rat IEC can produce IL-6 after stimulation by TGF-β[64], prostaglandin E2 (PGE2), lipopolysaccharide[65] and cholera toxin alone or together with IL-1α and TNF-α[66]. TGF-β and PGE2 (see below) are particularly interesting in that it is known that human and rat IEC lines can produce TGFβ and PGE2, suggesting an autocrine regulation of IL-6 production by these mediators[67–69]. TGF-β itself can be up-regulated by IL-2. Freshly isolated human IEC and a human intestinal cancer cell line (Caco2) produce constitutively monocyte-chemoattractant protein 1 (MCP-1)[70]. *In vitro*, mRNA for MCP-1 can be up-regulated by IL-1α and down-regulated by steroids. These observations on IEC cytokine secretion lead to the concept of epithelial cells regulating mucosal response to antigen and antibody production (e.g. TGF-β and IL-6 production) and in the recruitment of leukocytes (e.g. IL-8 and MCP-1 production). The latter suggests IEC may act as 'watchdogs' for adverse events within the mucosa[71]. As described below, there is also evidence for monitoring of events by IEC within the intestinal lumen.

Freshly isolated human IEC, as well as stimulated IEC lines, express mRNA for the common γ chain of the IL-2 receptor and the specific IL-2 receptor, IL-4 receptor, IL-7 receptor and IL-9 receptor chains as determined by polymerase chain reaction[72]. The IL-2 and IL-15 receptors expressed in human IEC are functional[73]. Furthermore, rat IEC express functional IL-1 receptor, the homologue to the human type I IL-1 receptor, but not IL-1 type II receptors[74,75]. IEC are also able to synthesize prostanoids which, in turn, regulate immune functions. Cultured rabbit colonic IEC constitutively express PGE2, 6-keto-prostaglandin F1α (6-keto PGF1α), the stable metabolite of prostacyclin, thromboxane B2, prostaglandin D2 and prostaglandin F2α[76]. The expression of PGE2 can be up-regulated by bradykinin[77], and down-regulated by indomethacin and 5-aminosalicylic acid[76]. In a rat IEC line, IL-1α and TGF-β have been shown to up-regulate synthesis of prostacyclin[78]. PGE2 is particularly interesting in that it has direct effects on intestinal mononuclear cells and, indirectly, on IEC. PGE2 reduces IL-3 secretion by lamina propria mononuclear cells, inhibits the effect of T cells on the IEC barrier function and reduces IL-2 and IL-3 secretion by activated intestinal T cells lines[79].

IMMUNOSURVEILLANCE FUNCTIONS (FIGURE 9)

There is increasing evidence that IEC can function as non-professional antigen-presenting cells[80]. Similar to the vast majority of cells in the body, IEC express classical MHC class I molecules (HLA-A, B, C). MHC class I molecules function in the presentation of nine amino acid peptides to CD8+ T cells. These peptides are derived from the degradation of intracellular (cytoplasmic) proteins which are transported by the transporter associated with antigen presentation (TAP) to the MHC class I/β_2-microglobulin heterodimer in the endoplasmic reticulum. As a result, MHC class I molecules sample the intracellular environment and, as such, CD8-bearing lymphocytes are concerned with monitoring the intracellular health of a cell such as a virally infected or a transformed IEC. Interestingly, IEC also express MHC class II, as shown in several species[81–83]. MHC class II expression can be up-regulated by activated iIEL through IFN-γ[40,84,85]. In addition, IEC express non-classical MHC class I (class Ib or class I-like) molecules such as CD1d[86,87] and MHC chain-related gene products in humans[88] and CD1[89] and the thymus leukaemia antigen (TL) in mouse[90] (see Figure 6).

MHC class II molecules present 14–18 amino acid peptides to CD4-bearing lymphocytes. These peptides are acquired from the processing of extracellular proteins obtained by the APC through fluid phase and receptor-mediated endocytosis. As such, CD4-bearing lymphocytes are concerned with monitoring abnormal extracellular antigen exposures. MHC class II molecules expressed by IEC are functional, suggesting that CD4+ iIEL, which are prominent in the colon, may be regulated by luminal antigen. For example, mouse enterocytes can present soluble antigens *in vitro* to CD4+ T cells, and this presentation can be inhibited by anti-class II antibodies[82]. In a human *in-vitro* model an intestinal epithelial cell line

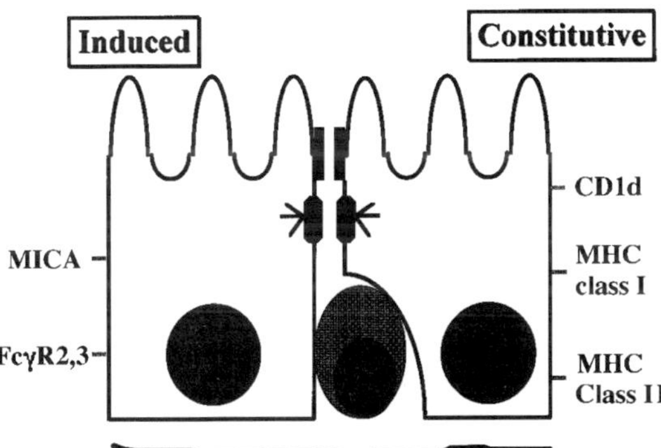

Figure 9 Immunosurveillance functions of IEC: A variety of molecules that are expressed by IEC either constitutively or upon induction are indicated and discussed in the text

that expresses MHC class II after induction with IFN-γ stimulates iIEL in an allogeneic system[40]. Antibody inhibition experiments confirmed that this stimulation was MHC class II-mediated, despite the fact that the iIEL preparations used consisted of 90% CD8+ T cells. In this model system colonic iIEL were used, making it likely that this proliferation reflected the CD4+ colonic iIEL which are uncommon in small intestine[91]. As shown in an *in-vitro* model, rat IEC are able to present antigen to T cells[18]. Rat IEC are able to induce proliferation of T cells in a mixed lymphocyte reaction (MLR), but only when co-incubated with either macrophages or supernatant from stimulated macrophages[92], suggesting the absence of important co-stimulatory factors on rat IEC. Recent studies in T84 model systems suggest MHC class II presentation by IEC is polarized with uptake occurring apically and basolaterally, but presentation occurring only basolaterally[93].

One of the MHC class I-like molecules that is expressed in the human intestine is CD1d[86,87,94]. Although CD1d is expressed on the cell surface in association with β2m, similar to classical MHC class I, it may also be expressed on the cell surface of certain cell types in the absence of β2m. This appears to be the case for IEC which express β2m-associated and unassociated forms of CD1d (ref. 95, and unpublished data). A functional role for β2m-unassociated CD1d is unknown. It is possible that mouse CD1, which is the homologue of human CD1d, can be expressed only in co-association with β2m[96]. However, this again may depend on the cell type. In mouse model systems, β2m-associated CD1 appears to be a ligand for a subset of, so-called, natural or NK1.1+ T cells. These cells, when ligated by CD1d, secrete IL-4 and IFN-γ, which presumably plays a role in T cell differentiation[97]. NK1.1+ T cells are not present in mouse epithelium, and human iIEL from small intestine are CD16, CD56 and CD32 negative[98], making it unlikely that this specific type of regulatory pathway exists in human small intestine. Nonetheless, the importance of CD1d on IEC as a ligand for iIEL is strengthened by the fact that CD1d is recognized by iIEL *in vitro*, and CD1d on IEC is recognized by peripheral blood T cells (refs 99 and 100, and unpublished data). This suggests that a unique pathway of CD1d-mediated immunoregulation probably exists in the epithelial unit.

Recently, the human CD1 group has been shown to present lipid antigens from bacteria and mycobacteria[101], and the murine homologue of CD1 has been shown to present large (20–22 amino acids) peptides with hydrophobic amino acids and lipids in a presentable pathway distinct from MHC class I and class II[102,103]. These observations on potential CD1 antigen presentation are intriguing given the known importance of luminal bacteria in IBD pathogenesis and the obvious close proximity of the epithelial unit to luminal bacteria. This raises the fascinating possibility that IEC sample luminal bacterial antigens and present it through CD1d, which in turn functions in the development and/or activation of iIEL and the intestinal milieu.

Another MHC class Ib molecule, MICA, functions in another type of immunosurveillance. Based upon studies with *in-vitro* model systems, this molecule would appear to be induced on the cell surface of stressed IEC as a β2m-independent glycoprotein, whereupon it activates the cytolytic activity of the resident T cells expressing $\gamma\delta$-TCR[88,104]. Consistent with this hypothesis, the MICA gene contains heat-shock elements in its promoter. Whether this event occurs in IBD needs to be determined.

Finally, human IEC also express Fc receptors for IgG. Human rectal IEC have been shown to be induced to express all three isotypes of FcγR II (CD32) and FcγR III (CD64) as shown by PCR, *in-situ* hybridization and immunohistology[105]. Such receptors function in receptor-mediated endocytosis which direct antigen to an MHC class II pathway.

FUNCTIONAL RELATIONSHIP BETWEEN IEC AND iIEL IN IBD

Under normal (healthy) conditions, the epithelial unit is concerned with maintenance of barrier function and the regulation of responses to the normal luminal milieu. As such, a dialogue occurs between the IEC and iIEL that is communicated by cell surface interactions and soluble mediators. For example, as shown in Figure 10, $\gamma\delta$ iIEL secrete keratinocyte growth factor (KGF) which regulates IEC turnover and the IEC secretes soluble mediators such as TGF-β, IL-7 and IL-15, which regulate iIEL growth and differentiation. Under pathological circumstances, as may occur in IBD, a transition occurs in which activation of the IEC and iIEL is evident with expression of a new set of cytokines and membrane receptors. This includes, for example, chemokine production by IEC and IL-2 production of IFN-γ (involved in IEC activation), and granule proteins involved in IEC lysis (granzyme and perforin). Whether this state of activation emanates directly from IEC alterations and/or the presence of pathological luminal antigens is unknown. Regardless, this pathological state is associated with disruption of the barrier and further amplification of the injury. Although the pathological model emphasizes cellular activation, it is clear that mechanisms are also probably stimulated that represent attempts of epithelial restitution and down-regulation of the immune response relating to iIEL activation[106]. Ultimately, however, in IBD these reparative and down-regulatory pathways are only temporary measures, as cycles of relapse mark the natural history of this enigmatic condition.

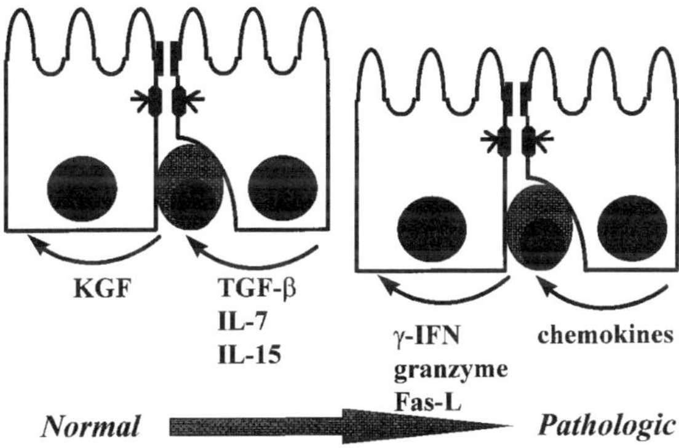

Figure 10 Relationship between IEC and iIEL in pathological conditions: For explanation of this figure, please see text. KGF (keratocyte growth factor), TGF-β (tumour growth factor-β), γ-IFN (γ-interferon), Fas-L (Fas ligand)

References

1. Blumberg RS, Stenson WF. The immune system. In: Yamada T, editor. Textbook of Gastroenterology. Philadelphia PA: JB Lippincott; 1995:111–40.
2. Blumberg RS, Yockey CE, Gross GG, Ebert EC, Balk SP. Human intestinal intraepithelial lymphocytes are derived from a limited number of T cell clones that utilize multiple $V\beta$ T cell receptor genes. J Immunol. 1993;150:5144–51.
3. Van Kerckhove C, Russel GJ, Deusch K *et al.* Oligoclonality of human intestinal intraepithelial T cells. J. Exp Med. 1992;175:57–63.
4. Madara JL. Epithelia: biologic principles of organization. In: Yamada T, editor. Textbook of Gastroenterology. Philadelphia, PA: JB Lippincott; 1995:141–57.
5. McKay DM, Perdue MH. Intestinal epithelial function: the case for immunophysiological regulation. Cells and mediators (1). Dig Dis Sci. 1993;38:1377–87.
6. McKay DM, Perdue MH. Intestinal epithelial function: the case for immunophysiological regulation. Implications for disease (2). Dig Dis Sci. 1993;38:1735–47.
7. Boismenu R, Havran WL. Modulation of epithelial cell growth by intraepithelial $\gamma\delta$ T cells. Science. 1994;266:1253–5.
8. Kaoutzani P, Colgan SP, Cepek KL *et al.* Reconstitution of cultured intestinal epithelial monolayers with a mucosal-derived T lymphocyte cell line. J Clin Invest. 1994;94:788–96.
9. Colgan SP, Resnick MB, Parkos CA *et al.* IL-4 directly modulated function of a model human intestinal epithelium. J Immunol. 1994;153:2122–9.
10. Allen C, Bell A, Mantle M, Pearson JP. The structure and physiology of gastrointestinal mucus. Adv Exp Med Biol. 1982;144:115–33.
11. Hermiston ML, Gordon JI. Inflammatory bowel disease and adenomas in mice expressing a dominant negative N-cadherin. Science. 1995;270:1203–7.
12. Podolsky DK, Kindon H, Lynch-Devaney K, Dignass A, Babyatsky M. Epithelium in inflammatory bowel disease: trefoil peptides at the interface. In: Tytgat GNJ, Bartelsman JFWM, van Deventer SJH, editors. Falk Symposium 85. Inflammatory Bowel Disease. Dordrecht; Kluwer; 1995:360–5.
13. Mashimo H, Wu DC, Podolsky DK, Fishman MC. Impaired defense of intestinal mucosa in mice lacking intestinal trefoil factor. Science. 1996;174:262–5.
14. Andoh A, Fujiama Y, Bamba T, Hosoda S. Differential cytokine regulation of complement C3, C4 and factor B synthesis in human intestinal epithelial cell line, Caco-2. J Immunol. 1993;151:4239–47.
15. Ouellette AJ, Greco RM, James M, Frederick D, Naftilan J, Fallon JT. Developmental regulation of cryptdin, a corticostatin/defensin precursor mRNA in mouse small intestinal crypt epithelium. J Cell Biol. 1989;108:1687–95.
16. Harwig SS, Eisenhauer PB, Chen NP, Lehrer RI. Cryptdins: endogenous antibiotic peptides of small intestinal Panteh cells. Adv Exp Med Biol. 1995;371A:251–5.
17. Eisenhauer PB, Harwig SS, Lehrer RI. Cryptdins: antimicrobial defensins of the murine small intestine. Infect Immun. 1992;60:3356–65.
18. Brandeis JM, Sayegh M, Gollan L, Blumberg RS, Carpenter CB. Rat intestinal epithelial cells present MHC allopeptides to primed T cells. Gastroenterology. 1994;197:1537–42.
19. Heyman M, Desjeux J-F. Antigen handling by intestinal epithelial cells. In Kaiserlian D, editor. Antigen Presentation by Intestinal Epithelial Cells. Austin, TX: Springer; 1996:1–19.
20. Casanova JE. Structure and function of the polymeric immunoglobulin receptor in epithelial cells. In: Kagnoff MF, Kiyono H, editors, Essential of Mucosal Immunology. San Diego, CA. Academic Press; 1996:201–14.
21. Mestecky J, Lue C, Russell MW. Selective transport of IgA. Cellular and molecular aspects. Gastroenterol Clin N Am. 1991;20:441–71.
22. Youngman KR, Fiocchi C, Kaetzel CS. Inhibition of IFN-gamma activity in supernatants from stimulated human intestinal mononuclear cells prevents up-regulation of the polymeric Ig receptor in an intestinal epithelial cell line. J Immunol. 1994;153:675–81.
23. Piskurich JF, France JA, Tamer CM, Willmer CA, Kaetzel CS, Kaetzel DM. Interferon-gamma induces polymeric immunoglobulin receptor mRNA in human intestinal epithelial cells by a protein synthesis dependent mechanism. Mol Immunol. 1993;30:413–21.
24. McGee DW, Aicher WK, Eldridge JH, Peppard JV, Mestecky J, McGhee JR. Transforming growth factor-beta enhances secretory component and major histocompatibility complex class I antigen expression on rat IEC-6 intestinal epithelial cells. Cytokine. 1991;3:543–50.

25. Kvale D, Brandtzaeg P. Constitutive and cytokine induced expression of HLA molecules, secretory component, and intercellular adhesion molecule-1 is modulated by butyrate in the colonic epithelial cell line HT-29. Gut. 1995;36:737–42.
26. Brandtzaeg P, Halstensen TS, Huitfeldt HS *et al*. Epithelial expression of HLA, secretory component (poly-Ig receptor), and adhesion molecules in the human alimentary tract. Ann NY Acad Sci. 1992;664:157–79.
27. Blumberg RS. One size fits all: nonclassical MHC fulfill multiple roles in epithelial function. Am J Physiol. 1998;274:G227–31.
28. Blumberg RS, Koss T, Story C *et al*. A major histocompatibility complex class I-related Fc receptor for IgG on rat hepatocytes. J Clin Invest. 1995;95:2397–402.
29. Israel EJ, Taylor S, Mizoguichi E, Bhan A, Blumberg RS, Simister NE. Expression of the major histocompatibility complex class I-like Fc receptor for IgG on the human intestinal epithelial cell. Immunology. 1997;92:69–74.
30. Christ AD, Lencer WI, Simister NE, Blumberg RS. Transcellular transport of IgG across model human intestinal epithelial cells (IEC): potential role of the IgG-receptor, FcRn. Gastroenterology. 1997;112:A950.
31. Greenwald BD, James SP. Immunology of inflammatory bowel disease. Curr Opin Gastroenterol. 1995;11:298–304.
32. Cepek KL, Parker CM, Madara JL, Brenner MB. Integrin $\alpha E\beta 7$ mediates adhesion of T lymphocytes to epithelial cells. J Immunol. 1993;150:3459–70.
33. Cepek KL, Shaw SK, Parker CM *et al*. Adhesion between epithelial cells and T lymphocytes mediated by E-cadherin and an integrin, $\alpha E\beta 7$. Nature. 1994;372:190.
34. Roberts AI, O'Connell SM, Ebert EC. Intestinal intraepithelial lymphocytes bind to colon cancer cells by HML-1 and CD11a. Cancer Res. 1993;53:1608–22.
35. Cerf-Bensussan N, Bégue B, Gagnon J, Meo T. The human intraepithelial lymphocyte marker HML-1 is an integrin consisting of a $\beta 7$ subunit associated with a distinctive α chain. Eur J Immunol. 1992;22:273–7.
36. Dogan A, Wang ZD, Spencer J. E-cadherin expression in intestinal epithelium. J Clin Pathol. 1995;48:143–6.
37. Guilford P, Hopkins J, Harraway J *et al*. E-cadherin germline mutations in familial gastric cancer. Nature. 1998;392:402–5.
38. Kvale D, Krajci P, Brandtzaeg P. Expression and regulation of adhesion molecules ICAM-1 (CD54) and LFA-3 (CD58) in human intestinal epithelial cell lines. Scand J Immunol. 1992;35:669–76.
39. Parkos CA, Colgan SP, Diamond MS *et al*. Expression and polarization of intracellular adhesion molecule-1 on human intestinal epithelia: consequences for CD11b/CD18-mediated interactions with neutrophils. Mol Med. 1996;2:489–505.
40. Hoang P, Crotty B, Dalton HR, Jewell DP. Epithelial cells bearing class II molecules stimulate allogeneic human colonic intraepithelial lymphocytes. Gut. 1992;33:1089–93.
41. Mayer L, Shlien R. Evidence for function of Ia molecules on gut epithelial cells in man. J Exp Med. 1978;166:1471–9.
42. Li Y, Yio XY, Mayer L. Human intestinal epithelial cell-induced CD8+ T cell activation is mediated through CD8 and the activation of CD8-associated p56lck. J Exp Med. 1995;182:1079–88.
43. Yio XY, Mayer L. Characterization of a 180-kDa intestinal epithelial cell membrane glycoprotein, gp180. A candidate molecule mediating T cell-epithelial cell interactions. J Biol Chem. 1997;272: 12786–92.
44. Toy LS, Yio XY, Lin A, Honig S, Mayer L. Defective expression of gp180, a novel CD8 ligand on intestinal epithelial cells, in inflammatory bowel disease. J Clin Invest. 1997;100:2062–71.
45. Flier SJ, Underhill LH. The tumor necrosis factor ligand and receptor families. N Engl J Med. 1996;334:1717–25.
46. Strater J, Wellisch I, Riedl S *et al*. CD95 (APO-1/Fas)-mediated apoptosis in colon epithelial cells: a possible role in ulcerative colitis. Gastroenterology. 1997;113:160–7.
47. O'Connell J, Bennett MW, O'Sullivan GC, Collins JK, Shanahan F. The Fas counterattack: a molecular mechanism of tumor immune privilege. Mol Med. 1997;3:294–300.
48. Ye G, Barrera C, Fan X, Gourley WK, Crowe SE, Ernst PB, Reyes VE. Expression of B7-1 and B7-2 costimulatory molecules by human gastric epithelial cells: potential role in CD4+ T cell activation during *Helicobacter pylori* infection. J Clin Invest. 1997;99:1628–36.
49. Liang Q, Schürmann G, Betzler M, Meuer SC. Activation and signaling status of human lamina propria T lymphocytes. Gastroenterology. 1991;101:1529–36.

50. Pirzer UC, Schürmann G, Post S, Betzler M, Meuer SC. Differential responsiveness to CD3-Ti vs. CD2-dependent activation of human intestinal T lymphocytes. Eur J Immunol. 1990;20:2339–42.

51. Qiao L, Schürmann G, Autschbach F, Wallich R, Meuer SC. Human intestinal mucosa alters T-cell reactivities. Gastroenterology. 1993;105:814–19.

52. Ebert EC, Roberts AI, Brolin RE, Nagase H. The action and physical features of an immuno-suppressive factor produced by colon cancer cells. In: McDermott RP, editor. Inflammatory Bowel Disease: current status and future approach. Amsterdam: Elsevier; 1988:48–54.

53. Ebert EC, Roberts AI, Devereux D, Nagase H. Selective immunosuppressive action of a factor produced by colon cancer cells. Cancer Res. 1990;50:6158–61.

54. Christ AD, Colgan SP, Probert CSJ, Balk SP, Blumberg RS. CD3 mediated proliferation of human lymphocytes is modulated by soluble factor(s) from a human intestinal epithelial cell (IEC) line. Gastroenterology. 1996;110:A883.

55. Llana T, Bell RG. Characterization of an inhibitory factor derived from epithelial cells of the small intestine. Reg Immunol. 1993;5:18–27.

56. Mayrhofer G. Absorption and presentation of antigens by epithelial cells of the small intestine: hypotheses and predictions relating to the pathogenesis of coeliac disease. Immunol Cell Biol. 1995;73:433–9.

57. Eckmann L, Jung HC, Schurer-Maly C *et al.* Differential cytokine expression by human intestinal epithelial cell lines: regulated expression of interleukin 8. Gastroenterology. 1993;105:1689–97.

58. Schuerer-Maly CC, Eckmann L, Kagnoff MF, Falco MT, Maly FE. Colonic epithelial cell lines as a source of interleukin-8: stimulation by inflammatory cytokines and bacterial lipopoly-saccharide. Immunology. 1994;81:85–91.

59. Eckmann L, Kagnoff, Fierer J. Epithelial cells secrete the chemokine interleukin-8 in response to bacterial entry. Infect Immun. 1993;61:4569–74.

60. Fierer J, Eckmann L, Kagnoff M. IL-8 secreted by epithelial cells invaded by bacteria. Infect Agents Dis. 1993;2:255–8.

61. Jung HC, Eckmann L, Yang SK *et al.* A distinct array of proinflammatory cytokines is expressed in human colon epithelial cells in response to bacterial invasion. J Clin Invest. 1995;95:55–65.

62. Watanabe M, Ueno Y, Yajima T *et al.* Interleukin 7 is produced by human intestinal epithelial cells and regulates the proliferation of intestinal mucosal lymphocytes. J Clin Invest. 1995;95:2945–53.

63. Panja A, Siden E, Mayer L. Synthesis and regulation of accessory/proinflammatory cytokines by intestinal epithelial cells. Clin Exp Immunol. 1995;100:298–305.

64. McGee DW, Beagley KW, Aicher WK, McGhee JR. Transforming growth factor-beta enhances interleukin-6 secretion by intestinal epithelial cells. Immunology. 1992;77: 7–12.

65. Meyer TA, Noguchi Y, Ogle CK *et al.* Endotoxin stimulates interleukin-6 production in intestinal epithelial cells. A synergistic effect with prostaglandin E2. Arch Surg. 1994;129:1290–4.

66. McGee DW, Elson CO, McGhee JR. Enhancing effect of cholera toxin on interleukin 6 secretion by IEC-6 intestinal epithelial cells: mode of action and augmenting effect of inflammatory cytokines. Infect Immun. 1993;61:4637–44.

67. Anzano MA, Rieman D, Prichett W, Bowen-Pope DF, Greig R. Growth factor production by human colon carcinoma cell lines. Cancer Res. 1989;49:2898.

68. Koyama S, Podolsky DK. Differential expression of transforming growth factors α and β in rat intestinal epithelial cells. J Clin Invest. 1989;83:1768.

69. Coffey RJ, Goustin AS, Sonderquist AM *et al.* Transforming growth factor α and β expression in human colon cancer cell lines; implications for an autocrine model. Cancer Res. 1987;47:4590.

70. Reinecker HC, Loh EY, Ringler DJ, Mehta A, Rombeau JL, MacDermott RP. Monocyte-chemoattractant protein I gene expression in intestinal epithelial cells and inflammatory bowel disease. Gastroenterology. 1995;108:40–50.

71. Eckmann L, Kagnoff MF, Fierer J. Intestinal epithelial cells as watchdogs for the natural immune system. Trends Microbiol. 1995;3:118–20.

72. Reinecker HC, Podolsky DK. Human intestinal epithelial cells express functional cytokine receptors sharing the common gamma c chain of the interleukin 2 receptor. Proc Natl Acad Sci. 1995;92:8353–7.

73. Ciacci C, Mahida YR, Dignass A, Koizumi M, Podolsky DK. Functional interleukin-2 receptors on intestinal epithelial cells. J Clin Invest. 1993;92:527–32.

74. Sutherland DB, Varilek GW, Neil GA. Identification and characterization of the rat intestinal epithelial cell (IEC-18) interleukin-1 receptor. Am J Physiol. 1994;266:C1198–203.

75. McGee DW, Vitkus SJ, Lee P. The effect of cytokine stimulation on IL-1 receptor mRNA expression by intestinal epithelial cells. Cell Immunol. 1996;168:276–80.

76. Hata Y, Ota S, Nagata T, Uehara Y, Terano A, Sugimoto T. Primary colonic epithelial cell culture of the rabbit producing prostaglandins. Prostaglandins. 1993;45:129–41.

77. LeDuc LE, Brown L, Vidrich A. Bradykinin and FMLP stimulate prostanoid production by adult rabbit colonocytes in culture. Am J Physiol. 1994;267:G778–85.

78. Gilbert RS, Reddy ST, Targan S, Herschman HR. TGFβ 1 augments expression of the TIS10/ prostaglandin synthase-2 gene in intestinal epithelial cells. Cell Mol Biol Res. 1994;40:653–60.

79. Barrera S, Lai J, Fiocchi C, Roche JK. Regulation by prostaglandin E2 of interleukin release by T lymphocytes in mucosa. J Cell Physiol. 1996;166:130–7.

80. Mayrhofer G. Absorption and presentation of antigens by epithelial cells of the small intestine. hypothesis and predictions relating to the pathogenesis of coeliac disease. Immunol Cell Biol. 1995;73:433–9.

81. Kaiserlian D. Murine epithelial cells express Ia molecules antigenically distinct from those of conventional antigen-presenting cells. Immunol Res. 1991;10:360–4.

82. Kaiserlian D, Vidal K. Revillard JP. Murine enterocytes can present soluble antigen to specific class II restricted CD4+ T cells. Eur J Immunol. 1989;19:1513.

83. Olivier M, Berthon P, Salmon H. Localisation immunohistochimique dans l'intestine de proc des composantes cellulaires et humorales de la réponse immunitaire. Vet Res. 1994;25:57–65.

84. Cerf-Bensussan N, Quaroni A, Kurnick JT, Bhan AK. Intraepithelial lymphocytes modulate Ia expression by intestinal epithelial cells. J Immunol. 1984;32:2244–52.

85. Lowes JR, Radwan P, Proddle JD, Jewel DP. Characterisation and quantification of mucosal cytokine that induces epithelial histocompatibility locus antigen-DR expression in inflammatory bowel disease. Gut. 1992;33:315–19.

86. Blumberg RS, Terhorst C, Bleicher P *et al.* Expression of a nonpolymorphic MHC class I-like molecule, CD1D, by human intestinal epithelial cells. J Immunol. 1991;147:2518–24.

87. Canchis PW, Bhan AK, Landau SB, Yang L, Balk SP, Blumberg RS. Tissue distribution of the non-polymorphic major histocompatibility complex class I-like molecule, CD1d. Immunology. 1993;80:561–5.

88. Bahram S, Bresnahan M, Geraghty DE, Spies T. A second lineage of mammalian major histocompatibility complex class I genes. Proc Natl Acad Sci USA. 1994;91:6259–63.

89. Bleicher PA, Balk SP, Hagen SJ, Blumberg RS, Flotte TJ, Terhorst C. Expression of murine CD1 on gastrointestinal epithelium. Science 1990;250:679–82.

90. Hershberg R, Eghtesady P, Brorson K, Modlin R, Kronenberg M. Expression of the thymus leukemia antigen (TL) on intestinal epithelial cells and intestinal epithelial lymphocytes. FASEB J. 1990;4:A1864.

91. Beagley KW, Fujihashi K, Lagoo AS *et al.* Differences in intraepithelial lymphocyte T cell subsets isolated from murine small versus large intestine. J Immunol. 1995;154:5611–19.

92. Li XC, Almawi W, Jevnikar A, Tucker J, Zhong R, Grant D. Allogeneic lymphocyte proliferation stimulated by small intestine-derived epithelial cells. Transplantation. 1995;60:82–9.

93. Hershberg RM, Framson PE, Nwepon GT. Intestinal epithelial cells use two distinct pathways for HLA class II antigen processing. J Clin Invest. 1997;100:204–10.

94. Blumberg RS, Gerdes D, Chott A, Procelli SA, Balk SP. Structure and function of the CD1 family of MHC-like cell surface proteins. Immunol Rev. 1995;147:1–29.

95. Balk SP, Burke S, Polischuk JE *et al.* Beta 2-microglobulin-independent MHC class 1b molecule expressed by human intestinal epithelium. Science. 1994;265:259–62.

96. Brutkiewicz RR, Bennink JR, Yewdell JW, Bendelac A. TAP-independent β2-microglobulin-dependent surface expression of functional mouse CD1.1. J Exp Med. 1995;182:1913–19.

97. Bendelac A, Lantz O, Quimby ME, Yewdell JW, Bennink JR. CD1 recognition by mouse NK1+ T lymphocytes. Science. 1995;268:863–5.

98. Balk SP, Stevens C, Polischuk JE *et al.* Composition of T cell receptor/CD3 complex in human intestinal intraepithelial lymphocytes: lack of FcεRIg chain. Int Immunol. 1995;7:1237–41.

99. Balk SP, Ebert EC, Blumenthal RL *et al.* Oligoclonal expansion and CD1 recognition by human intestinal intraepithelial lymphocytes. Science.1991;253:1411–15.

100. Panja A, Blumberg RS, Balk SP, Mayer L. CD1d is involved in T cell-intestinal epithelial cell interaction. J Exp Med. 1993;178:1115–19.

101. Bendelac A. CD1: Presenting unusual antigens to unusual T lympocytes. Science. 1995;269:185–6.
102. Castaño AR, Tangri S, Miller JEW *et al.* Peptide binding and presentation by mouse CD1. Science. 1995;269:223–6.
103. Joyce S, Woods AS, Yewdell JW *et al.* Natural ligand of mouse CD1d1: cellular glycosylphosphatidylinositol. Science. 1998;279:1541–4.
104. Groh V, Steinle A, Bauer S, Spies T. Recognition of stress-induced MHC molecules by epithelial $\gamma\delta$ cells. Science. 1998;2789:1737–40.
105. Hussain LA, Kelly CG, Hecht EM, Fellowes R, Jourdan M, Lehner T. The expression of Fc receptors for immunoglobulin G in human rectal epithelium. AIDS. 1991;5:1089–94.
106. Morales V, Christ A, Watt S *et al.* Biliary glycoprotein (BGP:CD66a) functions as an inhibitory coreceptor for activation of human intestinal intraepithelial lymphocytes (iIEL). Gastroenterology. 1998;114:A1044.

20
Cytokines and intestinal epithelial cells

T. ANDUS, G. ROGLER, V. GROSS and J. SCHÖLMERICH

FUNCTIONS OF INTESTINAL EPITHELIAL CELLS

The epithelium of the human intestine is a continuously renewing single layer of absorptive and secretory cells arising from the proliferative zone of undifferentiated stem cells in the Lieberkühn crypts[1-4]. The differentiated enterocytes are spread over the surface of the villi, whereas the proliferating mucus-secreting goblet cells are located predominantly in the crypts. The classical functions of the epithelium are absorption and secretion of fluids, electrolytes, and nutrients, and the maintenance of the primary physiological barrier against potentially pathogenic microorganisms and antigens in the gut lumen.

Intestinal epithelial cells (IEC) play a key role in protection in the gastrointestinal mucosa, the largest surface of the body (Figure 1). They build the first

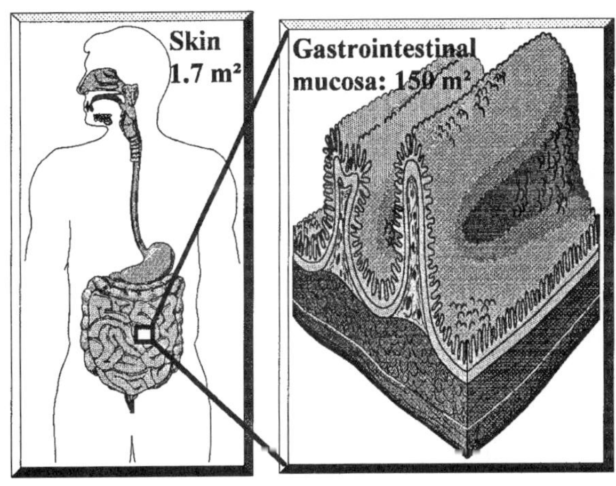

Figure 1 Functions of intestinal epithelial cells: cytokines

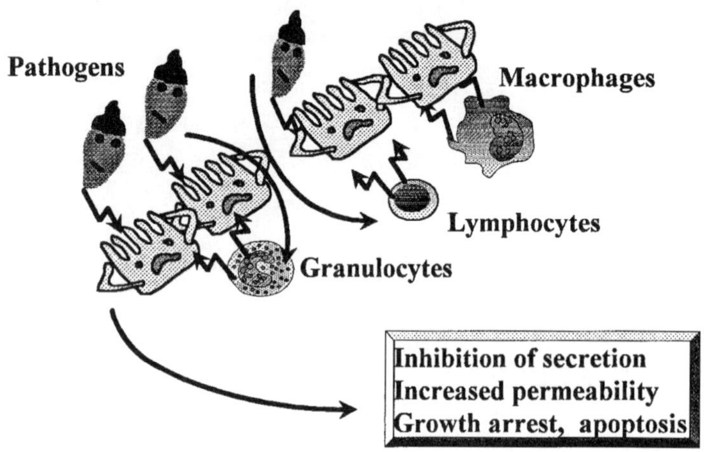

Figure 2 Role of intestinal epithelial cells during inflammation – old concept: IEC are passive target.

line of defence against pathogenic organisms and antigens and simultaneously facilitate the absorption of large amounts of nutrition[5]. Initially, the barrier function of IEC had been regarded as a mostly passive one (Figure 2).

However, recently we have learnt that IEC have more functions. IEC secrete protective and microbicidal products such as intestinal trefoil factor[6–8], complement components[9–11] and cryptdins[5,12] into the lumen. In addition, IEC produce the polymeric immunoglobulin (Ig) receptor that is essential for the transport of IgA from the lamina propria into the lumen[13–15]. Furthermore, IEC have regulatory functions for the classical immune system. They express adhesion molecules important in the homing of T cells and other leukocytes[16–19], and probably modulate T cell functions in a paracrine way[20–23]. Furthermore, IEC may play an important role as non-professional antigen-presenting cells by expressing classical MHC class I and class II and non-classical MHC class I molecules on the cell surface[24–27]. IEC produce and secrete cytokines, either constitutively or after bacterial challenge, and they express cytokine receptors[22,28–52]. Cytokines are an important class of mediator molecule involved in this regulation[53]. A complex network of cytokines and other mediators must be constantly balanced to get exactly the right amount of pro- and anti-inflammatory mediators for the actual situation[54]. Lastly, IEC initiate and control mucosal inflammation by a complex interaction with other inflammatory cells such as lymphocytes[20–23] and macrophages[55–58] (Figure 3). Taken together, IEC can be regarded as 'watchdogs' of the intestinal immune system (Figure 4)[59].

PRIMARY CULTURES OF HUMAN IEC

The study of the functions of IEC have been hampered for a long time by the fact that IEC rapidly undergo apoptosis after isolation from mucosal tissue[60]. The main reason for the rapid death of IEC is the fact that termination of the

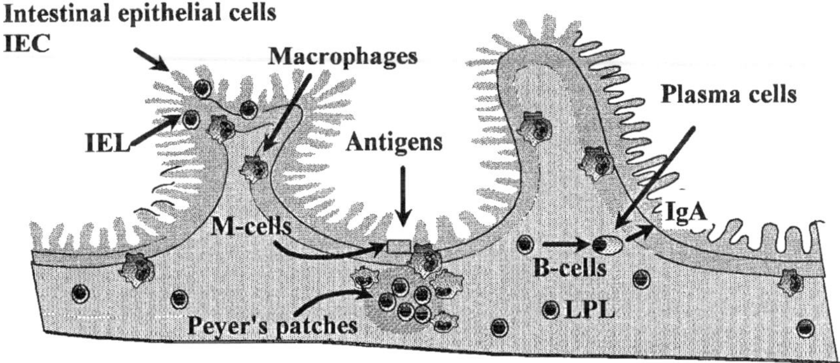

Figure 3 Network of inflammatory cells in the intestinal mucosa. IEL = intraepithelial lympho-cytes, LPL = lamina propria lymphocytes

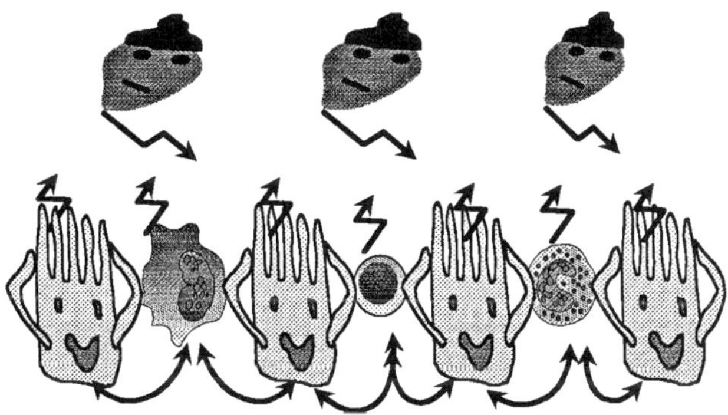

Figure 4 Role of intestinal epithelial cells during inflammation. New concept: IEC are 'watch-dogs' of the immune system

interactions between normal epithelial cells and the extracellular matrix induces apoptosis of the epithelial cells[61,62]. This phenomenon is mediated by $\beta1$-integrins[60] and interleukin-1 converting enzyme[63], and is called 'anoikis'[62]. To prevent anoikis we seeded IEC on collagen-coated permeable membranes and supplied them with just enough medium to cover the cells with a liquid film, so that the cells were provided with medium only from the bottom (Figure 5). We assume that under these conditions IEC were forced to contact the matrix closely in a way similar to the *in-vivo* situation.

With this new method of long-term culture of IEC on collagen-coated filter membranes, we did studies with human IEC in primary cultures[64]. More than 90% of the IEC isolated from colonic or ileal biopsies after culture were viable as determined by trypan blue exclusion. The yield of the viable cells isolated from surgical specimens was about 10^7 cells/specimen, and from biopsies in the range from 1 to 5×10^5/6 biopsies.

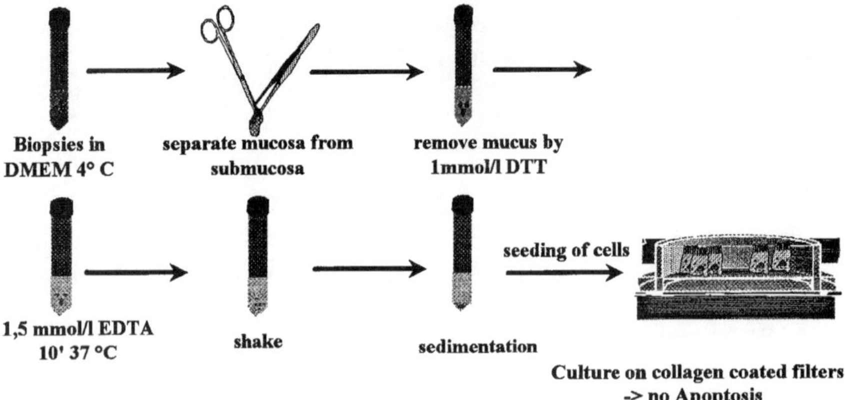

Figure 5   Flow chart of the isolation and culture of human intestinal epithelial cells

PURITY OF HUMAN IEC CULTURES

IEC primary cultures obtained by this method usually consist of more than 90% of IEC. This has been shown by immunocytochemistry and by flow cytometry. The freshly isolated IEC were analysed by flow cytometry using the FITC-labelled Ber-EP4 antibody, which recognizes a 34 kDa and a 49 kDa glyco-protein on human epithelial cells (Figure 6). Antibodies against macrophages (PE-labelled CD33), T cells (Tri-Color-labelled CD3), and B cells (Tri-Color-labelled CD19) were used to determine contaminating cells. The cell population comprised more than 90% IEC (Figure 6). Always less than 10% were of non-epithelial origin, including macrophages ($< 4\%$) and lymphocytes ($< 5\%$) (Figure 6). FITC-labelled isotype-matched antibody is shown as control.

INTEGRITY OF HUMAN IEC CULTURES

The structural and morphological integrity of the cells was shown by light microscopy, transmission and scanning electron microscopy. Some IEC cultured for 14 days formed partial monolayers. However, the cells did not form a con-tinuous monolayer with intercellular contacts, but were round, single cells some-times connected by extracellular material. Some of the cells did not adjust their apical/basolateral orientation to the new environment; they maintained their original polarity, which resulted in random positioning of the microvilli in the well. Sometimes cells were obviously seeded 'upside-down' or were lying on the lateral membrane.

Functional characterization was performed by measurement of alkaline phos-phatase. Some cultures could be extended up to 50 days (data not shown). Alkaline phosphatase, a marker enzyme for IEC, increased during the early phase of culture and reached a plateau after 4 days. Thereafter it remained con-stant over 50 days in culture. Considering that alkaline phosphatase is produced

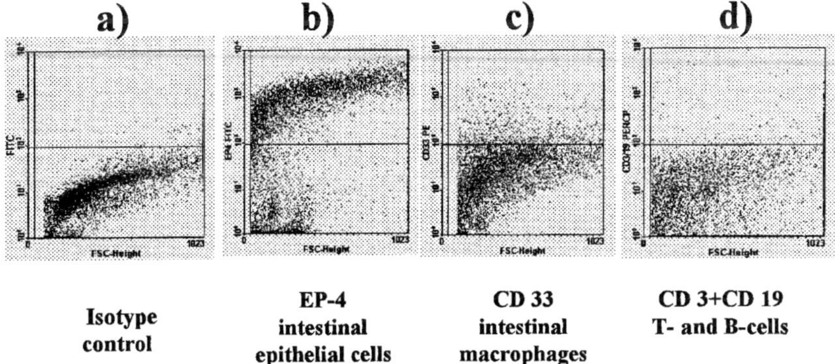

Figure 6 Flow cytometric characterization of colonic epithelial cells. Cells were moved from the filter membrane by aspiration and stained with the indicated antibodies. They were analysed with a FACScan flow cytometer by a triple fluorescence technique. (**a**) Isotype control for the FITC channel. Isotype control for the orange- and red channel also revealed no positive cells (not shown). (**b**) More than 90% of the intact cells after 7 days of culture were positive for the epithelial marker EP4. In the lower left corner of the dot plot debris is visible (circle). (**c**) Less than 4% of the cells were positive for the intestinal macrophage marker CD33. (**d**) Less than 2% of the cells were positive for T- and B-cell markers (CD3 and CD19 respectively)

PROLIFERATION AND APOPTOSIS OF HUMAN IEC

DNA synthesis as a marker of proliferation was determined by the incorporation of [^{3}H]thymidine into newly synthesized DNA of freshly isolated epithelial cells and of cells cultured for 1, 3, or 7 days. Independent from the culture period small amounts of ^{3}H-tritiated thymidine were incorporated. At all time-points IEC incorporated only 15% of [^{3}H]thymidine (2736 ± 604 cpm/10^5 cells versus 17 943 ± 1525 cpm/10^5 cells) compared with the rapidly growing HT-29 cell line, indicating a much lower rate of proliferation.

A low proliferation rate was also observed by flow cytometry cell cycle analysis. Uptake of propidium iodide into DNA after 3 days in culture showed that 82% of the epithelial cells rested in the G_0/G_1 phase, 8% were in S phase, and 10% were in the G_2 phase or M phase (data not shown). For comparison we measured uptake of propidium iodide in peripheral blood mononuclear cells, which showed no proliferation, and of cultured human intestinal fibroblasts, which showed a strong proliferation with a high percentage of cells in the S phase and G_2/M phase. The number of IEC did gradually decrease during culture. It was not possible to passage the cells. On the other hand, the normal life span of IEC *in vivo* is about 48 h[65]. Therefore, our culture conditions temporarily protect the cells from natural death by apoptosis. This is an interesting finding, which may be important for the understanding of apoptosis and cancerogenesis.

PRODUCTION OF CYTOKINES BY HUMAN IEC IN PRIMARY CULTURE

IEC produced the chemokines interleukin-8 (IL-8) and macrophage chemo-attractive protein 1 (MCP-1) but not IL-1 or IL-6 under our culture conditions[66,67]. Both IL-8 and MCP-1 production could be stimulated by IL-1, IL-6, tumour necrosis factor alpha (TNF-α), and by fetal calf serum[66]. IL-10 did not change the production of IL-8 in human epithelial cells in primary cultures. The IL-1-induced stimulation of the production of IL-8 was found to be mediated by nuclear factor κB, since we found an activation of nuclear factor κB by electrophoretic mobility shift assays[68]. Furthermore we demonstrated the presence of activated nuclear factor κB in intestinal epithelial cells by the use of an antibody, which reacts only with activated nuclear factor κB[69]. Interestingly, the production of IL-8 was significantly inhibited by IFN-γ[70]. This is in contrast to the finding that the production of IL-8 is stimulated by IFN-γ in the IEC line HT-29-19A[52]. This indicates that results obtained from experiments with transformed and dedifferentiated cell lines should be used with care.

Total RNA extracted from freshly isolated epithelial cells of five colonic surgical specimens was subjected to Northern blot analysis to screen for IL-1β, IL-1ra, IL-6, and IL-8 expression. Since the epithelial cell preparations contained some (< 10%) non-epithelial cells, RNA from lamina propria mononuclear cells (LPMNC) was isolated from the same surgical specimens for comparison. The production of IL-8 by IEC was significantly lower than the production of IL-8 by LPMNC isolated from the same patients. However, IEC primary cultures produced larger amounts of the anti-inflammatory cytokine IL-1ra compared to LPMNC from the same patients (Figure 7). From the data available it can be

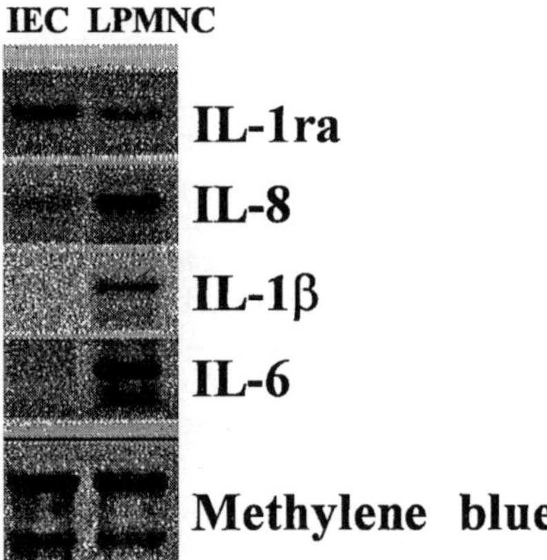

Figure 7 Northern blot analysis of cytokine mRNA in human colonic epithelial cells. Of the total RNA extracted from IEC or LPMNC, 25 μg were separated in an agarose gel containing 1% formaldehyde, transferred to nylon membranes, and hybridized with [^{32}P]dCTP-labelled cDNA fragments from IL-1β-, IL-1ra-, IL-6-, and IL-8-cDNA. Methylene blue staining was performed to document equal amounts of RNA. I = intestinal epithelial cells; LPMNC = lamina propria mononuclear cells; IL-1 = interleukin-1β, IL-1ra = interleukin-1 receptor antagonist, IL-6 = interleukin-6, IL-8 = interleukin-8

concluded that IEC produce a more anti-inflammatory pattern of cytokines compared to LPMNC.

IEC from patients with inflammatory bowel disease (IBD) produced significantly more cytokines than those from non-inflamed mucosa of healthy persons. The cytokine production by IEC correlated with the macroscopic and microscopic degree of inflammation in patients with IBD.

SUMMARY

We established a method for the long-term culture of structurally and functionally active IEC. This allowed the determination of some immunomodulatory functions of IEC, such as the production of cytokines, and may be helpful for the further study of IEC functions in IBD and colon carcinogenesis.

Acknowledgements

This study was supported by the Deutsche Forschungsgemeinschaft (An 168/3-1, and An 168/3-2) and by the Wilhelm-Sander-Stiftung.

References

1. Tidball CS. The nature of the intestinal epithelial barrier. Am J Dig Dis. 1971;16:745–67.
2. Gordon JI. Intestinal epithelial differentiation: new insights from chimeric and transgenic mice. J Cell Biol. 1989;108:1187–94.
3. Podolsky DK. Regulation of intestinal epithelial proliferation: a few answers, many questions. Am J Physiol. 1993;264:G179–86.
4. Potten CS, Booth C, Pritchard DM. The intestinal epithelial stem cell: the mucosal governor. Int J Exp Pathol. 1997;78:219–43.
5. Christ AD, Blumberg RS. The intestinal epithelial cell: immunological aspects. Springer Semin Immunopathol. 1997;18:449–61.
6. Suemori S, Lynch-Devaney K, Podolsky DK. Identification and characterization of rat intestinal trefoil factor: tissue- and cell-specific member of the trefoil protein family. Proc Natl Acad Sci USA. 1991;88:11017–21.
7. Wright NA, Poulsom R, Stamp G et al. Trefoil peptide gene expression in gastrointestinal epithelial cells in inflammatory bowel disease. Gastroenterology. 1993;104:12–20.
8. Dignass A, Lynch DK, Kindon H, Thim L, Podolsky DK. Trefoil peptides promote epithelial migration through a transforming growth factor beta-independent pathway. J Clin Invest. 1994;94:376–83.
9. Andoh A, Fujiyama Y, Bamba T, Hosoda S. Differential cytokine regulation of complement C3, C4, and factor B synthesis in human intestinal epithelial cell line, Caco-2. J Immunol. 1993;151:4239–47.
10. Andoh A, Fujiyama Y, Sumiyoshi K, Sakumoto H, Bamba T. Interleukin 4 acts as an inducer of decay-accelerating factor gene expression in human intestinal epithelial cells. Gastroenterology. 1996;111:911–18.
11. Moon R, Parikh AA, Szabo C, Fischer JE, Salzman AL, Hasselgren PO. Complement C3 production in human intestinal epithelial cells is regulated by interleukin 1beta and tumor necrosis factor alpha. Arch Surg. 1997;132:1289–93.
12. Eisenhauer PB, Harwig SS, Lehrer RI. Cryptdins: antimicrobial defensins of the murine small intestine. Infect Immun. 1992;60:3556–65.
13. Kaetzel CS, Robinson JK, Chintalacharuvu KR, Vaerman JP, Lamm ME. The polymeric immunoglobulin receptor (secretory component) mediates transport of immune complexes across epithelial cells: a local defense function for IgA. Proc Natl Acad Sci USA. 1991;88:8796–800.
14. Brandtzaeg P, Berstad AE, Farstad IN et al. Mucosal immunity – a major adaptive defence mechanism. Behring Inst Mitt. 1997;1–23.

15. Hayashi M, Takenouchi N, Asano M *et al.* The polymeric immunoglobulin receptor (secretory component) in a human intestinal epithelial cell line is up-regulated by interleukin-1. Immunology. 1997;92:220–5.
16. Kaiserlian D, Rigal D, Abello J, Revillard JP. Expression, function and regulation of the intercellular adhesion molecule-1 (ICAM-1) on human intestinal epithelial cell lines. Eur J Immunol. 1991;21:2415–21.
17. Kvale D, Krajci P, Brandtzaeg P. Expression and regulation of adhesion molecules ICAM-1 (CD54) and LFA-3 (CD58) in human intestinal epithelial cell lines. Scand J Immunol. 1992;35:669–76.
18. Dippold W, Wittig B, Schwaeble W, Mayet W, Meyer zum Büschenfelde K. Expression of intercellular adhesion molecule 1 (ICAM-1, CD54) in colonic epithelial cells. Gut. 1993;34:1593–7.
19. Vainer B, Nielsen OH, Horn T. Expression of E-selectin, sialyl Lewis X, and macrophage inflammatory protein-1alpha by colonic epithelial cells in ulcerative colitis. Dig Dis Sci. 1998;43:596–608.
20. Joseph NE, Fiocchi C, Levine AD. Crohn's disease and ulcerative colitis mucosal T cells are stimulated by intestinal epithelial cells: implications for immunosuppressive therapy. Surgery. 1997;122:809–14.
21. Christ AD, Colgan SP, Balk SP, Blumberg RS. Human intestinal epithelial cell lines produce factor(s) that inhibit CD3-mediated T-lymphocyte proliferation. Immunol Lett. 1997;58:159–65.
22. Watanabe M, Ueno Y, Yajima T *et al.* Interleukin 7 is produced by human intestinal epithelial cells and regulates the proliferation of intestinal mucosal lymphocytes. J Clin Invest. 1995;95:2945–53.
23. Yamamoto M, Fujihashi K, Kawabata K, McGhee JR, Kiyono H. A mucosal intranet: intestinal epithelial cells down-regulate intraepithelial, but not peripheral, T lymphocytes. J Immunol. 1998;160:2188–96.
24. Geppert TD, Lipsky PE. Antigen presentation by cells that are not of bone marrow origin. Reg Immunol. 1989;2:60–71.
25. Kearsey JA, Stadnyk AW. Class II MHC expression on rat intestinal intraepithelial lymphocytes. Immunol Lett. 1997;55:63–8.
26. Keren DF. Antigen processing in the mucosal immune system. Semin Immunol. 1992;4:217–26.
27. Ruemmele FM, Gurbindo C, Mansour AM, Marchand R, Levy E, Seidman EG. Effects of interferon gamma on growth, apoptosis, and MHC class II expression of immature rat intestinal crypt (IEC-6) cells. J Cell Physiol. 1998;176:120–6.
28. McGee DW, Elson CO, McGhee JR. Enhancing effect of cholera toxin on interleukin-6 secretion by IEC-6 intestinal epithelial cells: mode of action and augmenting effect of inflammatory cytokines. Infect Immun. 1993;61:4637–44.
29. Varilek GW, Neil GA, Bishop WP. Caco-2 cells express type I interleukin-1 receptors: ligand binding enhances proliferation. Am J Physiol. 1994;267:G1101–7.
30. Woywodt A, Neustock P, Kruse A *et al.* Cytokine expression in intestinal mucosal biopsies. *In-situ* hybridisation of the mRNA for interleukin-1 beta, interleukin-6 and tumour necrosis factor-alpha in inflammatory bowel disease. Eur Cytokine Netw. 1994;5:387–95.
31. Gross V, Andus T, Daig R, Aschenbrenner E, Schölmerich J, Falk W. Regulation of interleukin-8 production in a human colon epithelial cell line (HT-29). Gastroenterology. 1995;108:653–61.
32. Gibson P, Rosella O. Interleukin 8 secretion by colonic crypt cells *in vitro*: response to injury suppressed by butyrate and enhanced in inflammatory bowel disease. Gut. 1995;37:536–43.
33. Jung HC, Eckmann L, Yang SK *et al.* A distinct array of proinflammatory cytokines is expressed in human colon epithelial cells in response to bacterial invasion. J Clin Invest. 1995;95:55–65.
34. McGee DW, Bamberg T, Vitkus SJ, McGhee JR. A synergistic relationship between TNF-alpha, IL-1 beta, and TGF-beta 1 on IL-6 secretion by the IEC-6 intestinal epithelial cell line. Immunology. 1995;86:6–11.
35. Reinecker HC, Podolsky DK. Human intestinal epithelial cells express functional cytokine receptors sharing the common gamma c chain of the interleukin 2 receptor. Proc Natl Acad Sci USA. 1995;92:8353–7.
36. Jarry A, Vallette G, Branka JE, Laboisse C. Direct secretory effect of interleukin-1 via type I receptors in human colonic mucous epithelial cells (HT29-C1.16E). Gut. 1996;38:240–2.
37. Kolios G, Robertson DA, Jordan NJ *et al.* Interleukin-8 production by the human colon epithelial cell line HT-29; modulation by interleukin-13. Br J Pharmacol. 1996;119:351–9.
38. Mahida YR, Makh S, Hyde S, Gray T, Borriello SP. Effect of *Clostridium difficile* toxin A on human intestinal epithelial cells: induction of interleukin 8 production and apoptosis after cell detachment. Gut. 1996;38:337–47.

39. Mascarenhas JO, Goodrich ME, Eichelberger H, McGee DW. Polarized secretion of IL-6 by IEC-6 intestinal epithelial cells: differential effects of IL-1 beta and TNF-alpha. Immunol Invest. 1996;25:333–40.

40. McGee DW, Vitkus SJ, Lee P. The effect of cytokine stimulation on IL-1 receptor mRNA expression by intestinal epithelial cells. Cell Immunol. 1996;168:276–80.

41. Reinecker HC, MacDermott RP, Mirau S, Dignass A, Podolsky DK. Intestinal epithelial cells both express and respond to interleukin 15. Gastroenterology. 1996;111:1706–13.

42. Madrigal EL, McManus R, Byrne B *et al.* Human small intestinal epithelial cells secrete interleukin-7 and differentially express two different interleukin-7 mRNA transcripts: implications for extrathymic T-cell differentiation. Hum Immunol. 1997;58:83–90.

43. Seydel KB, Li E, Swanson PE, Stanley SL Jr. Human intestinal epithelial cells produce proinflammatory cytokines in response to infection in a SCID mouse-human intestinal xenograft model of amebiasis. Infect Immun. 1997;65:1631–9.

44. Weinstein DL, O'Neill BL, Metcalf ES. *Salmonella typhi* stimulation of human intestinal epithelial cells induces secretion of epithelial cell-derived interleukin-6. Infect Immun. 1997;65:395–404.

45. Yamada K, Shimaoka M, Nagayama K, Hiroi T, Kiyono H, Honda T. Bacterial invasion induces interleukin-7 receptor expression in colonic epithelial cell line, T84. Eur J Immunol. 1997;27:3456–60.

46. Yang SK, Eckmann L, Panja A, Kagnoff MF. Differential and regulated expression of C-X-C, C-C, and C-chemokines by human colon epithelial cells. Gastroenterology. 1997;113:1214–23.

47. Yu Y, Chadee K. *Entamoeba histolytica* stimulates interleukin 8 from human colonic epithelial cells without parasite-enterocyte contact. Gastroenterology. 1997;112:1536–47.

48. Casola A, Estes MK, Crawford SE *et al.* Rotavirus infection of cultured intestinal epithelial cells induces secretion of CXC and CC chemokines. Gastroenterology. 1998;114:947–55.

49. Fusynyan RD, Quinn JJ, Ohno Y, MacDermott RP, Sanderson IR. Butyrate enhances interleukin (IL)-8 secretion by intestinal epithelial cells in response to IL-1beta and lipopolysaccharide. Pediatr Res. 1998;43:84–90.

50. Li CK, Seth R, Gray T, Bayston R, Mahida YR, Wakelin D. Production of proinflammatory cytokines and inflammatory mediators in human intestinal epithelial cells after invasion by *Trichinella spiralis*. Infect Immun. 1998;66:2200–6.

51. Schulte R, Autenrieth IB. *Yersinia enterocolitica*-induced interleukin-8 secretion by human intestinal epithelial cells depends on cell differentiation. Infect Immun. 1998;66:1216–24.

52. Warhurst AC, Hopkins SJ, Warhurst G. Interferon gamma induces differential upregulation of alpha and beta chemokine secretion in colonic epithelial cell lines. Gut. 1998;42:208–13.

53. Rogler G, Andus T. Cytokines in inflammatory bowel disease. World J Surg. 1998;22:382–9.

54. Andus T, Daig R, Vogl D *et al.* Imbalance of the interleukin 1 system in colonic mucosa – association with intestinal inflammation and interleukin 1 receptor antagonist genotype 2. Gut. 1997;41:651–7.

55. Nathens AB, Rotstein OD, Dackiw AP, Marshall JC. Intestinal epithelial cells down-regulate macrophage tumor necrosis factor-alpha secretion: a mechanism for immune homeostasis in the gut-associated lymphoid tissue. Surgery. 1995;118:343–50.

56. Rogler G, Andus T, Aschenbrenner E *et al.* Alterations of the phenotype of colonic macrophages in inflammatory bowel disease. Eur J Gastroenterol Hepatol. 1997;9:893–9.

57. Napolitano LM, Buzdon MM, Shi HJ, Bass BL. Intestinal epithelial cell regulation of macrophage and lymphocyte interleukin 10 expression. Arch Surg. 1997;132:1271–6.

58. Ohno Y, Lee J, Fusunyan RD, MacDermott RP, Sanderson IR. Macrophage inflammatory protein-2: chromosomal regulation in rat small intestinal epithelial cells. Proc Natl Acad Sci USA. 1997;94:10279–84.

59. Eckmann L, Kagnoff MF, Fierer J. Intestinal epithelial cells as watchdogs for the natural immune system. Trends Microbiol. 1995;3:118–20.

60. Sträter J, Wedding U, Barth RFE, Koretz K, Elsing C, Möller P. Rapid onset of apoptosis *in vitro* follows disruption of β1-integrin/matrix interactions in human colonic crypt cells. Gastroenterology. 1996;110:1776–84.

61. Ruoslahti E, Reed JC. Anchorage dependence, integrins, and apoptosis. Cell. 1994;77:477–8.

62. Frisch SM, Francis H. Disruption of epithelial cell matrix interactions induces apoptosis. J Cell Biol. 1994;124:619–26.

63. Boudreau N, Sympson CJ, Werb Z, Bissel MJ. Suppression of ICE and apoptosis in mammary epithelial cells by extracellular matrix. Science. 1995;267:891–3.

64. Rogler G, Daig R, Aschenbrenner E *et al*. Establishment of long term primary cultures of human intestinal epithelial cells. Lab Invest. 1998;7:1–2.
65. Weiser MM, Ryzowicz S, Soroka CJ, Albini B. Synthesis of intestinal basement membrane. Immunol Invest. 1989;18:417–30.
66. Rogler G, Daig R, Vogl D, Gross V, Schölmerich J, Andus T. Induction of the secretion of MCP-1 and MIP-1α in primary cultures of human intestinal epithelial cells by fetal calf serum. Gastroenterology. 1998;112:A1076 (abstract).
67. Rogler G, Daig R, Vogl D, Gross V, Schölmerich J, Andus T. Intestinal epithelial cells secrete an anti-inflammatory cytokine profile in culture. Gastroenterology. 1998;112:A1076 (abstract).
68. Rogler G, Vogl D, Falk W, Gross V, Schölmerich J, Andus T. The induction of the secretion of IL-8 in primary human colonic intestinal epithelial cells is mediated by NF-κB. Gastroenterology. 1998;114:A1071 (abstract)
69. Rogler G, Vogl D, Andus T, Knüchel R, Schölmerich J, Gross V. Transcription factor NF-kappa B is activated in macrophages and epithelial cells of inflamed intestinal mucosa. Gastroenterology. 1998;115:1–14.
70. Rogler G, Vogl D, Falk W, Gross V, Schölmerich J, Andus T. Interferon gamma downregulates IL-8 secretion from primary human colonic epithelial cells. Gastroenterology. 1998;114:A1070 (abstract).

21
Gastrointestinal permeability in Crohn's disease – clinical relevance

H. LOCHS

The phenomenon of gastrointestinal permeability is defined by the fact of passive permeation of molecules or particles through the wall of the gastrointestinal tract. This excludes all active transport which is the major mechanism by which luminal contents are taken up into the blood. However, there is a physiological degree of leakiness of the intestinal wall which leads to intact permeation of macromolecules like proteins or particles like viruses, bacteria and fungi, from the intestinal lumen to the bloodstream.

Translocation of bacteria has been described in several animal species and seems to play an important role in the development of septicaemia in animals[1]. In rats, for example, the intestinal barrier is quite tight under normal conditions. However, if the animal suffers a major blood loss or trauma, massive translocation of bacteria has been described[1,2]. An adequate supply of substrates for the intestinal mucosa as well as luminal nutrition appears to be crucial for maintaining the intestinal barrier function under such conditions[3].

The degree to which permeation of bacteria takes place in humans is not yet completely clear[4]. However, permeation of macromolecules is a normal phenomenon in humans. Oral intake of animal proteins or other macromolecules leads to the appearance of these molecules, to a certain extent, in the peripheral blood[5].

Physiologically, the intestinal barrier is strictly regulated. Disturbances of the barrier function are therefore a very sensitive parameter for changes in the GI tract. Inflammation of the intestinal tract, for example, is followed by an increase in intestinal permeability[6].

Many drugs, like NSAIDs, also increase gastrointestinal permeability[7]. Due to the sensitivity of permeability to various influences, its measurement has been used as a diagnostic parameter for inflammatory diseases of the GI tract. Inflammation of the intestinal tract, for example, is followed by an increase in intestinal permeability.

MEASUREMENT OF INTESTINAL PERMEABILITY

To measure intestinal permeability in the clinical setting, it was necessary to develop tests with probes that would not be actively transported in the intestine, and would not be metabolized but excreted in the urine to a constant and high degree[6,8]. Furthermore, ideally these probes should have different molecular sizes since permeability is related to the molecular size of the probe[6]. From these prerequisites, a number of substances has been selected for permeability tests. Most investigations have been performed with PEG, [51Cr]EDTA, lactulose, rhamnose, mannitol or cellubiose. Since chromium EDTA has to be detected by its radioactive label, the various carbohydrates have been preferred for clinical use[6,8,9]. Most authors use different sugars and combine two sugar probes, one smaller molecule, like mannitol, and one bigger molecule, like lactulose. Subsequently, an index is calculated from the relationship of the two sugars. The lactulose–mannitol index or the lactulose–rhamnose index are the most commonly used indices for determination of intestinal permeability[6-8]. The test itself is easy to perform for the patient. Patients drink a test solution, which contains about 2–10 g of each sugar and collect their urine for 5–24 hours. Detection of the sugars is then performed by HPLC or gas chromatography[6]. The duration of urine collection is important since it allows a certain degree of differentiation between small bowel and colon permeability[10].

Recently, a new test has been described using sucrose to estimate the gastro-duodenal permeability[11,12]. This test can be combined with other sugar tests allowing measurement of the permeability of the stomach, the small intestine and, to some degree, also the colon, separately, with one procedure.

CLINICAL DATA

Patients with CD frequently have increased intestinal permeability[8]. The reason for this increase is not known. One explanation is that this increase is only the expression of the ongoing inflammation in the intestine. If this were the case, one would expect that permeability would be high in active disease and return to normal after successful treatment.

Initially, patients with active CD have been investigated before and after acute-phase treatment. Sanderson *et al.*[13] and Teahon *et al.*[14] demonstrated that therapy with elemental diets for six weeks to treat an active phase of CD was accompanied by a significant reduction of intestinal permeability as well as a reduction in the CDAI. They concluded that nutrition with an elemental diet reduced the inflammation of the intestinal tract and therefore improved the intestinal barrier. Similar results could be demonstrated for treatment with corticosteroids[15]. However, intestinal permeability is only normalized in some of the patients at the end of successful active-phase treatment. In an analysis, we showed that those patients who have elevated intestinal permeability after successful active-phase treatment do relapse within the next six months whereas those patients in whom permeability is completely normalized stay in remission. Therefore, intestinal permeability might constitute an excellent parameter to predict relapse in patients with CD after active-phase treatment.

In a similar investigation, we tested patients who were in remission for a minimum of six months. In this group, roughly 50% had significantly increased intestinal permeability. Follow-up showed that these patients had a significantly higher relapse rate than the patients with normal intestinal permeability[8]. Therefore, measuring intestinal permeability constitutes a good parameter to estimate the risk of relapse in patients with quiescent CD as well as after successful active-phase treatment.

Furthermore, studies in families of CD patients demonstrated that relatives also have increased intestinal permeability[16,17]. From these studies, it was concluded that disturbance of the intestinal barrier function might even be a genetically determined factor which consequently leads to the development of CD. These family studies, however, have not been confirmed in all cases[18]. Therefore, the question has to be raised whether increased intestinal permeability in families of Crohn's patients might indicate a subgroup of patients and relatives with a certain genetic predisposition or whether it might be caused by environmental factors or infections. These two hypotheses have been investigated and some evidence for both has been found. Yacyshyn *et al.*[19] have also studied intestinal permeability in families of Crohn's patients. They found that 67% of patients and 54% of relatives had significantly elevated permeability. They also investigated the expression of CD45RO and found that approximately the same number of patients and relatives had a high expression of CD45RO. Consequently, they correlated the high expression of CD45RO and increased permeability. They found that, in patients, there was an 80% positive correlation whereas, in relatives, there was a 100% positive correlation. This finding could indicate that those family members who have a high expression of CD45RO have an increased intestinal permeability and might even have increased risk for the development of CD. These studies certainly need further confirmation. However, if this proves to be true, intestinal permeability might be an excellent marker to screen for genetic susceptibility for CD easily.

In another study, spouses of patients with CD were investigated[20]. It was found that, from a big group of families, 27 spouses who had no known disease connected to increased permeability did have increased permeability. The percentage was as high as the incidence of elevated permeability in relatives in other studies. This finding would, of course, support the interpretation that there are either environmental or infectious agents which increase permeability. Whichever hypothesis is eventually confirmed, it seems that increases in intestinal permeability do parallel the development of CD and might eventually lead to the initiating factor, be it genetic or environmental.

From initial studies, one could also conclude that increases in intestinal permeability might allow differentiation between CD and ulcerative colitis. However, in studies where urine samples were collected at several time intervals, it was eventually demonstrated that patients with CD excreted the majority of markers within the first few hours whereas patients with ulcerative colitis excreted the markers later on[10]. Therefore, when the urine was collected for only five hours, patients with CD had increased levels of the markers whereas patients with ulcerative colitis excreted the markers later on. After 24 h, this difference was eliminated[10].

GASTRODUODENAL PERMEABILITY

While the initial studies were performed with markers for the intestinal permeability, a specific test for gastroduodenal permeability has been developed recently, using sucrose[11]. Using the sucrose test, Wyatt *et al.*[21] demonstrated that patients with CD do have elevated gastroduodenal permeability compared with healthy controls. They then performed gastroscopy in all these patients and found that the majority of patients had gastritis, either *Helicobacter*-associated or Crohn's-specific gastritis[22].

When they differentiated between the group with normal gastroscopy and histology and the group with inflammation, they found that only those patients with gastric inflammation had elevated gastroduodenal permeability. Therefore, the sucrose permeability test is an excellent parameter to diagnose gastric involvement in patients with CD. This might be of importance since the clinical symptoms in these patients are often non-specific. Recently, it has been shown that patients with CD frequently have a Crohn's-specific gastritis which does respond to active-phase treatment[21]. Taking this into account, the sucrose test might allow the successful treatment of CD patients with non-specific symptoms if they have increased gastric permeability.

SCIENTIFIC IMPLICATIONS

Since changes in gastroduodenal and intestinal permeability seem to be involved in the pathogenesis as well as the clinical manifestations of CD, several scientific conclusions can be made. Permeability testing might allow the selection of subgroups with a certain genetic background. It might also allow the better definition of the efficacy of new therapeutic methods. If permeability is measured in the isolated intestinal mucosa in Ussing chambers, specific transmitters can be used to disturb the barrier function. In such a model, therapeutic agents can be tested. This would be an excellent method to evaluate the therapeutic value of new substances, avoiding animal experiments.

In summary, the ability to measure gastrointestinal permeability has clinical and scientific advantages. It allows the estimation of the risk of relapse in patients with CD. It is also a very sensitive parameter for the evaluation of the efficacy of a treatment. Furthermore, by this method, subgroups of patients with different genetic backgrounds might be selected. For scientific research, it seems to offer a means to investigate therapeutic strategies without the need for animal experiments.

References

1. Deitch EA, Winterton J, Li M, Berg R. The gut as a portal of entry for bacteremia. Ann Surg. 1987;6:681–92.
2. Deitch EA, Winterton J, Berg R. Effect of starvation, malnutrition, and trauma on the gastrointestinal tract flora and bacterial translocation. Arch Surg. 1987;122:1019–24.
3. Wesley JA. Nutrition and translocation. J Parent Ent Nutr. 1990;14:170S–4S.
4. Sedman PC, Macfie J, Sagar P *et al.* The prevalence of gut translocation in humans. Gastroenterology. 1994;107:643–9.

5. Tagesson C, Andersson PA, Andersson T, Bolin T, Kallberg M, Sjodahl R. Passage of molecules through the wall of the gastrointestinal tract. Measurement of intestinal permeability to polyethylene glycols in the 634–1338 Dalton range (PEG 1000). Scand J Gastroenterol. 1983;18(4):481–6.
6. Travis S, Menzies I. Intestinal permeability: functional assessment and significance. Clin Sci. 1992;82:471–88.
7. Bjarnason I, Smethurst P, Fenn ChG, Lee CE, Menzies IS, Levi J. Microprostol reduces indomethacin-induced changes in human small intestinal permeability. Dig Dis Sci. 1989;3:407–11.
8. Wyatt J, Vogelsang H, Hübl W, Waldhoer T, Lochs H. Intestinal permeability and the prediction of relapse in Crohn's disease. Lancet. 1993;341:1437–9.
9. Sanderson IR, Walker WA. Uptake and transport of macromolecules by the intestine: Possible role in clinical disorders (an update). Gastroenterology. 1993;104:622–39.
10. Oriishi T, Sata M, Toyonag A, Sasaki E, Tanikawa K. Evaluation of intestinal permeability in patients with inflammatory bowel disease using lactulose and measuring antibodies to lipid A. Gut. 1995;36(6):891–6.
11. Sutherland LR, Verhoef M, Wallace JL, Rosendaal van G, Crutcher R, Meddings JB. A simple non-invasive marker of gastric damage: sucrose permeability. Lancet. 1994;343:998–1000.
12. Meddings JB, Sutherland LR, Byles NI, Wallace JL. Sucrose: A novel permeability marker for gastroduodenal disease. Gastroenterology. 1993;104:1619–26.
13. Sanderson IR, Boulton P, Menzies I, Walker-Smith JA. Improvement of abnormal lactulose/rhamnose permeability in active Crohn's disease of the small bowel by an elemental diet. Gut. 1987;28:1073–6.
14. Teahon K, Smethurst P, Pearson M, Levi AJ, Bjarnason I. The effect of elemental diet on intestinal permeability and inflammation in Crohn's disease. Gastroenterology. 1991;101:84–9.
15. Lochs H, Wyatt J, Reinsch W et al. Clinical relevance of intestinal permeability in active Crohn's disease. Gastroenterology. 1994;106:A722.
16. Hollander D, Vadheim CM, Brettholz E, Petersen GM, Delahunty Th, Rotter JI. Increased intestinal permeability in patients with Crohn's disease and their relatives. Ann Intern Med. 1986;105:883–5.
17. Hollander D. Permeability in Crohn's disease: altered barrier functions in healthy relatives? Gastroenterology. 1993;104:1848–73.
18. May GR, Sutherland LR, Meddings JB. Is small intestinal permeability really increased in relatives of patients with Crohn's disease? Gastroenterology. 1993;104:1627–32.
19. Yacyshyn BR, Meddings JB. CD45RO expression on circulating CD 19+ B cells in Crohn's disease correlates with intestinal permeability. Gastroenterology. 1995;108:132–7.
20. Brett BT, Savage K, Caplin ME, Khan K, Pounder RE, Dhillon AP. Lymphocyte sub-populations in Helicobacter pylori (HP) gastritis, low-grade gastric malt lymphoma and high grade gastric lymphoma. Gastroenterology. 1198;114A:3860.
21. Wyatt J, Oberhuber G, Pongratz S et al. Increased gastric and intestinal permeability in patients with Crohn's disease. Am J Gastroenterol. 1997;92:1891–6.
22. Püspök A, Oberhuber G, Wyatt J et al. Gastroduodenal permeability in Crohn's disease. Eur J Clin Invest. 1998;28:67–71.

22
Injury and healing in the epithelium

A. U. DIGNASS and H. GOEBELL

REPAIR OF GASTROINTESTINAL EPITHELIAL INJURY

The epithelium of the alimentary tract represents a crucial barrier between a broad spectrum of noxious substances present in the lumen of the gut and the individuum. Rapid resealing of this barrier following injuries is essential to preservation of normal homeostasis. Recent observations have demonstrated the ability of the gastrointestinal tract to re-establish the continuity of the surface epithelium rapidly after extensive destruction[1-4]. Currently, it is believed that epithelial continuity is re-established in three phases. First, epithelial cells adjacent to or just beneath the injured surface migrate into the wound to cover the denuded area. This process has been termed epithelial restitution and occurs both *in vitro* and *in vivo*[1-5]. It does not require cell proliferation. Intestinal epithelial restitution occurs within minutes to hours *in vivo* and *in vitro*. Secondly, epithelial cell proliferation is necessary in order to replenish the decreased cell pool and finally, maturation of initially proliferating and undifferentiated epithelial cells takes place in order to maintain the different functional activities of the intestinal epithelium. It has to be emphasized that the described separation of intestinal epithelial wound healing into distinct steps is rather artificial and extremely simplified. The three phases will overlap and distinct phases may not be observed *in vivo*. Nevertheless, the above-described model is helpful in order to better understand the physiology of intestinal repair mechanisms.

MODULATION OF THE INTESTINAL EPITHELIUM

Gastrointestinal epithelial cells are highly dynamic with complete turnover every 24–96 hours[6,7] The proliferative compartment of epithelial cells is localized in the crypt region and is segregated from a gradient of increasingly differentiated cells present along the vertical axis of the functional villus compartment. The balance of proliferative activity with both commitment to differentiation and loss of mature cells from the villus tips requires exquisite mechanisms to regulate this complex system.

The epithelial cell population of the alimentary tract is modulated and regulated by a number of factors that are present within the lumen, the epithelium itself or the underlying lamina propria. Modulating factors present in the lumen may include dietary compounds, products of alimentary secretion, secreted regulatory peptides and constituents or products of the intestinal microflora. Important factors modulating epithelial cells within the epithelium include various regulatory peptides produced by epithelial cells, locally acting hormones, products of intestinal epithelial lymphocytes and local cell–cell interactions. Factors produced within the lamina propria and the basal lamina include a spectrum of regulatory peptides expressed by various constituents of the lamina propria, extracellular matrix factors, neurotransmitters and nerval interactions. In addition, dying or injured cells will release a variety of mediators including regulatory peptides, phospholipids and adenine nucleotides. This chapter will focus mainly on the important modulatory effects of regulatory peptides on intestinal epithelial cell populations and their presumed role in inflammatory bowel disease (IBD).

REGULATORY PEPTIDES AND MODULATION OF INTESTINAL EPITHELIUM

A broad spectrum of structurally distinct regulatory peptides has been identified within the mucosa of the gastrointestinal tract[8–29]. These regulatory peptides, conventionally designated as growth factors and cytokines, play an essential role in regulating differential epithelial cell functions in order to preserve normal homeostasis and integrity of the intestinal mucosa.

Peptide growth factors encompass a group of peptides that are usually characterized by a relatively low molecular weight (< 25 kDa). These regulatory peptides exert their effects over a short or intermediate range of action through binding to specific high-affinity cell surface receptors present on the relevant target cells. In contrast to classical peptide hormones, peptide growth factors tend to act locally on adjacent cells (paracrine or juxtacrine action) or on the same cell in which they are expressed (autocrine action)[30]. The term cytokines has recently been used increasingly to describe a number of regulatory peptides which are variously identified as peptide growth factors, interleukins, interferons and colony-stimulating factors. It should be emphasized that the distinction between peptide growth factors and other peptide signalling molecules, notably cytokines, is often arbitrary, and that these terms are essentially interchangeable.

Although enormous progress has been made in the understanding and characterization of growth factor action in the gastrointestinal tract, the full variety of peptide growth factors that play a role within the intestinal mucosa has not yet been completely defined. Nevertheless, there is an increasing appreciation of the diversity of these factors in general, and the importance of several specific peptides produced within the intestinal mucosa. Several distinct peptide families have now been recognized to modulate different properties of the resident cell populations within the gastrointestinal tract (Figure 1). Peptide growth factors have been shown to play an important role in the modulation of cell proliferation, cell differentiation, angiogenesis, inflammation, gastrointestinal defence

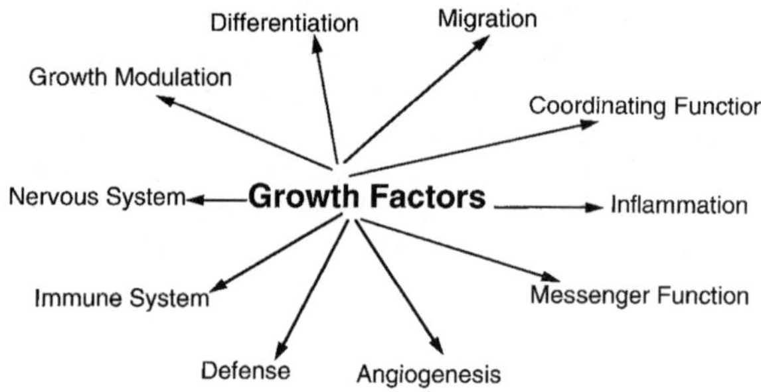

Figure 1 Regulatory peptides exert multifunctional activities within the intestinal mucosa

mechanisms and intestinal wound healing in gastrointestinal cell populations both *in vitro* and *in vivo*[9–13,15,18,19,21,24,26–29,31–39]. Furthermore, growth factors may serve as important messengers between the intestinal mucosa and the enteric nervous and enteric immune system[40–42].

The identification and characterization of numerous peptide growth factors has led to the recognition of a network of interrelated factors within the intestinal mucosa (Figure 2). The constituents of this network generally possess multiple functional properties and exhibit pleiotropism in their cellular sources and targets. As a result, this network is highly redundant in many of its functional features. The multiplicity of individual growth factor action and redundancy in the regulatory growth factor (cytokine network) is found in several dimensions. First, each cell type appears to produce more than one growth factor or cytokine. Second, each peptide growth factor may be produced by multiple different cell populations within the gastrointestinal tract. Third, most or perhaps all cell populations seem to express receptors specific for more than one growth factor.

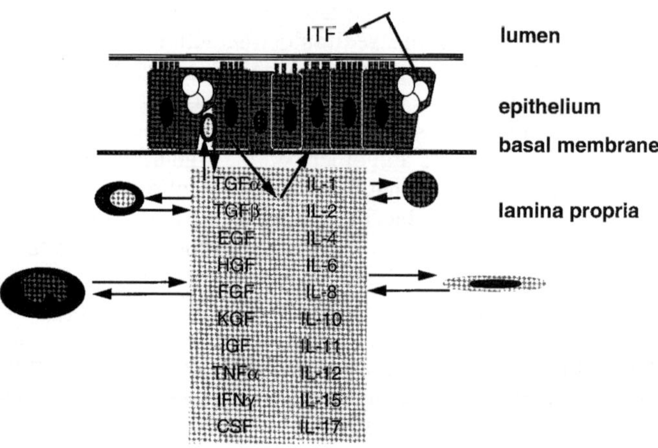

Figure 2 Intestinal mucosal cytokine interactions

Fourth, receptors for a single growth factor may be present on multiple different cell types. Thus, a single growth factor can exert a spectrum of different functional effects within a circumscribed region of the gastrointestinal tract. Fifth, functional effects of a certain growth factor may be modulated by copresence of other growth factors. Sixth, multiple structurally related members of a peptide growth factor family may interact with a single receptor (e.g. epidermal growth factor family peptides). Seventh, growth factors may modulate their own expression and also that of other growth factors and their receptors on various cellular targets.

Conveniently, peptide growth factors with relevance for inflammatory bowel disease can be classified into distinct growth factor families. These growth factor families include the transforming growth factor (TGF) β family, the epidermal growth factor (EGF) family, the fibroblast growth factor (FGF) family, the insulin-like growth factor (IGF) family, the colony-stimulating factors (CSF) and the trefoil factor family. In addition, hepatocyte growth factor/scatter factor, a peptide structurally unrelated to other characterized growth factors, and a broad spectrum of classical cytokines (interleukins and interferons) appear to play an important role in modulating intestinal epithelial cell function.

MODULATION OF EPITHELIAL WOUND HEALING BY REGULATORY PEPTIDES

The various effects of a number of growth factors on cell proliferation, migration, differentiation and angiogenesis suggest that these peptides are probably relevant factors for gastrointestinal repair mechanisms. Both *in-vitro* and *in-vivo* studies have demonstrated that several growth factors and cytokines can enhance epithelial cell restitution[1–4,32–34,43–45]. Recently, we could demonstrate that the growth factors and cytokines TGF-α, EGF, TGF-β, HGF, acidic and basic FGF, IL-1, IL-2 and interferon gamma (IFN-γ) enhance epithelial cell restitution in an *in-vitro* wounding model[11,13,15,41]. The results of these *in-vitro* studies are summarized in Figure 3. Growth factor-induced enhancement of epithelial restitution in this *in-vitro* model was independent of epithelial cell proliferation and was mediated through a TGF-β-dependent pathway. All cytokines that stimulated epithelial restitution enhanced the production of bioactive TGF-β. Addition of an immunoneutralizing antiserum against TGF-β to the culture medium could completely block the cytokine-induced enhancement of epithelial restitution. Interestingly, it appears that restitution-enhancing cytokines use different mechanisms to modulate TGF-β peptide levels. While TGF-α, EGF, IL-1, IFN-γ and HGF only increased the concentration of bioactive TGF-β, acidic and basic FGF, and also IL-2, enhanced both the bioactivation of TGF-β and the expression of TGF-β mRNA and production of latent TGF-β peptide. This might reflect a different mechanism, by which acidic and basic FGF and also IL-2 modulate the synthesis and bioactivation of TGF-β.

In contrast to the above-mentioned growth factors and cytokines which presumably act from the basolateral site of the epithelial surface, and which stimulate intestinal epithelial restitution through a common TGF-β-dependent pathway, members of the recently described trefoil factor family appear to stimulate

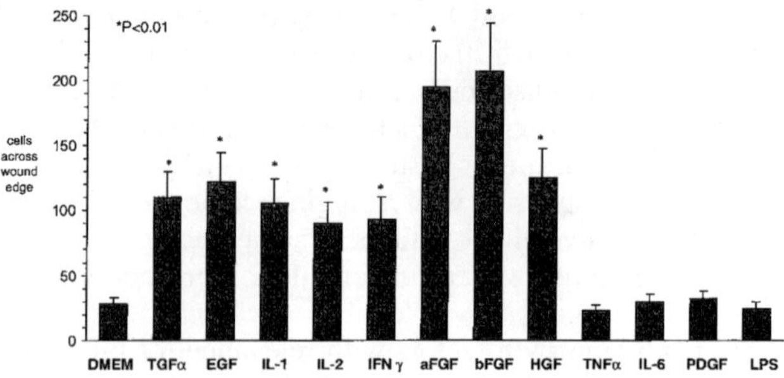

Figure 3 Various regulatory peptides stimulate epithelial cell restitution in an *in-vitro* wounding model

epithelial restitution in conjunction with mucin glycoproteins through a TGF-β-independent mechanism from the apical pole of the epithelium[12,46]. The trefoil factors are a family of recently recognized proteins expressed in a region-specific pattern throughout the gastrointestinal tract[47–55]. The members of this family share an array of structural features including most notably a highly conserved motif of six cysteine residues which leads to the formation of three intra-chain loops designated as the p domain. Members of the trefoil peptide family appear to be expressed in a region-specific pattern throughout the gastrointestinal tract in a manner which has been conserved through evolution. Thus, pS2 is normally expressed predominantly in gastric mucosa. The sP trefoil peptides are variously found in the distal stomach and pancreas, while intestinal trefoil factor is found in the small and large intestinal mucosa from the duodenum to the rectum. Although the high degree of evolutionary conservation of trefoil peptides and their abundance suggest that these peptides subserve important functions, insights into their physiological function are limited. It is notable that these peptides appear to be produced exclusively by goblet cells in the small and large intestine and their counterparts in other areas of the gastrointestinal tract which secrete them onto the luminal mucosal surface, presumably in conjunction with mucin glycoproteins. Therefore it has to be assumed that these peptides exert their most important function at the luminal–mucosal interface where they are most abundant. Indeed, the trefoil peptides are structurally well suited to survive in a functional state despite the inevitable exposure to the luminal proteases present throughout the gastrointestinal tract because of a high degree of resistance to protease digestion[23]. Although the physiological functions of these peptides remain to be clarified, trefoil factors have been found to stimulate proliferation of a number of colon cancer-derived cell lines and are presumed to play a role at sites of mucosal ulcerations in both the upper and lower gastrointestinal tract[55]. This might be of particular relevance for IBD. Recently, we have demonstrated that the trefoil peptides spasmolytic peptide and intestinal trefoil factor enhance epithelial restitution in an *in-vitro* model of epithelial injury[12]. In contrast to cytokine stimulation of intestinal epithelial restitution, which is mediated through enhanced TGF-β bioactivity[13,15], trefoil peptides stimulated epithelial restitution through a TGF-β-independent pathway, suggesting that trefoil peptides which are secreted onto the luminal surface of the gastrointestinal epithelium may act through mechanisms distinct from those which act at the basolateral site of the epithelium. In addition, trefoil peptides in conjunction with mucin glycoproteins are also able to protect model intestinal epithelia against a panel of deleterious agents present in the gastrointestinal lumen, including acid, bacterial products and lectins, by formation of a protective continuous gel on the mucosal surface[23]. Furthermore, exogenously administered trefoil peptides could protect gastric mucosa against experimentally induced gastritis, providing further evidence that these peptides may contribute to surface mucosal defence[17]. Intestinal trefoil factor (ITF)-deficient mice generated by gene knockout technology demonstrate impaired mucosal wound healing and die from extensive colitis after oral administration of dextran sulphate sodium, an agent that causes mild epithelial injury in wild-type mice. ITF-deficient mice are characterized by poor epithelial regeneration after injury, suggesting a central role for ITF in the maintenance and repair of the intestinal mucosa.

MODULATION OF EPITHELIAL CELL PROLIFERATION BY REGULATORY PEPTIDES

In addition to their potent effects on epithelial restitution, a number of growth factors also act as potent modulators of epithelial cell proliferation *in vitro*[9–11,15,21,28,40,56]. The most important modulators of intestinal epithelial cell proliferation include EGF and TGF-α, which act as potent stimulators of intestinal epithelial proliferation, and TGF-β, which inhibits intestinal epithelial cell proliferation and plays an important counterbalancing role in the regulation of intestinal epithelial cell proliferation. TGF-β inhibits cell proliferation of nearly all epithelial cell populations that have been examined[57–60]. TGF-β is also a very potent inhibitor of intestinal epithelial cell proliferation overriding the stimulatory effects of other stimulatory peptides. Interestingly, TGF-α, IL-2 and the FGF family members, acidic and basic FGF and KGF, induce a coordinated sequential induction of TGF-β which may be important to inhibit unrestrained cell growth[11,15,28,40]. Recently, we have demonstrated that the growth factors and cytokines IL-2, acidic and basic FGF, KGF and HGF stimulate epithelial cell proliferation two- to three-fold [11,15,40]. The growth-stimulating effect of these factors is rather moderate compared to the effects of EGF and TGF-α, which stimulate epithelial cell proliferation five- to ten-fold in several intestinal epithelial cell lines *in vitro*[21]. Nevertheless, it has to be considered that these factors may act in an additive or even synergistic fashion which may potentiate their single effects. Notably, only one factor present in the intestinal mucosa, TGF-β, has been identified to inhibit epithelial cell proliferation, thus providing a mechanism to counterbalance the effects of proliferative factors present within the intestinal mucosa and to inhibit unrestrained cell growth.

MODULATION OF INTESTINAL REPAIR BY NON-PEPTIDE FACTORS

In addition to the potent modulation of intestinal epithelial wound healing by regulatory peptides, we could recently demonstrate that intestinal epithelial wound healing is also modulated by non-peptide factors including adenine nucleotides and phospholipid derivatives that are released by disrupted or dying cells[61,62]. Recent studies showed that the adenine nucleotides ADP and ATP promote epithelial restitution and inhibit epithelial cell proliferation *in vitro*[61]. As adenine nucleotides exhibit only limited toxicity *in vivo*, and are available in large quantities at low cost, further studies are warranted to assess the potential benefit of adenine nucleotides in the modulation of epithelial injury *in vivo*.

The naturally occurring phospholipid lysophosphatidic acid (LPA) also significantly enhanced the migration of IEC-6 cells *in vitro*[62]. Further experiments suggest that enhancement of migration by LPA is mediated through a TGF-β-independent and pertussis toxin-sensitive and -insensitive G protein signalling cascades. In addition, LPA significantly inhibited IEC-6 cell proliferation through a TGF-β-independent pathway. Additional studies revealed that characterized pertussis toxin-sensitive and -insensitive G protein signalling cascades are not critical for the effects of LPA on IEC-6 cell proliferation. These findings suggest that LPA may modulate intestinal epithelial wound healing by enhancement of intestinal epithelial cell migration and by inhibition of intestinal epithelial proliferation through TGF-β-independent pathways. Thus, exogenous administration of LPA may provide a new approach to modulate intestinal injury.

References

1. Feil W, Wentzl E, Vattay P, Starlinger M, Sogukoglu R, Schiessel R. Repair of rabbit duodenal mucosa after acid injury *in vivo* and *in vitro*. Gastroenterology. 1987; 92:1973–86.
2. Lacy ER. Epithelial restitution in the gastrointestinal tract. J Clin Gastroenterol. 1988; 10(Suppl.):72–7.
3. Moore R, Carlson S, Madara JL. Rapid barrier restitution in an *in-vitro* model of intestinal epithelial injury. Lab Invest. 1989;60:237–44.
4. McCormack SA, Viar MJ, Johnson LR. Migration of IEC-6 cells: a model for mucosal healing. Am J Physiol. 263G:426–35.
5. Rutten MJ, Ito S. Morphology and electrophysiology of guinea pig gastric mucosal repair *in vitro*. Am J Physiol. 1983;244G:171–82.
6. Lipkin M, Sherlock P, Bell B. Cell proliferation kinetics in the gastrointestinal tract of man. II. Cell renewal in stomach, ileum, colon and rectum. Gastroenterology. 1963;45:721–9.
7. Potten CS, Kellet M, Roberts SA, Rew DA, Wilson GD. Measurement of *in vivo* proliferation in human colorectal mucosa using bromodeoxyuridine. Gut. 1992;33:71–8.
8. Dignass AU, Podolsky DK. Growth factors in inflammatory bowel disease. In: Fiocchi C, editor. Cytokines in Inflammatory Bowel Disease. Austin, TX: RG Landes; 1996;137–55.
9. Barnard JA, Beauchamp RD, Coffey RJ, Moses HL. Regulation of intestinal epithelial cell growth by transforming growth factor β. Proc Natl Acad Sci USA. 1989;86:1578–82.
10. Coffey RJ, Goustin AJ, Soderquist AM. Transforming growth factors α and β expression in human colon cancer lines. Cancer Res. 1987;47:4590–4.
11. Dignass AU, Lynch Devaney K, Podolsky DK. Hepatocyte growth factor/scatter factor modulates intestinal epithelial cell proliferation and migration. Biochem Biophys Res Commun. 1994;202:701–9.
12. Dignass AU, Lynch-Devaney K, Kindon H, Thim L, Podolsky DK. Trefoil peptides promote epithelial restitution through a TGFβ-independent pathways. J Clin Invest. 1994;94:376–83.
13. Dignass AU, Podolsky DK. Cytokine modulation of intestinal epithelial cell restitution: central role of transforming growth factor β. Gastroenterology. 1993;105:1323–32.
14. Dignass AU, Podolsky DK, Rachmilewitz D. NOx generation by cultured small intestinal epithelial cells. Dig Dis Sci. 1995;40:1859–65.
15. Dignass AU, Tsunekawa S, Podolsky DK. Fibroblast growth factors modulate intestinal epithelial cell growth and migration. Gastroenterology. 1994;106:1254–62.

16. Ciacci C, Lind SE, Podolsky DK. Transforming growth factor β regulation of migration in wounded rat intestinal epithelial monolayers. Gastroenterology. 1993;105:93–101.
17. Babyatsky MW, DeBeaumont M, Thim L, Podolsky DK. Oral trefoil peptides protect against ethanol- and indomethacin-induced gastric injury in rats. Gastroenterology. 1996;110:489–97.
18. Babyatsky MW, Rossiter G, Podolsky DK. Expression of transforming growth factor α and β in colonic mucosa in inflammatory bowel disease. Gastroenterology. 1996;110:975–84.
19. Jaffe DL, Koyama S, Podolsky DK. Expression of multiple insulin-like growth factor II (IGF II) transcripts in adult rat intestinal epithelial cells. Gastroenterology. 1990;98:A659.
20. Koyama S, Podolsky DK. Differential expression of transforming growth factors α and β in rat intestinal epithelial cells: mirror-image gradients from crypt to villus. J Clin Invest. 1989;83:1768–73.
21. Kurokawa M, Lynch K, Podolsky DK. Effects of growth factors on an intestinal epithelial cell line: transforming growth factor β inhibits proliferation and stimulates differentiation. Biochem Biophys Res Commun. 1987;142:775–82.
22. Mashimo H, Wu D-C, Podolsky DK, Fishman MC. Impaired defense of intestinal mucosa in mice lacking intestinal trefoil factor. Science. 1996;274:262–5.
23. Kindon H, Pothoulakis C, Thim L, Lynch-Devaney K, Podolsky DK. Trefoil peptide protection of intestinal epithelial barrier function: cooperative interaction with mucin glycoprotein. Gastroenterology. 1995;109:516–23.
24. New BA, Yeoman LC. Identification of basic growth factor sensitivity and receptor and ligand expression in human colon tumor cell lines. J Cell Physiol. 1992;150:320–6.
25. Park JHY, McCusker RH, Vanderhoof JA, Mohammadpour H, Harty RF, Macdonald RG. Secretion of insulin-like growth factor II (IGF-II) and IGF-binding protein-2 by intestinal epithelial (IEC-6) cells: implications for autocrine growth regulation. Endocrinology. 1992;131:1359–68.
26. Park JH, Vanderhof JA, Blackwood D, Macdonald RG. Characterization of type I and type II insulin-like growth factor receptors in an intestinal epithelial cell line. Endocrinology. 1990;126:2998–3005.
27. Procaino F, Reinshagen M, Hoffmann P et al. Protective effect of epidermal growth factor in an experimental model of colitis in rats. Gastroenterology. 1994;107:12–17.
28. Suemori S, Ciacci C, Podolsky DK. Regulation of transforming growth factor expression in rat intestinal epithelial cell lines. J Clin Invest. 1991;87:2216–21.
29. Zimmermann EM, Sartor RB, McCall RD, Pardo M, Bender D, Lund PK. Insulin-like growth factor I and interleukin 1β messenger RNA in a rat model of granulomatous enterocolitis and hepatitis. Gastroenterology. 1993;105:399–409.
30. Sporn MB, Roberts AB. Autocrine secretion – 10 years later. Ann Intern Med. 1992;117:408–14.
31. Anzano MA, Rieman D, Prichett W. Growth factor production by human colon carcinoma cell lines. Cancer Res. 1989;49:2898–904.
32. Basson MD, Modlin JM, Flynn SD, Jena BP, Madri JA. Independent modulation of enterocyte migration and proliferation by growth factors, matrix proteins and pharmalogic agents in an in-vitro model of mucosal healing. Surgery. 1992;112:299–308.
33. Basson MD, Modlin JM, Madri JA. Human enterocyte (Caco-2) migration is modulated in vitro by extra-cellular matrix composition and epidermal growth factor. J Clin Invest. 1992;90:15–23.
34. Blay J, Brown KD. Epidermal growth factor promotes the chemotactic migration of cultured rat intestinal epithelial cells. J Cell Physiol. 1985;24:107–12.
35. Challacombe DN, Wheeler EE. Trophic action of epidermal growth factor on human duodenal mucosa cultured in vitro. Gut. 1991;32:991–3.
36. Daig R, Andus T, Aschenbrenner E, Falk W, Schölmerich J, Gross V. Increased interleukin 8 expression in the colon mucosa of patients with inflammatory bowel disease. Gut. 1996;38:216–22.
37. Hoosein NM, Brattain DF, McKnight MK. Characterization of the inhibitory effects of transforming growth factor β on a human colon carcinoma cell line. Cancer Res. 1987;47:2950–4.
38. Johnson GR, Saeki T, Gordon AW, Shoyab M, Salomon DS, Stromberg K. Autocrine action of amphiregulin in a colon carcinoma cell line and immunocytochemical localization of amphiregulin in human colon. J Cell Biol. 1992;118:741–51.
39. Takacs L, Kovacs EJ, Smith MR, Young HA, Durum SK. Detection of Il-1 alpha and Il-1 beta gene expression by in situ hybridization. Tissue localization of Il-2 mRNA in the normal C57BLB/6 mouse. J Immunol. 1988;141:3081–95.
40. Ciacci C, Mahida YR, Dignass A, Koizumi M, Podolsky DK. Functional interleukin-2 receptors on intestinal epithelial cells. J Clin Invest. 1993;92:527–32.

41. Dignass AU, Podolsky DK. Interleukin 2 modulates intestinal epithelial cell function *in vitro*. Exp Cell Res. 1996;225:422–9.
42. Hoffmann P, Zeeh JM, Lakshmanan J, Eysselein VE. Transforming growth factor alpha immunoreactive nerve fibers in the rat and mouse intestinal tract. Soc Neurosci. 1994;14:A699.
43. Paimela H, Goddard PJ, Carter K *et al.* Restitution of frog gastric mucosa *in vitro*: effect of fibroblast growth factor. Gastroenterology. 1993;104:1337–45.
44. Silen W. Gastric mucosal defense and repair. In: Johnson LR, editor. Physiology of the Gastrointestinal Tract. New York: Raven Press; 1987:1044–69.
45. Nusrat A, Delp C, Madara J. Intestinal epithelial restitution. J Clin Invest. 1992;89:1501–11.
46. Playford RJ, Marchbank T, Chinery R *et al.* Human spasmolytic polypeptide is a cytoprotective agent that stimulates cell migration. Gastroenterology. 1995;108:108–16.
47. Thim L. A new family of growth factor-like peptides. FEBS Lett. 1989;250:85–90.
48. Thim L, Woldike HF, Nielsen PF *et al.* Characterization of human and rat intestinal trefoil factor produced in yeast. Biochemistry. 1995;34:4757–64.
49. Tomasetto C, Rio M-C, Gautier G. hSP, the domain-duplicated homolog of pS2 protein, is co-expressed with pS2 in stomach but not in breast carcinoma. EMBO J. 1990;9:407–14.
50. Wright NA, Poulsom R, Stamp G *et al.* Trefoil peptide gene expression in gastrointestinal epithelial cells in inflammatory bowel disease. Gastroenterology. 1993;104:12–20.
51. Podolsky DK, Lynch Devaney K, Stow JL *et al.* Identification of human intestinal trefoil factor. Goblet cell-specific expression of a peptide targeted for apical secretion. J Biol Chem. 1993;268:6694–702.
52. Podolsky DK, Kindon H, Lynch-Devaney K, Dignass A, Babyatsky M. Epithelium in inflammatory bowel disease: trefoil peptides at the interface. In: Tytgat GNJ, Bartelsman JFWM, van Deventer SJH, editors. Inflammatory Bowel Diseases. Dordrecht: Kluwer; 1995:360–5.
53. Sands BE, Ogata H, Lynch-Devaney K, DeBeaumont M, Ezzell RM, Podolsky DK. Molecular cloning of rat intestinal trefoil factor gene. J Biol Chem. 1995;270:9353–61.
54. Suemori S, Lynch-Devaney K, Podolsky DK. Identification and characterization of rat intestinal trefoil factor: tissue- and cell-specific member of the trefoil protein family. Proc Natl Acad Sci USA. 1991;88:11017–21.
55. Sands BE, Podolsky DK. The trefoil peptide family. Annu Rev Physiol. 1996;58:253–73.
56. Cordon-Cardo C, Vlodavsky I, Haimovitz-Friedmann A, Hicklin D, Fuks Z. Expression of basic fibroblast growth factor in normal human tissues. Lab Invest. 1990;63:832–40.
57. Barnard JA, Lyons RM, Moses HL. The cell biology of transforming growth factor β. Biochim Biophys Acta. 1990;1032:79–87.
58. Sporn MB, Roberts AB, Wakefield LM, Assoian RK. Transforming growth factor-β: biological function and chemical structure. Science. 1986;233:532–4.
59. Roberts AB, Sporn MB. The transforming growth factor-βs. In: Sporn MB, Roberts AB, editors. Peptide Growth Factors and their Receptors. I. New York: Springer-Verlag: 1991:417–72.
60. Massague J. The transforming growth factor β family. Annu Rev Cell Biol. 1990;6:597–641.
61. Dignass AU, Becker A, Spiegler S, Goebell H. Adenine nucleotides modulate gastrointestinal epithelial repair mechanisms *in vitro*. Eur J Clin Invest. 1998 (In press).
62. Sturm A, Becker A, Goebell H, Dignass AU. Modulation of intestinal epithelial cell restitution and proliferation *in vitro* by lysophosphatidic acid. Gastroenterology. 1998:114:A1184.

Section VI
Endotoxin and IBD

23
Detection of endotoxin in IBD

K. R. GARDINER

INTRODUCTION

While the aetiology of inflammatory bowel disease (IBD) remains unknown, much has been learned about the pathogenesis of IBD from intensive studies of patients and from animal models. Current thinking is that the development of IBD requires a genetic predisposition reflected in either an impaired intestinal mucosal barrier, an inappropriate immune response or an impaired healing capacity allowing persistent immune activity against normal intestinal flora[1,2].

The evidence that the normal enteric flora play a crucial role in the pathogenesis of IBD has been comprehensively reviewed by Sartor[3,4]. The major components of this argument are the predilection of IBD for the distal intestine (the site of the highest luminal bacterial concentration), the resemblance of IBD to enterocolonic infections, the response of Crohn's disease to altering luminal bacterial concentrations (antibiotic administration and faecal diversion) and the increased systemic immune response to luminal bacteria[3–5].

Which component of the bacterial flora (living bacteria or bacterial products) is the main culprit is not clear. The microecology of the distal ileum and colon is complex with over 200 bacterial strains[3]. In the colon, anaerobes such as *Bacteroides*, *Peptostreptococcus*, *Clostridia* and bifidobacteria outnumber aerobes (coliforms) by 1000:1. Anaerobes are also present in the distal ileum but are rare in the proximal intestine. Bacteriological findings in patients with ulcerative colitis have ranged from a normal flora to increased numbers of group D streptococci and coliforms to the presence of invasive *Escherichia coli*[6–8]. A decrease in the number of anaerobic Gram-negative organisms and of protective lactobacilli has been described in patients with active ulcerative colitis[9,10]. Increased numbers of anaerobic Gram-negative and coccoid rods have been reported in patients with small bowel Crohn's disease[11–13] and increases in *Escherichia coli* and *Bacteroides fragilis* in colonic Crohn's disease[7,14]. In patients with active Crohn's disease a significant reduction in bifidobacteria and lactobacilli has been found – two species which are generally regarded as beneficial for the host[14,15]. Gorbach *et al.*[16] investigated the relationship between faecal microbial ecology and disease activity. They found that the flora in patients with mild to moderate ulcerative colitis was very similar to that of healthy individuals. However those with Crohn's disease and severe ulcerative colitis had increased numbers of coliforms in their stools[16].

In addition to quantitative disturbances, qualitative abnormalities in the faecal flora have also been described in IBD. A number of studies have shown that *E. coli* from patients with ulcerative colitis have greater adhesive properties than those isolated from controls[8,17,18]. Cooke[19] reported that *E. coli* isolated from patients with ulcerative colitis included a larger proportion that produced haemolysin and necrotoxin than those from controls or other patients with diarrhoeal disease.

The luminal bacteria produce chemotactic formylated oligopeptides (such as FMLP) and cell-wall polymers such as lipopolysaccharide (LPS, endotoxin) and peptidoglycan–polysaccharide (PG-PS complexes). These bacterial products are known to be potent activators of inflammatory cells resulting in the secretion of soluble inflammatory mediators that are capable of enhancing mucosal permeability, recruiting immune effector cells and establishing a self-perpetuating inflammatory response[4].

The aim of this chapter is to review the evidence that endotoxins cross the intestinal wall in IBD (translocate) and to investigate the role that translocating endotoxin has in the initiation or aggravation of the inflammatory process in these diseases.

WHAT ARE ENDOTOXINS?

Endotoxins are the lipopolysaccharide (LPS) constituents (molecular weight approx. 400 000–4 000 000 daltons) of the outer membrane of Gram-negative bacteria. Three well-defined regions of the LPS molecule have been described: (a) *an O-specific side chain* which is highly immunogenic, consists of repeating oligosaccharide units and shows considerable variation between serotypes of the same species; (b) *a core oligosaccharide* which shows only minor structural variability between serotypes; and (c) *lipid A* which is thought to mediate most of the biological effects of endotoxin such as pyrogenicity, activation of phagocytic cells, activation of coagulation factors, nephrotoxicity and hepatotoxicity[20]. LPS functions as a hydrophobic barrier for the bacterium, restricting the entry of noxious substances such as bile salts, digestive enzymes and certain antibiotics, enabling it to evade host-defence factors such as complement, lysozyme and cationic proteins[21]. Endotoxins are released by Gram-negative bacteria during autolysis, after exposure to cell-membrane toxins or antibiotics, during rapid growth and when essential nutrients are depleted from the environment[22]. During growth *in vitro*, bacteria constantly shed outer membrane fragments[23] that contain a high concentration of endotoxins; bacterial strains differ in their rate of endotoxin shedding[24]. Released endotoxins are thought to be responsible for most, if not all, of the pathophysiological effects associated with Gram-negative sepsis[25]. Lipopolysaccharides bind to a number of circulating plasma proteins such as high-density lipoproteins and lipopolysaccharide binding protein (LBP). LBP is a 60 kDa acute-phase glycoprotein which binds avidly to lipid A, so facilitating the binding of LPS molecules to monocytes via the CD14 receptor and augmenting cytokine production[26–28].

METHODS OF ENDOTOXIN DETECTION

Endotoxin has been detected by radioimmunoassay using a specific bacterial antigen (*E. coli* 0111)[29–31], by measuring biological endotoxin activity using the qualitative *Limulus* gelation assay[32–37] or the quantitative *Limulus* amoebocyte lysate assay[38–43] and by two-dimensional gas chromatography with electron capture[44].

The radioimmunoassay described detected endotoxin from *E. coli* 0111, endotoxin derived from bacterial species with cross-reactivity and other immunologically cross-reactive substances[29]. The *Limulus* gelation test (Figure 1) suffered from being qualitative, relatively insensitive and having a high incidence of false-positive results[45,46]. The development of the quantitative and highly sensitive *Limulus* amoebocyte lysate (LAL) assay was a significant advance[47]. This assay (Figure 2) is based on the activation by endotoxin of a proenzyme in the lysate derived from the blood cells (amoebocytes) of the horseshoe crab (*Limulus polyphemus*)[48]. Heat treatment of the plasma samples releases endotoxin from plasma proteins either present constitutively or released during the host acute-phase response (lipopolysaccharide binding protein, bactericidal/permeability-increasing protein, anti-endotoxin antibodies and high-density lipoproteins) that may bind endotoxin. Sonesson *et al.*[44] reported on the detection of endotoxin using a two-dimensional gas chromatographic technique.

The presence of endotoxin has also been sought using indirect methods such as the epinephrine skin test[49,50], the spontaneous formation of fibrin microclots[51], the consumption and subsequent increased production of anti-endotoxin or anti-lipid A antibodies[37,52] and the identification of increasing numbers of CD14 positive neutrophils and monocytes[53]. The EndoCAb ELISA developed by Barclay measures the concentration of antibodies to endotoxin core which are cross-reactive with endotoxins of a number of Gram-negative bacterial species

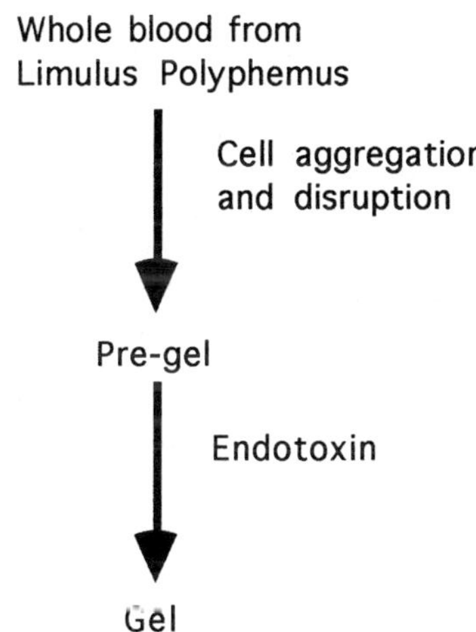

Figure 1 *Limulus* gelation test

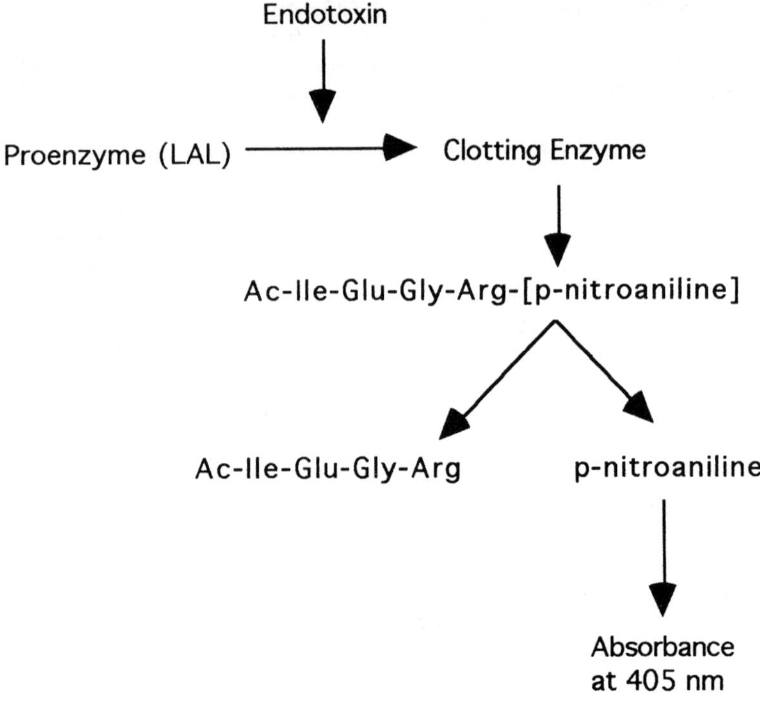

Figure 2 *Limulus*–amoebocyte–lysate (LAL) assay

and strains. Changes in EndoCAb may indicate endotoxin exposure even when endotoxin cannot be measured, and in many clinical situations EndoCAb may have prognostic value[52].

TRANSLOCATION OF ENDOTOXIN IN HEALTH AND DISEASE

Endotoxin is present in large quantities in the human gut without producing harmful effects[54]. Even the ingestion of milligram quantities of endotoxin fails to produce adverse reactions in healthy human volunteers[55]. The intestinal mucosa provides an effective barrier to these macromolecules through its intact mucosal surface (a monolayer of epithelial cells joined at tight junctions). However, even in physiological conditions, a quantitatively unimportant but immunologically important fraction of luminal antigens bypass this barrier and are absorbed by a process of transcytosis at specialized antigen transport mechanisms in the villous epithelium and particularly in Peyer's patches[56]. As a result small amounts of luminal endotoxin cross the intact intestine during health but are rapidly cleared by the reticuloendothelial system[32,57]. Specific antibody responses to endotoxins (endotoxin core) have been found in healthy subjects[43,58,59], indicating exposure of the immune system to these antigens.

Endotoxaemia of intestinal origin is thought to occur when there is an alteration in endotoxin translocation and/or detoxification[54]. If the gastrointestinal mucosa, portal circulation and hepatic reticuloendothelial system are intact, gut-derived endotoxin does not appear to give rise to detectable systemic endotoxaemia[54]. In contrast, clinical studies have shown that if the gut mucosal barrier is damaged (bacterial enteritis, colonoscopy, colonic carcinoma), the portal vein occluded or hepatic function impaired, systemic endotoxaemia results[46,47,60].

There appear to be three main routes of uptake of endotoxins into the systemic circulation: via the portal vein[32], by direct transmural absorption into the systemic blood stream[61] or via intestinal lymphatics and the thoracic duct[62].

TRANSLOCATION OF ENDOTOXINS IN EXPERIMENTAL IBD

Direct evidence

Portal endotoxaemia has been reported in experimental models of colitis in the rat (hapten-, acetic acid-, and ethanol-induced models)[63,64] and the guinea pig (carrageenan model)[65].

Systemic endotoxaemia has been observed in experimental models of colitis in the mouse (dextran sulphate sodium)[66], rat (hapten-, acetic acid- and ethanol-induced models)[63,64,67–69], rabbit (carrageenan- and formalin-lipopolysaccharide-induced)[31,70] and dog (spontaneous haemorrhagic enterocolitis)[45]. Systemic endotoxaemia has been found to correlate positively with portal endotoxaemia[64], severity of the colitis[31,67,68] and of the systemic response (serum concentrations of lactate and α_2-macroglobulin)[69].

Indirect evidence

There is evidence of a specific systemic antibody response to endotoxin in the trinitrobenzenesulphonic acid (TNBS) rat model of colitis with an initial reduction in both IgG and IgM antibodies to the endotoxin core with a subsequent increase but no change in IgG and IgM antibodies to tetanus toxoid[69]. This is thought to represent a consumption of antibody by translocating endotoxin followed by a B cell response and increased antibody production[69]. Antibody concentrations against the antigens of enteric bacterial flora are also easily demonstrated in colitic C3H/HeJBir mice, whereas normal mice have relatively little or no antibody[71].

Further evidence of transmigration of endotoxin across the inflamed intestinal wall is the high expression of membrane-bound CD14, a receptor for lipopolysaccharide, by inflammatory macrophages from the inflamed intestine in the dextran sulphate sodium model of ulcerative colitis in the mouse[53].

TRANSLOCATION OF ENDOTOXINS IN CLINICAL IBD

Direct evidence

Radioimmunoassay

Circulating immunoreactive endotoxin was detected in very high concentrations in two patients suffering from ulcerative colitis with a radioimmunoassay technique utilizing *E. coli* 0111 as the antigen[29]. Aoki[30], using a similar radioimmunoassay technique, reported systemic endotoxaemia in 62% of patients with ulcerative colitis ($n = 61$) and 43% patients with Crohn's disease ($n = 7$). Higher concentrations of endotoxin were detected during active disease. In 12 endotoxaemic patients with ulcerative colitis, endotoxaemia disappeared following surgical excision of diseased intestine[30].

Unspecified biological method

Studies from the Soviet Union reported systemic endotoxaemia in 70% of patients with active ulcerative colitis ($n = 77$) using a biological method which they did not specify[72,73].

Limulus *gelation test*

Liehr[34] reported an incidence of endotoxaemia of 64% in hospitalized patients with Crohn's disease ($n = 11$) and 50% in patients with ulcerative colitis ($n = 4$) using the *Limulus* gelation test. Using the same technique, Auer *et al.*[33] reported systemic endotoxaemia in 80% of patients with Crohn's disease ($n = 33$) in association with B cell-lymphocytosis, and Colin *et al.*[35] reported endotoxaemia in 68% of patients with Crohn's disease ($n = 11$) and 63% of patients with ulcerative colitis ($n = 11$). Endotoxaemia was demonstrated in all patients with active disease and was found to correlate positively with disease activity and intestinal ulceration[35].

Systemic and portal endotoxaemia were detected in one of two patients with ulcerative colitis undergoing colectomy using the *Limulus* gelation test (sensitivity 1 ng/ml)[32]. In another study of patients with ulcerative colitis ($n = 8$) undergoing colectomy, portal endotoxaemia was found in 38% and systemic endotoxaemia in 12% before bowel mobilization (*Limulus* gelation test: sensitivity 100 pg/ml); portal and systemic endotoxaemia were detected in 50% during mobilization[36]. Colonoscopy has also been reported to precipitate systemic endotoxaemia (*Limulus* gelation test) in patients with ulcerative colitis ($n = 4$); there was a 25% incidence of sytemic endotoxaemia prior to, and a 100% incidence after, colonoscopy in these patients[74].

In contrast, Kruis and colleagues[37] detected systemic endotoxaemia in only 2.5% of patients with Crohn's disease ($n = 40$) and 3% of patients with ulcerative colitis ($n = 23$) using the *Limulus* gelation test (sensitivity 10 pg/ml). They found, however, a raised titre of antibodies against lipid A (passive haemolysis test), the toxic moiety of the endotoxin molecule, in patients with Crohn's disease. This latter finding indicates that there was, in fact, increased exposure to the endotoxin molecule in these patients. In another study[75], none of 15 patients with IBD (Crohn's disease $n = 7$; ulcerative colitis $n = 8$) undergoing colonoscopy were found to have systemic endotoxaemia using a *Limulus* gelation test (sensitivity 1 ng/ml). The low sensitivity of the assay and a lower inflammatory activity in their patients may explain their divergent findings (all patients who had a temperature $> 37°C$ or who were on therapy were excluded).

LAL *assay*

Wellmann and colleagues were the first to use a quantitative *Limulus* assay (sensitivity 20 pg/ml) to detect systemic endotoxaemia in patients with IBD[38,39].

In a group of 125 outpatients with IBD, 13% of patients with Crohn's disease ($n = 97$) and 29% of patients with ulcerative colitis ($n = 28$) were positive for circulating endotoxin[39]. There was a significant positive correlation between systemic endotoxaemia and measures of disease activity. In a group of 12 patients hospitalized with a clinical relapse of IBD (Crohn's disease $n = 8$, ulcerative colitis $n = 4$), all were endotoxaemic[38]. In a further study investigating the treatment of systemic endotoxaemia in Crohn's disease, 94% of patients with severe disease ($n = 18$) had circulating endotoxins[40]. The same group compared the detection of systemic endotoxaemia by the simultaneous determination of plasma elastase/α_1-proteinase-inhibitor and *Limulus*–amoebocyte–lysate reactivity in patients with Crohn's disease[41]. They reported a parallelism between elastase/α_1-proteinase inhibitor and *Limulus*–amoebocyte–lysate reactivity for 15/16 patients with active Crohn's disease. Systemic endotoxaemia was reported in 44% of patients with Crohn's disease ($n = 16$) using a quantitative *Limulus* assay[42]. Baldassano *et al.*[76] measured endotoxin using the LAL assay in a group of patients with active ($n = 8$) and quiescent ($n = 5$) Crohn's disease and reported a mean endotoxin concentration of 16 pg/ml. Engström *et al.*[77] found mesenteric endotoxaemia in one of three patients undergoing proctocolectomy for ulcerative colitis using a LAL assay. Liao *et al.*[78] have reported that patients with quiescent Crohn's disease ($n = 57$) do not have significantly elevated systemic endotoxin concentrations compared with controls (LAL assay).

Gardiner *et al.*[43] measured systemic endotoxin concentrations using a quantitative LAL assay in IBD patients with quiescent and active disease. In IBD patients requiring hospitalization for acute relapse, systemic endotoxaemia was demonstrated in 88% of patients with ulcerative colitis ($n = 25$), 75% with indeterminate colitis ($n = 8$) and 94% of those with Crohn's disease ($n = 31$). In a group of outpatients with inactive disease, systemic endotoxaemia was demonstrated in 33% of patients with ulcerative colitis ($n = 33$) and 9% of those with Crohn's disease[63]. Systemic endotoxaemia was found to correlate positively with anatomical extent and clinical activity of ulcerative colitis[43].

There is limited information on portal endotoxaemia in IBD, with only 10 reports of portal sampling in patients with ulcerative colitis, of which four were positive; and no reports regarding Crohn's disease.

Reduction in systemic endotoxaemia is associated with resolution of disease relapse[30,38,40,41]; with restoration to normal of plasma protein and serum iron concentrations[38,72]; and with reduction in indices of disease activity[38].

Indirect evidence

Epinephrine skin test

Bowen and Kirsner[49] were the first to suggest that 'bacterial endotoxins by direct action or perhaps *via* a hypersensitivity mechanism, may contribute to the necrotizing tissue reaction of fulminant ulcerative colitis', and possibly to the extraintestinal complications of these diseases. This hypothesis was then investigated using the epinephrine (adrenaline) skin test as an indication of circulating endotoxin in patients with IBD and in controls. The epinephrine skin test was positive for circulating endotoxin in 50% of patients with ulcerative colitis ($n = 68$) and 60% of patients with Crohn's disease ($n = 38$). Patients with positive tests were more severely ill than those with negative tests. The epinephrine skin test was always positive in the presence of extraintestinal complications of ulcerative colitis. In addition, the tests became negative after clinical improvement. In the control group ($n = 90$), 2% had positive epinephrine skin tests (one with leprosy; one with rheumatoid arthritis). Bowen and Kirsner[49] concluded that an endotoxin-like substance or bacterial endotoxin is absorbed from the inflamed intestine in IBD, and drew attention to its presence in more active disease.

Gilbert and Ravelo[50] also utilized this epinephrine skin test. They injected rabbits intradermally with adrenaline followed by the intravenous injection of sera from patients ($n = 20$) with active ulcerative colitis. Initial haemorrhage and vascular congestion at the dermal injection site were followed by haemorrhagic necrosis in all animals. The similarity of these lesions to the Shwartzman and Thomas phenomena led these authors to conclude that circulating endotoxins were present in active ulcerative colitis (100%).

Fibrin microclots

Spontaneous formation of radially orientated microclots (an indication of endotoxaemia) was observed in the blood of 81% of patients with active Crohn's disease ($n = 16$) and 50% of patients with active ulcerative colitis ($n = 14$)[51].

Endotoxin-induced monocyte superoxide production

Baldassano et al.[76] have shown that the ability of serum from patients with Crohn's disease to prime normal monocytes to produce superoxide anions was lost after lipopolysaccharide was removed from the serum using polymyxin, thus providing further indirect evidence of systemic endotoxaemia.

Antibodies to specific lipopolysaccharides

Zeitz et al.[59] measured circulating antibody concentrations against lipopolysaccharides purified from three different E. coli strains (E. coli 0119, 075, 014) in patients with Crohn's disease and healthy controls. Ten out of 27 patients with Crohn's disease had no complement-fixing antibodies against the E. coli lipopolysaccharides, whereas all ($n = 20$) healthy individuals had anti-lipopolysaccharide antibodies. In six of 27 patients with Crohn's disease they found rapidly changing titres of anti-lipopolysaccharide antibodies not paralleled by changes in anti-tetanus toxoid antibody[59], suggesting that there was depletion of circulating anti-lipopolysaccharide antibodies as the serum passed inflamed intestinal mucosa.

Antibodies to endotoxin core

Gardiner et al.[43] found a significant increase in the plasma concentrations of antibodies (IgG) to the endotoxin core (EndoCAb assay) in patients with active Crohn's disease compared with healthy controls or patients with ulcerative colitis. The plasma anti-endotoxin core antibody concentration correlated positively with systemic endotoxaemia. Analysis of these results according to distribution of the disease showed the highest IgG endotoxin core antibody concentrations were found in patients with small bowel Crohn's disease. Intermediate concentrations were found in patients with Crohn's disease of both large and small intestines and the lowest concentrations in those with colonic inflammation only. As might have been predicted, patients with indeterminate colitis had intermediate plasma IgG endotoxin core antibody concentrations as this group probably contained patients with ulcerative colitis and patients with Crohn's disease. The finding that plasma IgG endotoxin core concentration was highest in patients with small intestinal Crohn's disease may be explained by the much greater permeability of the mucosal barrier of the small intestine (130-fold) to macromolecules compared with that of the colon[79]. With regard to IgA, plasma concentration of IgA to endotoxin core was non-significantly increased in patients with Crohn's disease (107.3 ± 20.5 median units) and ulcerative colitis (93.0 ± 24.2) in comparison with healthy controls (61.3 ± 15.7)[63,80].

Antibodies to lipid A

Schüßler and his colleagues reported a significant elevation in the titre of antibodies to lipid A in Crohn's disease patients ($n = 18$) compared with patients with ulcerative colitis ($n = 28$), acute enteritis ($n = 24$) and healthy controls ($n = 68$)[81–84]. Serum antibodies to lipid A in titres up to 1:256 were detected in 39% of patients with Crohn's disease ($n = 18$), 100% of patients with ulcerative colitis ($n = 3$) but also in 10% of controls ($n = 100$)[85]. Kruis et al.[37] found that lipid A antibody titres were significantly higher in Crohn's disease patients ($n = 40$) than in controls ($n = 42$) or patients with ulcerative colitis ($n = 23$). Titres of anti-lipid A antibody were significantly higher during active disease. These findings were confirmed in a subsequent larger study which showed in addition that anti-lipid A antibodies frequently disappeared after total removal of the inflamed bowel or after ampicillin therapy[86]. More recently, Oriishi et al[87] reported that blood IgG and IgA anti-lipid A antibody concentrations were significantly higher in patients with Crohn's disease ($n = 14$) than in healthy controls ($n = 12$) or in patients with ulcerative colitis ($n = 12$). IgA anti-lipid A antibody concentration was significantly higher in patients with ulcerative colitis than in controls.

However, increased circulating anti-lipid A antibodies have not been found in all studies[59,88,89]. Mattsby-Baltzer et al.[88] found lower levels of IgG anti-lipid A antibodies in patients with IBD (ulcerative colitis $n = 46$; Crohn's disease $n = 38$) than in blood donors. Nolan et al.[89] found that the titre of IgA anti-lipid A antibody was not raised in any of nine patients with Crohn's disease. Zeitz et al.[59] found complement-fixing haemolytic antibodies against free lipid A in four of 20 healthy individuals and in only three of 27 patients with Crohn's disease[59]. It was thought that these findings of low or reduced concentrations of anti-lipid A antibody may reflect consumption of the antibodies due to increased invasion of bacterial antigen[59,88].

T cell clones reactive to lipopolysaccharide

Circulating and gut-derived lymphocyte populations from patients with IBD have an increased proliferation when exposed to lipopolysaccharides[90].

CD14 positive immune cells in intestinal wall

Intestinal inflammation in IBD is characterized by an influx of large numbers of CD14-positive neutrophils and monocytes[53,91,92]. The persistence of CD14 positivity in these cells suggests that these cells continue to be exposed to translocating endotoxin.

Colonic expression of bactericidal/permeability-increasing protein (BPI)

BPI competitively binds to the lipid A terminal of LPS and has been shown to inhibit various endotoxin-induced biological effects[93]. Mucosal levels of BPI are increased in patients with both ulcerative colitis and Crohn's disease, which is thought to be a response to endotoxin translocation[93].

CLINICAL SIGNIFICANCE OF SYSTEMIC ENDOTOXAEMIA IN IBD

Assay of circulating endotoxin in animal models and clinical studies of IBD confirms that translocation of endotoxin is a frequent occurrence in the presence of active intestinal inflammation. Antibody studies are more difficult to interpret as there may be both increased production of antibodies against bacterial products (endotoxin, endotoxin-core, lipid A) following exposure to these antigens as well as consumption of these antibodies and rapidly changing levels during active disease[59,69]. However, the weight of the evidence from animal model and clinical studies is that systemic bacterial antigenaemia occurs in IBD. The degree of exposure to bacterial products appears to depend on disease activity (endotoxin, lipid A), disease extent (endotoxin) and the presence of intestinal ulceration (endotoxin).

The next logical question is what this finding of endotoxaemia in IBD means: (a) is it a measure of gut leakiness, (b) does it contribute to intestinal inflammation in IBD or (c) does it contribute to systemic inflammation?

Is endotoxaemia a measure of gut leakiness?

Gut barrier function can be measured by the demonstration of translocation of enteric bacteria (as well as bacterial products) to extraintestinal sites or by showing increased passive penetration of the intestinal barrier by non-charged macromolecules (permeability)[94]. The findings of bacterial translocation, increased intestinal permeability, intestinal protein loss, increased circulating antibodies to enteric bacteria and dietary antigens and increased circulating immune complexes in patients with IBD confirm that there is dysfunction of the gut mucosal barrier[94].

Does endotoxin contribute to the intestinal inflammation?

This question will be addressed by considering what effect luminal or circulating endotoxins have on the intestine:

Effect of endotoxin on the intact intestine

As noted earlier, endotoxins are present in large quantities within the gut. There is no evidence that these bacterial antigens induce intestinal inflammation at physiological concentrations.

Effect of luminal endotoxin on the inflamed intestine

Studies in two experimental models of colitis provide evidence that luminal endotoxin exacerbates intestinal inflammation[66,70]. Høtta *et al.*[70] induced colitis in the rabbit by injection of lipopolysaccharide in Freund's adjuvant into the footpad, followed by further weekly subcutaneous injections for 3 weeks to induce lipopolysaccharide sensitization. The rabbits were then subjected to intra-colonic instillation with 1% formalin and lipopolysaccharide. A colitis developed which was characterized by mucosal petechial haemorrhage and ulceration. Repeat lipopolysaccharide enemas maintained the colitis for over 1 month[70].

Lange *et al.*[66], using the dextran sulphate sodium mouse model of colitis, found that the Lps[n] genotype (indicating sensitivity to lipopolysaccharide) developed earlier-onset and more persistent intestinal bleeding than occurred in Lps[d] mice (hyporesponsive to lipopolysaccharide). Responsiveness to lipopolysaccharide was seen to augment colonic inflammation in response to dextran sulphate sodium.

Effect of circulating endotoxins on the intestinal wall

Parenteral administration of endotoxin to experimental animals results in endothelial cell damage, increased vascular permeability, vascular congestion and microthrombi in the venules and capillaries of the lamina propria of the intestine in association with mucosal necrosis, intestinal bleeding and diarrhoea[95–98].

Using a freeze–fracture technique, Walker and Porvaznik[99] demonstrated a disruption of the tight junctional complexes of the intestinal epithelium in 5% of mice following an intraperitoneal injection of endotoxin. Intravenous administration of endotoxin to experimental animals has also been shown to increase intestinal permeability to $[^{51}Cr]$EDTA[100] and to increase the translocation of viable microbes to mesenteric lymph nodes[101] and systemic blood[102].

A phenomenon analogous to flare-ups in IBD can be induced in rats with PG-PS granulomatous colitis, in which, 20 days after intramural injection of the caecum with PG-PS, intravenous endotoxin injection resulted in a more severe colitis[103]. In human volunteers, administration of a single dose of endotoxin increased intestinal permeability to lactulose and mannitol[104].

Two major lessons emerge from this review of experimental studies. Firstly, luminal and systemically administered endotoxins exacerbate experimental IBD. Secondly, parenterally administered endotoxin produces changes in the intestinal miocrovasculature and increases gut permeability. The finding that endotoxin administration itself can damage the gut mucosal barrier suggests that if sufficient endotoxin enters the systemic circulation, then endotoxaemia can become self-sustaining. Indeed, Caridis *et al.*[105] observed that, following a lethal injection of endotoxin, animals die with more endotoxin in their livers than was injected.

Does endotoxin contribute to the systemic inflammatory response?

It has been suggested that systemic endotoxaemia contributes to disease activity, development of toxic megacolon, abnormalities of liver function and other extraintestinal manifestations of IBD[30,34,35,38]. Certainly endotoxin administration to human volunteers or experimental animals has been shown to cause many of the systemic findings in IBD: fever, tachycardia, chills, release of stress hormones, activation of monocyte/macrophage procoagulant activity and complement system as well as the release of vasoactive amines and platelet-activating factor[106].

There is also some supporting evidence from animal studies. In the dextran sulphate sodium mouse model of colitis, mice sensitive to lipopolysaccharides (Lps^n) have a more severe systemic inflammatory response and higher mortality than those mice who are hyporesponsive[66].

Clinical evidence exists in two forms. First, the positive correlations of systemic endotoxin concentrations with clinical and laboratory indices of disease activity in IBD and with the presence of extraintestinal manifestations in IBD[30,35,38,39,43]. Secondly, a reduction in systemic endotoxaemia is associated with: (a) resolution of the disease process[30,38,40,41], (b) restoration to normal of plasma protein and serum iron concentrations[38,72], and (c) reduction in the indices of disease activity[38]. However, the decline in systemic endotoxin concentrations in association with an improvement in clinical and laboratory features may be due to intestinal healing and restitution of the gut mucosal barrier.

CONCLUSIONS

Translocation of endotoxin and other bacterial products does occur in IBD. These bacterial products exacerbate but do not initiate the intestinal inflammation. Systemic bacterial antigenaemia is likely to contribute to the systemic inflammatory response and extraintestinal manifestations associated with IBD. In view of the close and prolonged contact between luminal endotoxin and denuded mucosa, it is surprising that systemic sepsis occurs so rarely. This suggests that these patients have some degree of tolerance to translocating bacterial products. Tolerance to endotoxin is known to occur in experimental animals in response to repeated injections with loss of physiological and cytokine responses[107]. However, the mechanisms of LPS tolerance are not yet known. One might speculate that the increased production of anti-endotoxin core and anti-lipid A antibodies[37,43,81,83,84,87], the increased concentrations of endotoxin-binding mucosal and circulating proteins[93,108], and the down-regulation of CD14-positive macrophages to lipopolysaccharide[109] contribute to this endotoxin tolerance.

These conclusions provide a rationale to support additional therapy for patients with IBD with the aim of reducing the luminal load of bacteria and bacterial products. Systemic endotoxaemia has been successfully reduced in experimental models of IBD using enteral adsorbents, lactulose, paromomycin, glutamine[65,67,110,111] and parenteral taurolidine[110]. In clinical studies a combination of whole-gut lavage with saline and oral 5-aminosalicylic acid cleared LPS more rapidly in patients with active Crohn's disease in association with a more rapid resolution of the disease process[40].

Acknowledgements

My interest in this subject was stimulated and encouraged by Professor Brian J. Rowlands, Professor of Gastrointestinal Surgery, University of Nottingham. I would also like to acknowledge Dr Isla Halliday, lecturer in surgery, the Queen's University of Belfast, for her comments and suggestions on this chapter, as well as for her part in the design, execution and publication of our studies of the role of gut-derived endotoxins in inflammatory bowel disease.

References

1. Sartor RB. Current concepts of the etiology and pathogenesis of ulcerative colitis and Crohn's disease. Gastroenterol Clin N Am. 1995;24:475–507.
2. Elson CO, Sartor RB, Tennyson GS, Riddell RH. Experimental models of inflammatory bowel disease. Gastroenterology. 1995;109:1344–67.
3. Sartor RB. Microbial factors in the pathogenesis of Crohn's disease, ulcerative colitis, and experimental intestinal inflammation. In: Kirsner JB, Shorter RG, editors. Inflammatory Bowel Disease, 4th edn. Baltimore: Williams & Wilkins; 1995:96–124.
4. Sartor RB. Role of the enteric microflora in the pathogenesis of intestinal inflammation and arthritis. Aliment Pharmacol Ther. 1997;11 (Suppl. 3):17–23.
5. Gorbach SL. How the intestinal microflora causes inflammation in the gastrointestinal tract. In: Tytgat GNJ, Bartelsman JFWM, van Deventer SJH, editors. Inflammatory Bowel Diseases. Falk Symposium 85. Lancaster: Kluwer; 1995:556–60.
6. Seneca H, Henderson E. Normal intestinal bacteria in ulcerative colitis. Gastroenterology. 1950;15:34–9.
7. Keighley MRB, Arabi Y, Dimock F, Burdon DW, Allan RN, Alexander-Williams J. Influence of inflammatory bowel disease on the intestinal microflora. Gut. 1978;19:1099–104.
8. Dickinson RJ, Varian SA, Axon ATR, Cooke EM. Increased incidence of faecal coliforms with *in-vitro* adhesive and invasive properties in patients with ulcerative colitis. Gut. 1980;21:787–92.
9. Fabia R, Rajab AA, Johansson M-L *et al*. Impairment of bacterial flora in human ulcerative colitis and experimental colitis in the rat. Digestion. 1993;54:248–55.
10. Hartley MG, Hudson MJ, Swarbrick ET *et al*. The rectal mucosa-associated microflora in patients with ulcerative colitis. J Med Microbiol. 1992;36:96–103.
11. Bourgault A-M, Rosenblatt JE, Fitzgerald RH. *Peptococcus magnus*: a significant human pathogen. Ann Intern Med. 1980;93:244–8.
12. Wensinck F, Custers-van Lieshout LMC, Poppelaars-Kustermans PAJ, Schröder AM. The faecal flora of patients with Crohn's disease. J Hyg. 1981;87:1–12.
13. Ambrose NS, Young D, Burdon DW, Keighley MRB. Changes in intestinal flora in Crohn's disease. Br J Surg. 1982;69:681.
14. Giaffer MH, Holdsworth CD, Duerden BI. The assessment of faecal flora in patients with inflammatory bowel disease by a simplified bacteriological technique. J Med Microbiol. 1991;35:238–43.
15. Favier C, Neut C, Mizon C, Cortot A, Colombel JF, Mizon J. Fecal beta-d-galactosidase production and Bifidobacteria are decreased in Crohn's disease. Dig Dis Sci. 1997;42:817–22.
16. Gorbach SL, Nahas L, Plaut AG, Weinstein L, Patterson JF, Levitan R. Studies of intestinal microflora. V. Fecal microbial ecology in ulcerative colitis and regional enteritis: relationship to severity of disease and chemotherapy. Gastroenterology. 1968;54:575–87.
17. Burke DA, Axon AT. Adhesive *Escherichia coli* in inflammatory bowel disease and infective diarrhoea. Br Med J. 1988;297:102–4.
18. Hartley MG, Hudson MJ, Swarbrick ET, Gent AE, Hellier MD, Grace RH. Adhesive and hydrophobic properties of *Escherichia coli* from the rectal mucosa of patients with ulcerative colitis. Gut. 1993;34:63–7.
19. Cooke EM. Properties of strains of *Escherichia coli* isolated from the faeces of patients with ulcerative colitis, patients with acute diarrhoea and normal persons. J Pathol Bacteriol. 1968;95:101–13.
20. Morrison DC, Ryan JC. Endotoxin and disease mechanisms. Annu Rev Med. 1987;38:417–32.
21. Nakaido H, Nakae T. The outer membrane of gram-negative bacteria. Adv Microb Physiol. 1979;20:163–250.
22. Flynn PM, Shenep JL, Gigliotti F, Davis DS, Hildner WK. Immunolabelling of lipopolysaccharide liberated from antibiotic-treated *Escherichia coli*. Infect Immun. 1988;56:2760–2.
23. Hoekstra D, van der Laan JW, de Ly L, Witholt B. Release of outer membrane fragments from normally growing *Escherichia coli*. Biochim Biophys Acta. 1976;455:889–99.

24. Domenico P, Diedrich DL, Straus DC. Extracellular polysaccharide production by *Klebsiella pneumoniae* and its relationship to virulence. Can J Microbiol. 1985;31:472–8.
25. Rietschel ET, Schade U, Jensen M, Wollenweber H-W, Luderitz O, Greisman SG. Bacterial endotoxins: chemical structure, biological activity and role in septicaemia. Scand J Infect Dis. 1982 (Suppl. 31):8–21.
26. Couturier C, Haeffner-Cavaillon N, Caroff M, Kazatchkine MD. Binding sites for endotoxins (lipopolysaccharides) on human monocytes. J Immunol. 1991;147:1899–1904.
27. Schumann RR, Leong SR, Flaggs GW *et al.* Structure and function of lipopolysaccharide binding protein. Science. 1990;249:1429–31.
28. Martin TR, Mathison JC, Tobias PS *et al.* Lipopolysaccharide binding protein enhances the responsiveness of alveolar macrophages to bacterial lipopolysaccharide. J Clin Invest. 1992;90:2209–19.
29. Tai C, Tanaka S. Endotoxemia and clinical severity in ulcerative colitis. Geka. 1974;36:655–70.
30. Aoki K. A study of endotoxaemia in ulcerative colitis and Crohn's disease. I. Clinical Study. Acta Med Okayama. 1978;32:147–58.
31. Aoki K. A study of endotoxemia in ulcerative colitis and Crohn's disease. II. Experimental study. Acta Med Okayama. 1978;32:207–16.
32. Jacob AI, Goldberg PK, Bloom N, Degenshein GA, Kozinn PJ. Endotoxin and bacteria in portal blood. Gastroenterology. 1977;72:1268–70.
33. Auer IO, Wechsler W, Ziemer E, Malchow H, Sommer H. Immune status in Crohn's disease. 1. Leukocyte and lymphocyte subpopulations in peripheral blood. Scand J Gastroenterol. 1978;13:561–71.
34. Liehr H. The *Limulus* assay for endotoxaemia as applied in gastroenterology. In: Cohen E, editor. Biomedical Applications of the Horseshoe Crab (Limulidae). New York: Liss; 1979;309–20.
35. Colin R, Grancher T, Lemeland J-F *et al.* Recherche d'une endotoxinemie dans les enterocolites inflammatoires cryptogenetiques. Gastroenterol Clin Biol. 1979;3:15–19.
36. Palmer KR, Duerden BI, Holdsworth CD. Bacteriological and endotoxin studies in cases of ulcerative colitis submitted to surgery. Gut. 1980;21:851–4.
37. Kruis W, Schussler P, Weinzierl M, Galanos C, Eisenburg J. Circulating lipid A antibodies despite absence of systemic endotoxemia in patients with Crohn's disease. Dig Dis Sci. 1984;29:502–7.
38. Wellmann W, Fink PC, Schmidt FW. Whole-gut irrigation as anti-endotoxinaemic therapy in inflammatory bowel disease. Hepatogastroenterology. 1984;31:91–3.
39. Wellmann W, Fink PC, Benner F. Endotoxinamie bei entzundlichen Darmerkrankungen. Verh Ges Inn Med. 1984;90:827–9.
40. Wellmann W, Fink PC, Benner F, Schmidt FW. Endotoxaemia in active Crohn's disease. Treatment with whole gut irrigation and 5-aminosalicylic acid. Gut. 1986;27:814–20.
41. Fink PC, Suin de Boutemard C, Haeckel R, Wellmann W. Endotoxaemia in patients with Crohn's disease: a longitudinal study of elastase/a1-proteinase inhibitor and *Limulus*–amoebocyte–lysate reactivity. J Clin Chem Clin Biochem. 1988;26:117–22.
42. Busch J, Hammer M, Brunkhorst R, Wagner P. Endotoxinbestimmung bei entzundlich-rheumatischen Erkrankungen – Der einflusss nichtsteroidaler antiphlogistika auf die darmpermeabilitat. Z Rheumatol. 1988;47:156–60.
43. Gardiner KR, Halliday MI, Barclay GR *et al.* The significance of systemic endotoxaemia in inflammatory bowel disease. Gut. 1995;36:897–901.
44. Sonesson A, Larsson L, Andersson R, Adner N, Tranberg K-G. Use of two-dimensional gas chromatography with electron-capture detection for the measurement of lipopolysaccharides in peritoneal fluid and plasma from rats with induced peritonitis. J Clin Microbiol. 1990;28:1163–8.
45. Wessels BC, Gaffin SL, Wells MT. Circulating plasma endotoxin (lipopolysaccharide) concentrations in healthy and hemorrhagic enteric dogs: antiendotoxin immunotherapy in hemorrhagic enteric endotoxemia. J Am Anim Hosp Assoc. 1987;23:291–5.
46. van Deventer SJH, ten Cate JW, Tytgat GNJ. Intestinal endotoxemia. Clinical significance. Gastroenterology. 1988;94:825–31.
47. Fink PC, Lehr L, Urbaschek RM, Kozak J. *Limulus*–amoebocyte–lysate test for endotoxemia: investigations with a femtogram sensitive spectrophotometric assay. Klin Wochenschr. 1981;59:213–18.
48. Iwanaga S, Morita T, Harada T. Chromogenic substrate for horseshoe crab clotting enzyme. Its application for the assay of bacterial endotoxin. Haemostasis. 1978;7:183–8.

49. Bowen GE, Kirsner JB. Positive epinephrine skin test for 'circulating endotoxin' in inflammatory disease of the intestine. Am J Clin Pathol. 1965;44:642–7.

50. Gilbert AP, Ravelo GZ. Serum proteins and endotoxins in chronic ulcerative colitis. Dis Colon Rectum. 1968;11:124–6.

51. Juhlin L, Krause U, Shelley WB. Endotoxin-induced microclots in ulcerative colitis and Crohn's disease. Scand J Gastroenterol. 1980;15:311–14.

52. Barclay GR. Endogenous endotoxin-core antibody (EndoCAb) as a marker of endotoxin exposure and a prognostic indicator: a review. In: Levin J, Alving CR, Munford RS, Redl H, editors. Bacterial Endotoxins: Lipopolysacharides from genes to therapy. Proceedings of the 3rd Conference of the International Endotoxin Society. New York: Wiley; 1995;263–72.

53. Wozniak A, Van der Pol E, Doe WF. Inflammatory macrophages but not resident macrophages express membrane-bound CD14, a receptor for lipopolysaccharide in a mouse model of ulcerative colitis. Gastroenterology. 1995;108:A944.

54. Nolan JP. The role of intestinal endotoxins in gastrointestinal and liver diseases. In: van Deventer SJ, Sturk A, editors. Bacterial Endotoxins: Pathophysiological effects, clinical significance and pharmacological control. New York: Liss; 1988;147–59.

55. Emody L, Ralovich B, Barna K, Brasch G, Ternak G. Physiological effect of orally administered endotoxin to man. J Hyg Epidem Microb Immun. 1974;4:454–8.

56. Seidman E, Walker WA. Intestinal defenses. In: Kirsner JB; Shorter RG, editors. Inflammatory Bowel Disease. Philadelphia, PA: Lea & Febiger;1988:65–74.

57. Brearley S, Harris RI, Stone P, Keighley MRB. Endotoxin in portal blood – is it normal? Gut. 1984;25:A1178.

58. Mattsby-Baltzer I, Alving CR. Antibodies to Lipid A: occurrence in humans. Rev Infect Dis. 1984;6:553–7.

59. Zeitz M, Hopf U, Wust B et al. Absence of complement fixing antibodies against lipopolysaccharides from *Escherichia coli* in a subgroup of patients with Crohn's disease. Gut. 1987;28:1460–6.

60. Wilkinson SP, Moodie H, Stamatakis JD, Kakkar VV, Williams R. Endotoxaemia and renal failure in cirrhosis and obstructive jaundice. Br Med J. 1976;2:1415–18.

61. Ravin HA, Rowley D, Jenkins C, Fine J. On the absorption of bacterial endotoxin from the gastrointestinal tract of the normal and shocked animal. J Exp Med. 1960;112:783–92.

62. Daniele R, Singh H, Appert HE, Pairent FW, Howard JM. Lymphatic absorption of intraperitoneal endotoxin in the dog. Surgery. 1970;67:484–7.

63. Gardiner KR. Systemic endotoxaemia in inflammatory bowel disease and experimental colitis (MD thesis). Belfast: Queen's University; 1993.

64. Brand HS, Maas MAW, Bosma A et al. Experimental colitis in rats induces low-grade endotoxinemia without hepatobiliary abnormalities. Dig Dis Sci. 1994;39:1210–15.

65. Fujita T, Sakurai K. Efficacy of glutamine-enriched enteral nutrition in an experimental model of mucosal ulcerative colitis. Br J Surg. 1995;82:749–51.

66. Lange S, Delbro DS, Jennische E, Mattsby-Baltzer I. The role of the Lps gene in experimental ulcerative colitis in mice. APMIS. 1996;104:823–33.

67. Gardiner KR, Anderson NH, McCaigue MD, Erwin PJ, Halliday MI, Rowlands BJ. Adsorbents as anti-endotoxin agents in experimental colitis. Gut. 1993;34:51–5.

68. Gardiner KR, Anderson NH, Rowlands BJ, Barbul A. Colitis and colonic mucosal barrier dysfunction. Gut. 1995;37:530–5.

69. Neilly PJD, Gardiner KR, Kirk SJ et al. Endotoxaemia and cytokine production in experimental inflammatory bowel disease. Br J Surg. 1995;82:1479–82.

70. Høtta T, Yoshida N, Yoshikawa T, Sugino S, Kondo M. Lipopolysaccharide-induced colitis in rabbits. Res Exp Med. 1986;186:61–9.

71. Brandwein SI, McCabe RP, Dadrat A et al. Immunologic reactivity of colitis C3H/HeJBir mice to enteric bacteria. Gastroenterology. 1994;106:A656.

72. Kirkin BV, Fomin SA, Ivanov AF et al. Efficiency of hemosorption in treatment of patients with ulcerative colitis. Biomater Artif Cells Artif Org. 1987;15:271–9.

73. Kirkin BV. Hemosorption as part of combined treatment for nonspecific ulcerative colitis. Sov Med. 1988;3:7–10.

74. Kelley CJ, Ingoldby CJII, Blenkharn JI, Wood CB. Colonoscopy related endotoxemia. Surg Gynecol Obstet. 1985;161:332–4.

75. Kiss A, Ferenci P, Graninger W, Pamperl H, Potzi R, Meryn S. Endotoxaemia following colonoscopy. Endoscopy. 1983;15:24–6.

76. Baldassano RN, Schreiber S, Johnston RB, Fu RD, Muraki T, MacDermott RP. Crohn's disease monocytes are primed for accentuated release of toxic oxygen metabolites. Gastroenterology. 1993;105:60–6.
77. Engström L, Törngren S, Rohdin-Alm C. Peroperative endotoxin concentrations in portal and peripheral venous blood in patients undergoing right hemicolectomy for carcinoma. Eur J Surg. 1992;158:301–5.
78. Liao W, Lindgren S, Lindhagen T, Starck M, Florén CH. Plasma endotoxin in patients with quiescent Crohn's disease. J Intern Med. 1992;232:371–7.
79. Warshaw AL, Bellini CA, Walker WA. The intestinal mucosal barrier to intact antigenic protein. Difference between colon and small intestine. Am J Surg. 1977;13:55–8.
80. Gardiner KR, Rowlands BJ, Maxwell RJ, Barclay GR. Intestinal permeability. Gut. 1995;37:589.
81. Marget W, Schüßler P, Kruis W, Weinzierl M, Rindfleisch G. Is the pathogenesis of Crohn's disease similar to that of juvenile recurrent pyelonephritis? Infection. 1976;4:110–12.
82. Marget W, Schüssler P. Lipopolysaccharides in Crohn's disease. Lancet. 1976;2:97.
83. Schüßler P, Kruis W, Marget W. Lipoid-A-Antikörpertiter und O-Antikörpertiter bei enterocolitis Crohn, colitis ulcerosa und akuter enteritis. Med Klin. 1976;71:1898–902.
84. Schüßler P, Kruis W, Marget W. Lipoid-A-Antikörpertiter bei Morbus Crohn. Klin Wochenschr. 1976;54:1055–6.
85. Ramadori G, Hopf U, Galanos C, Eckardt R, Meyer zum Büschenfelde KH. Studies of circulating antibodies against lipid A in patients with chronic diseases of liver and gut. Hepatogastroenterology. 1980 (Suppl.): 305.
86. Kruis W, Schussler P, Weinzierl M. Circulating lipid A antibodies and their relationship to different clinical conditions of patients with Crohn's disease. Hepatogastroenterology. 1987;34:123–6.
87. Oriishi T, Sata M, Toyonaga A, Sasaki E, Tanikawa K. Evaluation of intestinal permeability in patients with inflammatory bowel disease using lactulose and measuring antibodies to lipid A. Gut. 1995;36:891–6.
88. Mattsby-Baltzer I, Fasth A, Jaup B, Kaijser B, Nilsson LÅ. Studies of antibodies to lipid A and Tamm-Horsfall in patients with inflammatory bowel disease. Scand J Gastroenterol. 1983;18:305–11.
89. Nolan JP, DeLissio MG, Camara DS, Feind DM, Gagliardi NC. IgA antibody to lipid A in alcoholic liver disease. Lancet. 1986;1:176–9.
90. Fiocchi C, Battisto J, Farmer R. Studies on isolated gut mucosal lymphocytes in inflammatory bowel disease. Detection of activated T-cells and enhanced proliferation to Staphylococcus aureus and lipopolysaccharides. Dig Dis Sci. 1981;26:728–36.
91. Grimm MC, Pavli P, van de Pol E, Doe WF. Evidence for a CD14+ population of monocytes in inflammatory bowel disease mucosa – implications for pathogenesis. Clin Exp Immunol. 1995;100:291–7.
92. Grimm MC, Pullman WE, Bennett GM, Sullivan PJ, Pavli P, Doe WF. Direct evidence of monocyte recruitment to inflammatory bowel disease mucosa. J Gastroenterol Hepatol. 1995;10:387–95.
93. Monajemi H, Meenan J, Lamping R et al. Inflammatory bowel disease is associated with increased mucosal levels of bactericidal/permeability-increasing protein. Gastroenterology. 1996;110:733–9.
94. Gardiner KR. Intestinal permeability in inflammatory bowel disease. In: Blum HE, Bode Ch, Bode JCh, Sartor RB, editors. Gut and the Liver. Falk Symposium 100. Lancaster: Kluwer; 1998:61–74.
95. Hsueh W, González-Crussi F, Arroyave JL. Platelet-activating factor: an endogenous mediator for bowel necrosis in endotoxemia. FASEB. 1987;1:403–5.
96. Mathan VI, Penny GR, Matn MM, Rowley D. Bacterial lipopolysaccharide-induced intestinal microvascular lesions leading to acute diarrhea. J Clin Invest. 1988;82:1714–21.
97. Hutcheson IR, Whittle BJ, Boughton-Smith NK. Role of nitric oxide in maintaining vascular integrity in endotoxin-induced acute intestinal damage in the rat. Br J Pharmacol. 1990;101:815–20.
98. Ciancio MJ, Vittiritti L, Dhar A, Chang EB. Endotoxin-induced alterations in rat colonic water and electrolyte transport. Gastroenterology. 1992;103:1437–43.
99. Walker RI, Porvaznik MJ. Disruption of the permeability barrier (zonula occludens) between intestinal epithelial cells by lethal doses of endotoxin. Infect Immun. 1978;21:655–8.

100. Fink MP, Antonsson JB, Wang H, Rothschild HR. Increased intestinal permeability in endo-toxic pigs. Arch Surg. 1991;126:211–18.
101. Deitch EA, Berg R, Specian R. Endotoxin promotes the translocation of bacteria for the gut. Arch Surg. 1987;122:185–90.
102. Souba WW, Herskowitz K, Klimberg VS *et al*. The effects of sepsis and endotoxemia on gut glutamine metabolism. Ann Surg. 1990;211:543–51.
103. Green KD, Sartor RB. Systemic lipopolysaccharide reactivates peptidoglycan–polysaccharide-induced intestinal inflammation in rats. Gastroenterology. 1988;94:A154.
104. O'Dwyer ST, Michie HR, Ziegler TR, Revhaug A, Smith RJ, Wilmore DW. A single dose of endotoxin increases intestinal permeability in healthy humans. Arch Surg. 1988;123:1459–64.
105. Caridis DT, Reinhold RB, Woodruff PWH, Fine J. Endotoxaemia in man. Lancet. 1972;2:1381–6.
106. Sturk A, van Deventer SJH, Wortel CH *et al*. Detection and clinical relevance of human endo-toxaemia. Z Med Lab Diagn. 1990;31:147–58.
107. Erroi A, Fantuzzi G, Mengozzi M *et al*. Differential regulation of cytokine production in lipopolysaccharide tolerance in mice. Infect Immun. 1993;61:4356–9.
108. Erwin PJ, Lewis H, Schumann RR, Gardiner KR, Halliday MI. The role of lipopolysaccharide binding protein in acute and chronic inflammation. J Endotoxin Res. 1996;3:21.
109. Rugtveit J, Nilsen EM, Bakka A, Carlsen H, Brandtzaeg P, Scott H. Cytokine profiles differ in newly recruited and resident subsets of mucosal macrophages from inflammatory bowel disease. Gastroenterology. 1997;112:1493–505.
110. Gardiner KR, Anderson NH, McCaigue MD, Erwin PJ, Halliday MI, Rowlands BJ. Enteral and parenteral antiendotoxin treatment in experimental colitis. Hepato-Gastroenterology. 1994;41:554–8.
111. Gardiner KR, Erwin PJ, Anderson NH, McCaigue MD, Halliday MI, Rowlands BJ. Lactulose as an anti-endotoxin agent in experimental colitis. Br J Surg. 1995;82:469–72.

Section VII
Diagnosis of IBD

24
Radiological investigation of IBD

K. HAUENSTEIN and C. SCHULZE

INTRODUCTION

Patients with inflammatory bowel disease (IBD) require prompt diagnosis and management, both to relieve their symptoms and to minimize potential complications. Until recently, ulcerative colitis (UC) and Crohn's disease (CD) were the two inflammatory bowel disorders most often diagnosed radiographically in central Europe. Increased global travel and immigration from developing countries as well as immunosuppression as a result of chemotherapy or acquired immunodeficiency syndrome (AIDS) have led to more widespread occurrence of enteritis and colitis. These disorders often simulate the clinical and radiological features of idiopathic inflammation of the gut[1]. Indeed, the number of possible enteric pathogens seems to expand each year, further complicating the diagnosis of various types of enterocolitis. Radiological studies are not usually the sole decisive examination in these patients, but they can play a crucial role in determining the initial site and extent of intestinal involvement, therapeutic response and follow-up of complications[2]. This chapter reviews the radiological approach to patients with IBD and provides differential diagnostic guidelines.

DIAGNOSTIC IMAGING TECHNIQUES

Abdominal plain film

Radiological evaluation of patients with suspected inflammatory processes affecting the alimentary tract typically begins with a plain abdominal film in the supine position[3]. Upright or decubitus views are obtained if there is the possibility of an obstructive process or perforation. The diagnostic yield of plain radiographs of the abdomen is 10% or less in terms of positive findings of clinical relevance[4]. Nevertheless, plain film of the abdomen can be most useful in establishing the diagnosis of toxic megacolon, intestinal infarction and bowel obstruction or perforation.

The calibre and mural thickness of the gut, mucosal fold pattern and haustral markings, and the intraluminal content of gas or faecal residue should be carefully evaluated on all plain abdominal films. Ancillary findings, such as nephrolithiasis, cholelithiasis, ankylosing spondylitis, sacroiliitis, and avascular necrosis of femoral heads, may be seen as important clues to the diagnosis of UC or CD.

Barium enema

Fluoroscopic evaluation of the colon during its opacification with contrast material is the principal radiological method of the detection of IBD. Barium enema, however, should not be used in suspected cases of fulminant colitis or toxic megacolon because of the inherent risk of perforation with intraperitoneal leakage of barium. Furthermore, the presence of barium in the colon may interfere with subsequent colonoscopy and the ability to obtain stool samples for culture.

Double-contrast colon examination is more accurate than the conventional barium enema for demonstrating subtle changes, such as mucosal granularity and superficial ulcerations; hence, it can detect both the presence and the extent of inflammatory processes much earlier. Double-contrast enema is the method of choice in patients who can tolerate adequate cleansing of their colon, whereas solid column barium enemas are more appropriate for debilitated patients in whom prompt diagnosis of gross bowel abnormalities is desired.

Computed tomography

Over the past decade, computed tomography (CT) has emerged as one of the most important imaging techniques for the evaluation of patients with gastro-intestinal disorders[5]. Although CT cannot depict mucosa of the gut with the same detail as colonoscopy or double-contrast radiography, it does offer several major advantages. It is non-invasive and accurate for detecting the intramural and intraperitoneal extent of intestinal involvement. The excellent soft-tissue discrimination of CT permits morphological evaluation of the bowel wall, its mesentery, peritoneal surfaces and adjacent organs. Therefore, CT is the recommended imaging procedure after the plain abdominal film for the evaluation of the following disorders: intra-abdominal abscesses, mesenteric ischaemia, bowel obstruction, typhlitis, pneumatosis, intestinal perforation, diverticulitis, and complicated appendicitis[6]. A complete survey of the abdomen and pelvis can be achieved in approximately 15 min with a minimum of patient preparation and cooperation. Whenever possible, both intravenous and oral contrast material are administered to enhance the visibility of bowel loops and mural vascularity. On CT, normal bowel wall measures 3–5 mm in thickness when the lumen is adequately distended. Most inflammatory processes cause mural thickening that appears to be homogeneous or shows a multilayered target sign owing to low density in the submucosa secondary to fat deposition or oedema. Segmental or diffuse circumferential thickening of the inflamed wall up to 20 mm may be seen, depending on the severity of the colitis[5].

Ultrasonography

Ultrasonography has become the initial cross-sectioning imaging procedure of choice in most cases of acute appendicitis and cholecystitis. Its applications are less clearly defined in the assessment of other infectious and inflammatory disorders of the abdomen. Nevertheless, intestinal pathology may be identified during screening abdominal sonography and prompt further investigation with CT, barium examination or endoscopy. Abnormal bowel wall as a result of infection or inflammation is typically thickened and may be homogeneous in echogenicity or show stratification. Real-time ultrasound imaging usually shows absent or diminished peristalsis of the involved segments owing to its rigidity from oedema or inflammation[7].

Magnetic resonance imaging

Magnetic resonance (MR) imaging has not been widely used for the evaluation of infectious and inflammatory disease of the gut because of artifacts caused by respiratory motion and peristalsis, inadequate intraluminal contrast agents and prolonged imaging times. Studies using fast pulse sequences and intravenous contrast agents (Gd-DTPA) have shown good correlation between MR findings and histopathological results in terms of bowel wall thickness, length of diseased colon, and severity of involvement in patients with inflammatory bowel disease[8]. Also, MR can display the course and extent of fistulas and sinus tracts in the sagittal and coronal as well as the standard axial plane[9]. At the present time, however, this technique offers relatively minor practical value for the evaluation of acute gastrointestinal inflammation.

Scintigraphy

Radionuclide scanning with indium-111-labelled leukocytes has proved useful in localizing the extent of inflammatory bowel disease in patients with fulminant colitis, in whom barium enema and colonoscopy may be contraindicated. Labelled white cells migrate to areas of active inflammation, including the intestinal mucosa of patients with active IBD. By demonstrating small bowel involvement in acutely ill patients with IBD, this scintigraphic method can assist in the different diagnosis of Crohn's disease from ulcerative colitis[10].

ULCERATIVE COLITIS

Ulcerative colitis is an inflammatory disease of unknown origin that primarily involves the colorectal mucosa but may later extend to other layers of the bowel wall. This disease is often manifested by an acute fulminating course associated with explosive diarrhoea, haematochezia and hypotension. In many instances, however, the inflammation becomes chronic in nature with intermittent periods of exacerbation.

Plain film features

Although the extent of UC is generally assessed by colonoscopy and barium enema, these procedures carry a significant risk of bowel perforation in severely ill patients. Considerable information can be gained from abdominal radiographs in such cases, however. The following plain film findings can be used to assess the severity and extent of the colitis: the amount and location of faecal residue, the appearance of the mucosal margins, the width and number of visible haustra, colonic calibre and thickness of colorectal wall. The presence of faecal residue provides a clue to the extent of the colitis. If no faecal residue is seen, the patient probably has an active pancolitis. If the residue extends down into the sigmoid colon, a limited proctitis is more likely. As a general rule, faecal residue is noted only proximal to the inflamed segment of the colon.

In active colitis, the colonic mucosal edge on plain films may be granular, indistinct or disrupted rather than having its normal smooth appearance. Only oedematous mucosal islands remain when there is extensive ulceration. Mottled-appearing intramural gas shadows indicate either extremely deep ulceration or transmural perforation with entrapped gas in pericolic soft tissues.

Widening of the haustral markings greater than 5–6 mm is an early manifestation of bowel wall oedema in UC; it is often more obvious on plain films than the mucosal granularity or ulceration it accompanies. Haustral thickness should be assessed only when there is an adequate amount of air in the colon because appearance of such markings may be misleading if the colon is collapsed or incompletely distended. Furthermore, the distal half of the colon may normally have decreased haustration, particularly among elderly patients with atonic or redundant colons.

The calibre of the air-filled colon, as seen on plain films, can provide a clue to the diagnosis of colitis. The diameter of the normal transverse colon is less than 5.5 cm. In chronic, burned-out UC, the colon becomes tubular and narrowed. In patients with fulminant colitis, a diameter greater than 6–7 cm suggests toxic megacolon with risk of perforation. Mural thickness can also be assessed by measuring the distance between the pericolic fat line and gas-filled lumen. Normally, it is less than 3–5 mm but can increase to more than 10 mm in chronic ulcerative or granulomatous colitis[11].

Barium enema features

In patients with known or suspected UC, barium enema is performed to confirm the clinical diagnosis, assess the extent and severity of disease, differentiate UC from CD and other colitides, follow the course of disease, and detect complications.

The earliest barium enema findings in UC are a granular mucosal pattern often accompanied by blunted haustral folds. The smooth, featureless mucosa seen on normal double-contrast colon examinations is replaced by a diffusely granular surface. With progressive disease, mucosal stippling can be observed. This stippling is caused by punctate barium collections filling crypt of Lieberkühn abscesses. As the ulcers of the crypt abscess breach the lamina propria and muscularis mucosae, they cause undermining of the less-resistant areolar tissue of the submucosa. The involved submucosa becomes necrotic, and the ulcers extend laterally causing further undermining, contained by the muscularis propria on the serosal side and by the muscularis mucosae on the lumen side of the colon. Initially the mucosal defect is small relative to the degree of undermining and produces a flask-like collar-button ulcer. As these ulcers enlarge and interconnect, the collar-button configuration is lost, and a network of residual islands of mucosa is produced. This inflamed oedematous mucosa protrudes above the surrounding areas of ulceration and gives a polypoid appearance. These are termed inflammatory pseudopolyps because they represent inflamed and swollen mucosa rather than new growths[11].

Ultrasound and computed tomography features

Inflammation limited to the colonic mucosa is not recognizable on cross-sectional imaging. When the bowel wall becomes oedematous, there is apparent mural thickening with preservation of mural stratification. The sonographic architecture of the different mural layers produces a target appearance, with mucosa, lamina propria and submucosa being echogenic and musculous mucosae and muscularis propria being hypoechoic. A similar target appearance can be seen on CT examinations of patients with chronic UC who have mural thickening and lumen narrowing. There is an inner ring of soft-tissue density; a middle ring of low attenuation resulting from widening and fatty infiltration of the submucosa; and a peripheral soft-tissue-density ring representing the muscularis propria. This target or double halo sign is not specific for UC; it has also been reported in CD, radiation enteritis, ischaemic colitis, infectious colitis, pseudomembranous colitis, and mesenteric venous thrombosis. Thinning of the colonic wall and luminal distension in toxic megacolon can be demonstrated on CT. Pneumatosis coli is more clearly visible on CT than on plain radiography or conventional barium studies[5,8].

CROHN'S DISEASE

Plain film features

Radiographic findings of small bowel obstruction can be seen in patients with CD. It is uncommon, however, to visualize the stenotic segment on plain film, but the dilated loops proximal to or between stenotic areas can be seen. When confined to the colon, CD has plain-film features similar to UC. An extended gas-filled stricture of the colon is suggestive of granulomatous colitis but it can also be present in carcinoma, healing ischaemic colitis and UC.

Enteroclysis features

The radiological signs of CD are well seen during enteroclysis. Ulceration is a frequent finding and may be seen as discrete ulcers, fissure ulcers, cobblestoning or longitudinal ulcers (Figure 1). Sinus tracks and fistulas are also well shown. Other radiological signs of small-intestinal CD include thickening of the valvulae conniventes, stricture formation, thickened intestinal wall and a right iliac fossa mass. Discontinuity of the disease process may be shown as asymmetry or skip lesions[11].

Barium enema features

The earliest pathological manifestation of CD in the small intestine is alteration of villous morphology with oedema, hyperplasia, clubbing, and inflammatory cell infiltrate, which produces mucosal granularity. This manifestation is frequently coexistent with enlargement of the submucosal lymphoid follicles,

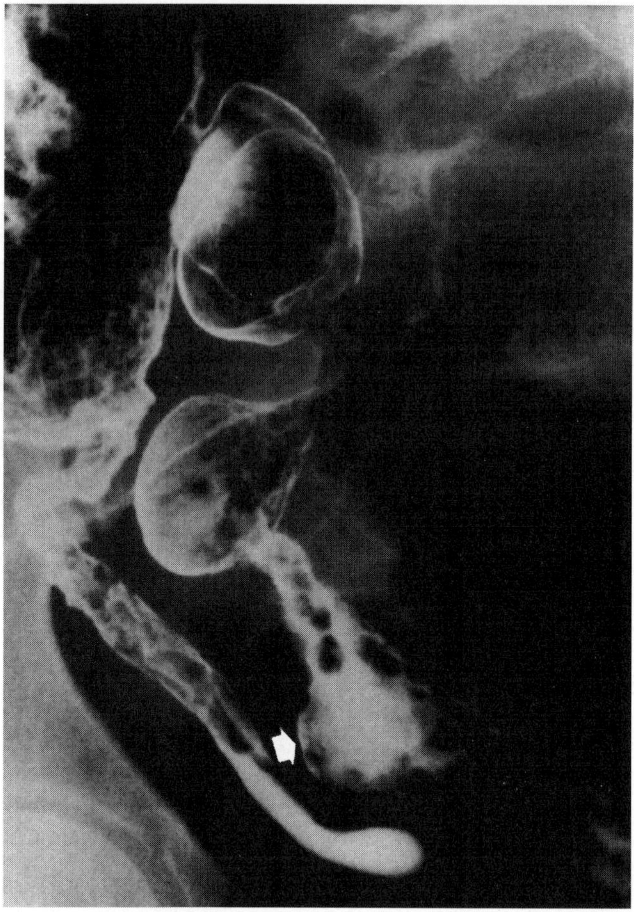

Figure 1 Crohn's disease. Widening of folds in the terminal ileum with granularity and ulcers (arrow). The appendix is also affected

which then cause 3–5-mm mucosal elevations visible on small bowel series. Enlarged lymphoid follicles are also the earliest manifestation of CD. As the lymphoid follicles enlarge, the overlying mucosa may ulcerate to produce the characteristic aphthous lesion. On barium studies, aphthae appear as small superficial collections of barium surrounded by a thin radiolucent halo that produces a target or bull's-eye appearance. On double-contrast studies, aphthae may be found scattered throughout the colon, on the edge of more severe disease, or in clusters of different sizes. These lesions are usually set on a background of normal mucosa, in contrast to the fine uniform granularity and ulcerations seen in early UC. Aphthous lesions may regress spontaneously, recur at various intervals or, more commonly, enlarge and deepen. As the aphthae expand, they become irregular in outline and lose their surrounding lucent halo. Adjacent ulcers may coalesce, forming a network of longitudinal linear ulcerations and transverse fissuring with oedematous intervening mucosa producing a raised cobblestone pattern[11].

Ultrasound features

The bowel wall thickening, caused by transmural inflammation and ultimately fibrosis in CD, is manifested sonographically as an eccentric target pattern with a wall thickness ranging from 0.5 to 1.8 cm. Involved segments show loss of mural stratification, appear rigid and poorly compressible, and show diminished or absent peristalsis on real-time ultrasound studies[7,8].

Computed tomography features

CT has had a dramatic impact on the management of patients with acute complications of CD. The palpation of an abdominal mass or separation of bowel loops on a small bowel study in these patients evokes a large differential diagnosis with significantly different prognostic and therapeutic implications: abscess, phlegmon, creeping fat or fibrofatty proliferation of the mesentery, thickening of the bowel wall, and enlarged mesenteric lymph nodes (Figure 2). CT can readily differentiate these extraluminal complications.

On CT, involved segments of gut show mural thickening ranging from 1.0 to 2.0 cm. The thickened bowel may have a homogeneous density or less frequently an inhomogeneous appearance. The target or double halo appearance may be due to oedema or fat in the submucosa. The sharp interface between bowel and mesentery is lost in creeping fat of the mesentery, and the attenuation value of this fat is elevated owing to the influx of inflammatory cells and fluid. With more severe disease, a phlegmon or abscess may form. Intra-abdominal

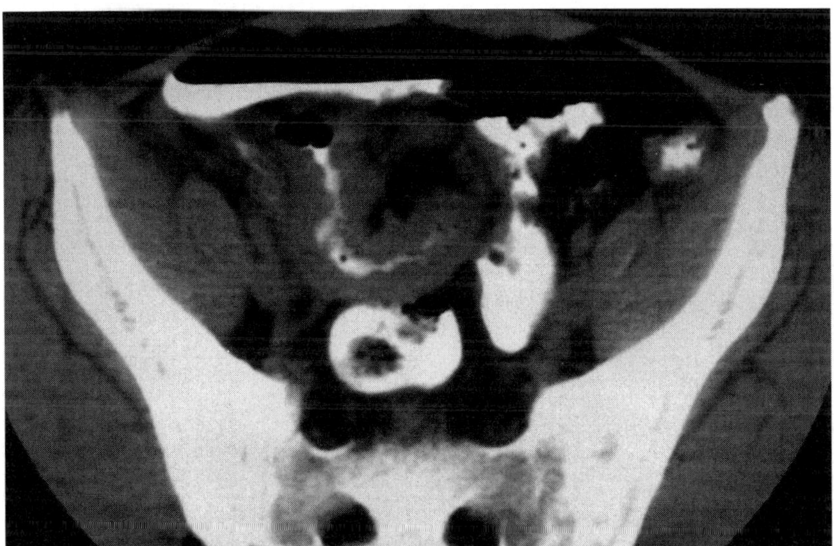

Figure 2   Markedly thickened small bowel wall on CT of patient with Crohn's disease

abscesses develop in about 15–20% of patients with Crohn's enteritis or ileo-colitis but are rare when only the colon is involved. Abscesses appear as circum-scribed, round or oval soft-tissue masses with a thick capsule often showing contrast enhancement, whereas the central area containing pus or necrotic mater-ial does not. Intracavitary gas is seen within the abscess in 40–50% of cases if there is intestinal communication or anaerobic micro-organisms are involved. CT can be used to guide percutaneous abscess drainage. CT is also helpful for evaluating perianal disease, enterocutaneous fistulas and sinus tract, and inter-loop abscess or intra-abdominal extension of inflammatory changes.

Magnetic resonance features

Fistula, a frequent complication of CD, may course to rare sites and exhibit unexpected symptoms, thus making clinical diagnosis difficult. Atypical presen-tations not only delay diagnosis but also result in the provision of inappropriate treatment. Unique fistulas with atypical presentations, including spinal, enterovenous, umbilical, duodenopancreatic, colobronchial, and gastrocolic fistulas, have been described in the literature[9]. MR imaging is an excellent method for demonstration of perirectal and perianal fistulous tracts and fluid-filled cavities in patients with IBD. The multiplanar capability of the method allows good definition of normal anatomy. The supralevator and infralevator compartments are well displayed on coronal and sagittal images.

Gadolinium DTPA-enhanced imaging improves the conspicuity and delin-eation of fistulous tracts and with complex fistulous systems (Figure 3). Distension of collapsed portions of the fistula and fluid compartments aids in delineation of the extent and ramifications of the system and thus results in increased confidence in the diagnosis.

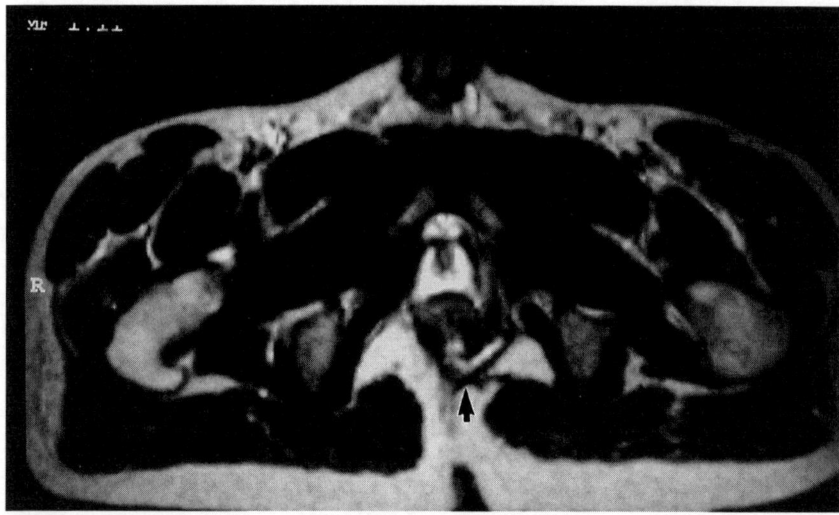

Figure 3 Axial T1-weighted image illustrating horseshoe extension in the intersphincteric space (arrow)

CONCLUSION

It can be stated that diagnostic radiology in inflammatory bowel diseases maintains its value in spite of improvements in sonography and endoscopy. Enteroclysis continues to be required for assessing the small intestine. In the acute abdomen, plain radiography and CT are capable of detecting complications early and allowing subsequent intervention. MR imaging is the method of choice for characterizing perianal fistulas.

References

1. Lavy A, Militianu D, Eidelman S. Diseases of the intestine mimicking Crohn's disease. J Clin Gastroenterol. 1992;15:17–24.
2. Thoeni RF, Margulis AR. Radiology in inflammatory disease of the colon. Invest Radiol. 1980;15:281–9.
3. Brazaitis MP, Dachman AH. The radiologic evaluation of acute abdominal pain of intestinal origin. Med Clin North Am. 1993;77:939–54.
4. Eisenberg RL, Heineken P, Hedgecock MW. Evaluation of abdominal radiology in the diagnosis of abdominal pain. Ann Surg. 1983;197:464–9.
5. Gore M, Balthazar EJ, Ghahremani GG, Miller FH. CT features of ulcerative colitis and Crohn's disease. Am J Roentgenol. 1996;167:3–15.
6. Balthazar EJ, Bimbaum BA, Yee J. Acute appendicitis: CT and US correlation in 100 patients. Radiology. 1994;190:31–7.
7. Solvig J, Ekberg O, Lindgren S, Floren CH, Nilsson P. Ultrasound examination of the small bowel: comparison with enteroclysis in patients with Crohn's disease. Abdominal Imaging. 1995;20:323–6.
8. Bagley AS, Semelka RC. Investigating bowel disease with ultrasound and MRI. Abdominal Imaging. 1994;19:403–4.
9. Tsui BCH, Cummings GE. Anorectal fistula: an unusual presentation in a Crohn's disease patient. J Emerg Med. 1997;15:39–43.
10. Khaw KI, Saverymuttu SH, Joseph AEA. Correlation of 111Indium WBC scintigraphy with ultrasound in the detection and assessment of inflammatory bowel disease. Clin Radiol. 1990;42:410–15.
11. Rioux M, Gagnon J. Imaging modalities in the puzzling world of inflammatory bowel disease. Abdominal Imaging. 1997;22:173–4.

25
The pancreas in Crohn's disease

M. LÖHR, A. THISTLETON, C. KUHN-THIEL, G. KLÖPPEL and
S. LIEBE

INTRODUCTION

Pancreatic changes associated with inflammatory bowel disease (IBD) are rare
events compared to other extraintestinal symptoms, such as skin or joint
lesions[1]. The first observation of an association of IBD with pancreatic changes
was made almost fifty years ago[2]. Gastroenterologists and a pathologist
described pancreatic changes in patients with ulcerative colitis. The pancreas
may be present with two symptomatic conditions in IBD, namely Crohn's
disease (CD): acute pancreatitis and exocrine pancreatic insufficiency.
Furthermore, asymptomatic elevation of pancreatic enzymes and pancreatic
autoantibodies may be observed. In general, reports on the pancreas in relation
to IBD are very rare[3,4]. This chapter will focus on pancreatic alterations which
have been described in association with Crohn's disease. The connection
between CD and the pancreas may be looked at from a different angle in the
future since autoimmune pancreatitis is emerging as a new entity that may represent a distinct form of pancreatitis to be found either on its own or linked to
autoimmune syndromes, including CD[5] (see below).

ACUTE PANCREATITIS

According to the few reports available, the incidence may vary between 1.5%[7]
and 5%[6]. To date, there is no in-depth investigation of the relationship between
episodes of acute pancreatitis and CD. Usually, these episodes were mild.
Recurrent attacks were rare. The pathogenetic link between acute pancreatitis
and CD is not known. Pancreatitis may represent the direct involvement of the
duodenum and papillary region[6,7], an extraintestinal manifestation of CD, or a
side-effect of drugs, either those routinely administered as base-line medication[8,9] or other immunomodulatory substances, e.g. azathioprine[10]. Furthermore,
additional autoimmune diseases, such as PSC or Sjögren's syndrome, should be
taken into account as they are known to be associated with a higher frequency of
(autoimmune) pancreatitis[11].

Reports on pancreatic calcification in conjunction with IBD, in this case ulcerative colitis, are extraordinarily rare[12]; whether this is a true causative linkage or attributable to the medication (azulfidine and corticosteroids) remains undetermined.

EXOCRINE PANCREATIC INSUFFICIENCY

Exocrine pancreatic insufficiency has been reported in 40% of the cases[18]. Since the detection of autoantibodies in pancreatic acini[13] and pancreatic juice proteins[14,15], there has been much debate about a distinct defect in the secretory capacity of the pancreas in CD. Employing the 'gold test' for exocrine pancreatic function, the secretin stimulation test[16], earlier studies indeed demonstrated an exocrine pancreatic insufficiency[17,18], however, its nature remains undetermined. In patients with manifestations of CD in the terminal ileum (ileitis terminalis), exocrine pancreatic insufficiency was more pronounced in those with moderate to severe disease[19]; however, there was no correlation for the entire group of patients with CD. With the advent of the faecal elastase-1 pancreatic function test[20], a non-invasive powerful tool is available that is good enough for routine screening for exocrine pancreatic insufficiency despite some draw-backs for mild disease[21,22]. This test needs to be explored in CD in order to screen patients routinely.

Our preliminary data show levels of < 200 U/g elastase-1 in faeces in 3/10 and levels of < 100 U/g in 1/10 unselected patients with CD; there was no correlation with disease activity in this small series. If investigated repeatedly, levels seem not to differ in relation to the disease activity in an individual patient.

ASYMPTOMATIC ELEVATION OF PANCREATIC ENZYMES

A small proportion of patients (8–16%) have hyperamylasaemia with no clinical signs of pancreatitis[3,23]. Further investigations in these patients using imaging techniques and ERCP revealed no morphological abnormalities. Whether this phenomenon represents a true pancreatic involvement of the underlying CD or is merely an effect of the medication remains to be clarified.

PANCREATIC AUTOANTIBODIES

Pancreatic autoantibodies were found in 27% of patients with CD[13]. Tissue damage in CD is immune mediated and more than one mechanism may be involved. Pancreatic autoantibodies are considered to represent a specific marker for CD[13]; however, in contrast to other immunologically mediated disorders, determination of autoantibodies in CD did so far not have an important role in clinical diagnosis. In light of these two clinical conditions of the pancreas which are associated with CD, acute pancreatitis and exocrine pancreatic insufficiency, it is mandatory to re-evaluate the role of autoantibodies although there is no conclusive evidence for a direct pathogenic role for these or any other autoantibody in CD[24].

Although it is an intriguing perspective to build a link between two epithelial linings, the gut mucosa and the pancreatic epithelial cell in CD, overall evidence

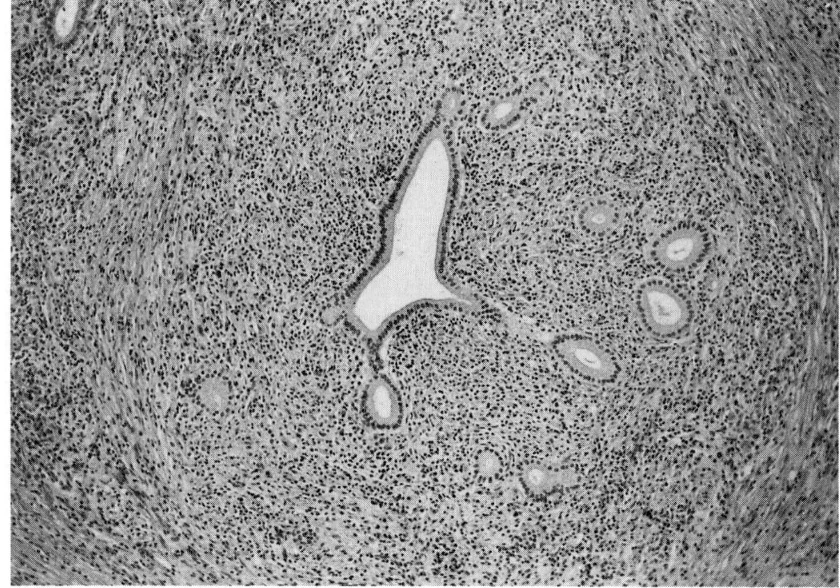

Figure 1 Histological appearance of a duct destructive chronic pancreatitis in a patient with Crohn's disease. Note the dense lymphocytic infiltrate and the absence of any calcifications

for a crossover autoimmunity or a causative relationship between CD and pancreatitis or exocrine pancreatic insufficiency is rather sparse.

AUTOIMMUNE PANCREATITIS

Recently, a patient with PSC and a special type of chronic pancreatitis has been reported[5]. The pancreatic pathology is made up by a dense lymphocytic periductular infiltration with destruction of the pancreatic ducts[5]. In this paper, 2/12 patients had CD and UC respectively (Figure 1), 1/12 Sjögren's syndrome, and 1/12 PSC[5]. Since PSC is known to be commonly associated with UC, the concomittant occurence of UC, PSC and chronic pancreatitis may be more frequent than so far recognized. This assumption is supported by the early report by Ball *et al.*[2] who found in a post mortem study of patients with UC pancreatic changes in more than half of the cases. Similar results might also be expected in patients with CD. These histological features had been noted already, then being called acute interstitial pancreatitis[25], and in 2/53 patients with 'hereditary' pancreatitis[26]. The serological evidence may be derived from the fact that, in another study of patients with idiopathic chronic pancreatitis and Sjögren's syndrome, antibodies against the lead enzyme of pancreatic duct cell, carbonic anhydrase type II[27], have been described[28–30]. A valuable study yet to be conducted would be to determine those antibodies in patients with IBD suspected to suffer from pancreatic involvement in order to assess the frequency of an autoimmune component in this disease.

References

1. Lembcke B, Kruis W, Sartor RB. Systemic Manifestations of IBD (Falk Symposium 98). Dordrecht: Kluwer Academic Publishers; 1997.
2. Ball WP, Baggenstoss AH, Bargen JA. Pancreatic lesions associated with chronic ulcerative colitis. Arch Pathol. 1950;50:345–8.
3. Tromm A, May B. Pankreasbeteiligung beim Morbus Crohn. In: Demling L, Editor, Extraintestinale Manifestationen des Morbus Crohn. Neu-Isenburg: LinguaMed Verlag; 1996:13–19.
4. Goebell H, Dignass AU. Chronic IBD and the pancreas. In: Lembcke B, Kruis W, Sartor RB, editors, Systemic Manifestations of IBD. The Pending Challenge for Subtle Diagnosis and Treatment. Dordrecht: Kluwer Academic Publishers; 1998:143–8.
5. Ectors N, Maillet B, Aerts R *et al.* Non-alcoholic duct destructive chronic pancreatitis. Gut. 1997;41:263–8.
6. Tromm A, Respondek M, Schwelger U, Kuntz HD, May B. Morbus-Crohn-assoziierte Pankreatitis: Gibt es eine neue extraintestinale Manifestation der Erkrankung? Z Gastroenterol. 1990;28:208–10.
7. Seyrig JA, Jian R, Madigliani R *et al.* Idiopathic pancreatitis associated with inflammatory bowel disease. Dig Dis Sci. 1985;30:1121–6.
8. Dobrilla G, Felder M, Chilovi F. Medikamentös induzierte Pankreatitis. Schweiz Med Wschr. 1985;115:850–8.
9. Block MB, Genant HK, Kirsner JB. Pancreatitis as an adverse reaction to salicylazosulfapyridine. N Engl J Med. 1970;282:380–2.
10. Löhr M. Pankreas: Gutachterliche Stellungnahme. In: Hahn EG, Riemann JF, Editors, Klinische Gastroenterologie. Z. Aufl. Stuttgart: Georg Thieme Verlag; 1996:1216–23.
11. Satori N, Löhr M, Basan B, Holle A, Liebe S. Pancreatitis in systemic scleroderma. Z Gastroenterol. 1997;35:667–70.
12. Ahmad M, Bauer W, Katz S. Ulcerative colitis, hyperamylasemia, and asymptomatic pancreatic calcifications: making the case for pancreatitis as an extra luminal manifestation. Am J Gastroenterol. 1997;92:2307–9.
13. Seibold F, Mörk H, Tanza S *et al.* Pancreatic autoantibodies in Crohn's disease: a family study. Gut. 1997;40:481–4.
14. Müller-Ladner U, Gross V, Andus T *et al.* Distinct patterns of immunoglobulin classes and IgG subclasses of autoantibodies in patients with inflammatory bowel disease. Eur J Gastroenterol Hepatol. 1996;8:579–84.
15. Stöcher W, Otte M, Ulrich S *et al.* Autoimmunity to pancreatic juice in Crohn's disease. Results of an autoantibody screening in patients with chronic inflammatory bowel disease. Scand J Gastroenterol. 1987;139:41–52.
16. Lankisch PG. Function tests in the diagnosis of chronic pancreatitis. Int J Pancreatol. 1993;14:9–20.
17. Hoppe-Seyler P, Holtermann D, Gerok W. Untersuchung der exokrinen Pankreasfunktion bei M. Crohn. Z Gastroenterol. 1981;19:570.
18. Angelini G, Cavallini G, Bovi P *et al.* Pancreatic function in chronic inflammatory bowel disease. Int J Pancreatol. 1988;3:185–93.
19. Hegnhøj J, Hansen CP, Rannem T *et al.* Pancreatic function in Crohn's disease. Gut. 1990;31:1076–9.
20. Katschinski M, Schirra J, Bross A, Göke B, Arnold R. Duodenal secretion and fecal excretion of pancreatic elastase-1 in healthy humans and patients with chronic pancreatitis. Pancreas. 1997;15:191–200.
21. Amann ST, Bishop M, Curington C, Toskes PP. Fecal pancreatic elastase-1 is inaccurate in the diagnosis of chronic pancreatitis. Pancreas. 1996;13:226–30.
22. Lankisch PG, Schmidt I, König H, Knollmann R, Löhr M, Liebe S. Faecal elastase-1: not helpful in diagnosing chronic pancreatitis with mild to moderate exocrine pancreatic insufficiency. Gut. 1998;42:551–4.
23. Katz S, Bank S, Greenberg RE, Lendvai S, Lesser M, Napolitano B. Hyperamylasemia in inflammatory bowel disease. J Clin Gastroenterol. 1988;10:627–30.
24. Shanahan F. Antibody 'markers' in Crohn's disease: opportunity or overstatement? Gut. 1997;40:557–8.
25. Kimura W, Ohtsubo K. Clinical and pathological features of acute interstitial pancreatitis in the aged. Int J Pancreatol. 1989;5:1–9.

26. Tomsik H, Grün R, Wagner E. Hereditäre Pankreatitis. Ergebn Inn Med Kinderheilk. 1992;60:1–64.
27. Sirica AE, Longnecker DS. Biliary and Pancreatic Ductal Epithelia. Pathobiology and Pathophysiology. New York: Marcel Dekker Inc.; 1997.
28. Nishimori I, Yamamoto Y, Okazaki K *et al.* Identification of autoantibodies to a pancreatic antigen in patients with idiopathic chronic pancreatitis and Sjögren's syndrome. Pancreas. 1994;9:374–81.
29. Kino-Ohsaki J, Nishimori I, Morita M *et al.* Serum antibodies to carbonic anhydrase I and II in patients with idiopathic chronic pancreatitis and Sjögren's syndrome. Gastroenterology. 1996;110:1579–86.
30. Cavallini G, Frulloni L, Bovo P, Di Francesco V, Filippini M. Carbonic anhydrase and primary chronic pancreatitis. Gastroenterology. 1997;112:1054–5.

26
Colonoscopy and laparoscopy in Crohn's disease in children

F. SCHIER and G. KÄHLER

INTRODUCTION

The diagnosis of Crohn's disease in children is based initially on clinical suspicion. The list of non-specific symptoms is long (Table 1) and the list of extraintestinal manifestations is endless[1,2]. Also, there is uneven regional involvement within the gastrointestinal tract (Table 2).

With these diffuse symptoms in mind, establishing the diagnosis is the primary goal. Traditionally, the diagnosis of Crohn's disease was made by inspection of the inner bowel wall (as far as possible) and examination of biopsies. In addition, contrast studies provided a two-dimensional image of the bowel. All these procedures were undertaken with the understanding that the whole gastrointestinal tract can be involved, the stomach as frequently as the rectum. The transverse colon was the area with the highest probability of encountering noticeable manifestations of Crohn's disease by endoscopy[3].

Table 1 Symptoms of Crohn's disease in children

	Percentage
Abdominal pain	75
Diarrhoea	65
Weight loss	65
Growth retardation	25
Nausea/vomiting	25
Perineal bleeding	20
Perirectal disease	15
Extraintestinal manifestations	25

From Reference 4.

Table 2 Regional involvement in Crohn's disease

71% upper GI	16% oesophagus
	46% fundus
	36% antrum
	7% duodenum
86% large bowel	71% transverse colon
	53% terminal ileum
	69% caecum
	60% sigmoid colon
	41% rectum

$n = 56$; endoscopic findings from Reference 3.

AIM

In childen, colonoscopy requires anaesthesia. We wondered whether this anaesthesia could be used for an additional laparoscopy.

PATIENTS AND METHODS

Crohn's disease was suspected in six children aged between 8 and 14 years. On ultrasound examination, wall thickening in the terminal ileum was diagnosed. The laparoscope was advanced through the umbilicus and a pair of forceps was inserted through the left anterior abdominal wall for bowel manipulation. With the laparoscope in place, the colonoscope was advanced. The bowel wall could thus be inspected simultaneously on two separate monitors.

RESULTS

There were no complications. The entry of the colonoscope into the terminal ileum was supported by the laparoscopy forceps. The intraoperative images did not match the preoperative impression. Preoperative ultrasonography was imprecise. In some children, thickening of the terminal ileum was diagnosed on ultrasound, although the terminal ileum was normal on colonoscopy. However, far more proximally there were stenotic segments, which had not been diagnosed on ultrasound. In other children, the terminal ileum appeared normal laparoscopically but intraluminally there were numerous lesions. In one child, colonoscopy had to be aborted in the transverse colon due to the presence of faeces. Laparoscopy was able to provide at least a complete overview of the whole gastrointestinal tract including the liver and spleen (Figures 1–3).

In the last three children, a lymph node biopsy was taken from the mesentery adjacent to the involved small bowel segment (Figure 2). In four children, the liver appeared indurated; therefore a biopsy was taken from a relevant area (Figure 3). Histological examination, however, yielded normal results. Technically, the intra-abdominal pressure rose intermittently to more than 20 mmHg due to the combined laparoscopy pressure and endoscopy insufflation. Anaesthesia times ranged from 25 to 55 min.

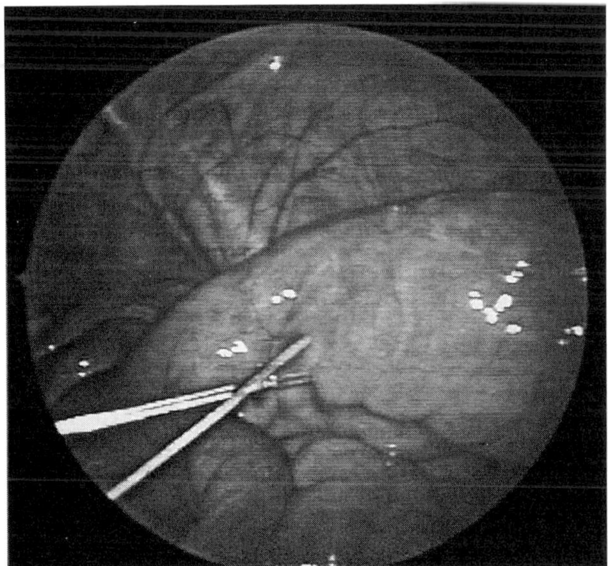

Figure 1 Small bowel. Normal segment (left) next to an affected segment with 'creeping fat' on the right

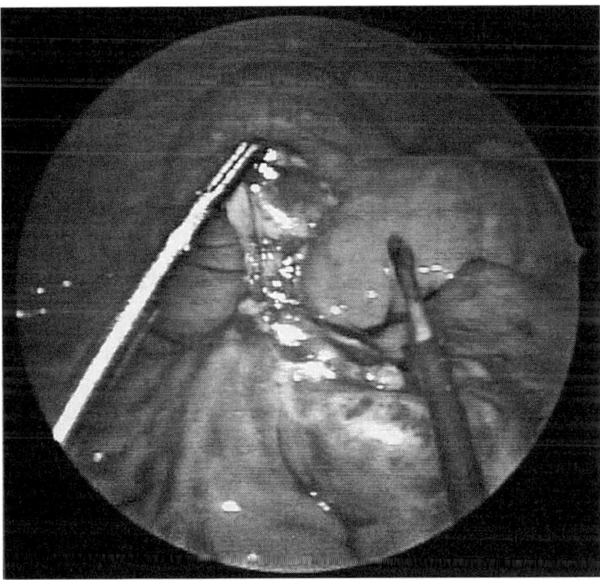

Figure 2 Lymph node biopsy from the mesentery adjacent to the affected small bowel segment

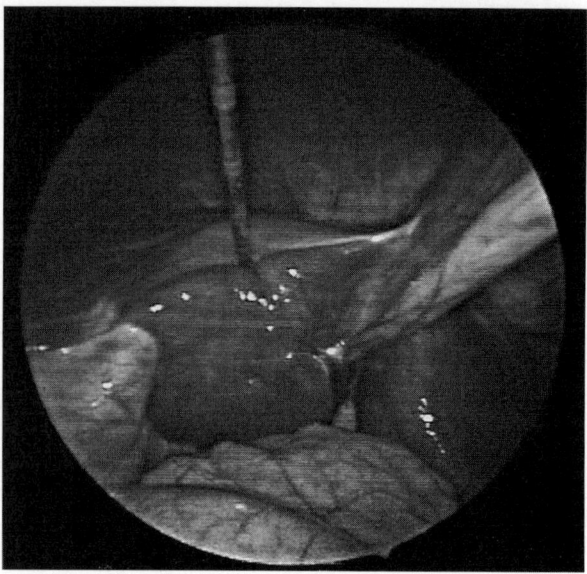

Figure 3 Liver biopsy during laparoscopy for Crohn's disease

DISCUSSION

The traditional diagnostic methods for Crohn's disease are limited to the inner aspect of the bowel. Colonoscopy allows examination of the colon and a small part of the ileum while the rest of the gastrointestinal tract remains unseen, although it may also be involved in the disease. Laparoscopy could fill this gap as it evaluates the whole abdominal cavity and can allow biopsies to be taken if deemed necessary. Transmural and segmental lesions are probably diagnosed better by laparoscopy than by colonoscopy. There is no disadvantage to the child as anaesthesia is required for both.

CONCLUSIONS

A laparoscopy yields additional information about the stage and the character of the disease. The diagnosis of Crohn's disease might therefore be established more firmly and earlier, allowing the initiation of appropriate therapy.

References

1. Hyams JS. Extraintestinal manifestations of inflammatory bowel disease. J Pediatr Gastroenterol Nutr. 1994;19:8–12.
2. Hyams JS. Crohn's disease in children. Pediatr Clin N Am. 1996;43:255–77.
3. Cameron DJ. Upper and lower gastrointestinal endoscopy in children and adolescents with Crohn's disease: a prospective study. J Gastroenterol Hepatol. 1991;6:355–8.
4. Hyams SJ. Crohn's disease. In: Wyllie R, Hyams SJ, editors, Pediatric Gastrointestinal Disease Management. Philadelphia, US: WB Saunders; 1993:746.

Section VIII
IBD and Malignancy

27
IBD: intestinal cancer risk and surveillance

E.-O. RIECKEN and H. SCHERÜBL

INTRODUCTION

Colorectal cancer has become well recognized as the most serious complication faced by patients with long-standing ulcerative colitis (UC) or Crohn's disease (CD). Although accounting for less than 1% of all colorectal cancers, it is the leading cause of long-term disease-related mortality in patients with UC.

CANCER RISK IN IBD

The incidence of colorectal carcinoma is substantially increased in patients with long-standing inflammatory bowel disease (IBD). Although this increased risk has been studied more extensively for UC, the association between colorectal cancer and CD is now acknowledged to be equal among patients with similar risk characteristics[1-7]. The best-defined risk factors are disease duration and anatomical extent. The cancer risk begins to rise appreciably after about 7–8 years of disease activity. Overall, the risk of colon cancer for those with pancolitis increases after 8–10 years of disease by 0.5–1% per person per year. Estimates of cancer incidence in UC vary widely. The cumulative incidence after 20 years is 5–13%. The risk for cancer also increases as the extent increases. Overall, the average relative risk of cancer is increased approximately 14-fold for patients with pancolitis and two- to three-fold for left-sided disease. Patients with only proctitis or procto-sigmoiditis have only a slightly increased risk. Epidemiological studies on cohorts with either extensive UC or extensive CD show that the relative cancer risks (18- and 19-fold, respectively) and the cumulative incidence rates (8% after 20 years and 9% after 22 years, respectively) are almost identical[7,8].

CHARACTERISTICS OF COLORECTAL CANCER IN IBD

Colorectal cancers that arise in patients with IBD differ in many ways from sporadic cancers[9,10]. Colorectal cancers in IBD are more uniformly distributed throughout the colon, are multiple in 12% of cases at the time of diagnosis and occur at much younger age than sporadic cancers (at a mean age of 43 years in UC and at a mean of 54 years in CD). The molecular pathogenesis of colitis-associated and sporadic colon cancer shows some interesting differences. Whereas mutations of the APC and p53 tumour-suppressor genes are common in both types of colon cancer, the sequence of the molecular alterations is different between the two types of cancer. In colitis-associated cancer p53 abnormalities can occur rather early in carcinogenesis, whereas in sporadic colon cancer this molecular alteration is typically a late event. Conversely, APC mutations are considered the earliest gatekeeper event in sporadic colon cancer, but in colitis cancer it is usually high-grade dysplasia or cancer that manifests changes in this gene. Other molecular changes such as abnormal DNA content (aneuploidy) and expression of the mucin-associated carbohydrate antigen sialosyl-Tn can occur early both in sporadic and colitis-associated carcinogenesis[10–13].

SURVEILLANCE AND PATIENT MANAGEMENT

To prevent or to make an early diagnosis of colorectal cancer surveillance is recommended in colitis (UC or CD) patients. Surveillance is started after 8–10 years' duration of pancolitis or after 12–15 years' duration of left-sided colitis. This consists of annual colonoscopies with mucosal biopsies taken from every 10 cm of flat mucosa and additionally from elevated lesions other than typical postinflammatory polyps. In left-sided UC sigmoidoscopy may be adequate. The aim is to identify dysplasia, a premalignant histological change[9,10].

The probability of finding colon cancer in colitic patients depends on the degree of dysplasia (see Table 1). If colonoscopy reveals high-grade dysplasia in flat mucosa, immediate colectomy reveals cancer in 42–67% of colectomy specimens. When a DALM (dysplasia associated with a lesion or mass) is the initial discovery, immediate surgery reveals carcinoma in 43% of such patients regardless of whether the DALM contains low-grade or high-grade dysplasia. When low-grade dysplasia is found on initial colonoscopy, 19% of patients already have cancer at the time of immediate colectomy. Conversely, the finding of no

Table 1 Frequency of colon cancer in colitic patients with different degrees of dysplasia

	Probability of finding cancer at colectomy	
Diagnosis	*Immediately*	*After some follow-up*
DALM	43% (17/40)	NA
High-grade dysplasia	42% (10/24)	32% (15/47)
Low-grade dysplasia	19% (3/16)*	8% (17/204)
Indefinite for dysplasia	NA	9% (9/95)
Negative for dysplasia	NA	2% (11/595)

* May reflect referral bias.
DALM = dysplasia-associated lesion or mass; NA = data not available.
Modified from ref. 14, with permission.

dysplasia is strongly predictive of a good immediate outcome; only 2% of these patients develop cancer during follow-up[14–16].

DYSPLASIA AND COLECTOMY

Cancer mortality in colitic patients is best reduced by prophylactic colectomy[17]. Colectomy should be performed immediately when a DALM or high-grade dysplasia is unequivocally diagnosed by two experienced pathologists. In case of low-grade dysplasia colectomy should be strongly recommended. The management of low-grade dysplasia is often considered more problematic. The histology should be confirmed by two expert gastrointestinal pathologists. Low-grade dysplasia may occur in up to 80% of long-standing colitis, and many patients opt for further surveillance instead of immediate colectomy. If a patient with low-grade dysplasia opts against colectomy, a control colonoscopy after 3–6 months is to be recommended, as the cancer risk is about 19%. Simple adenomatous polyps are considered incidental findings unrelated to the underlying colitis, and are managed as in the non-colitic patient.

Surveillance and colectomy do improve survival in colitic patients with cancer[17,18]. Giardiello and Bayless[19] and Choi *et al.*[20] showed that cancers found in the surveillance group were at an earlier tumour stage (67% at stage I or II) compared with the group without surveillance. The 5-year survival was 77–89% in the surveillance group versus 19–36% in the no-surveillance group. As these studies were non-randomized, retrospective and limited to small groups of patients, data from large series are much needed. Controlled prospective large trials on this important issue have not been performed, and because of practical and ethical reasons probably never will be performed.

MOLECULAR MARKERS

There are limitations to using dysplasia alone as a marker of the cancer-prone colon. As regards the molecular pathogenesis of colitis-associated cancer, several tumour suppressor genes or oncogenes could be envisaged as possible markers. The list of candidate premalignant markers includes global DNA hypomethylation, DNA aneuploidy, abnormal mucin expression, proto-oncogene mutations, suppressor gene mutations, loss of heterozygosity and microsatellite instability, TGF-βRII mutation and E-cadherin expression[10–13]. However, two of these markers have not yet been well studied in colitic patients. At present the most promising molecular tissue markers are mutations of p53, aneuploidy and sialysyl-Tn antigen. Future studies need to show whether immunohistochemical staining for p53 or sialosyl-Tn signifies more aggressive disease, and if these patients should be treated by colectomy. Alternative markers of malignancy which are objective, inexpensive and sensitive are still needed to improve morbidity and life expectancy. Screening for cancer in IBD would obviously much benefit from the availability of faecal DNA based tests for markers of cancer risk. Both endoscopic and molecular surveillance techniques should ultimately result in improved cancer-related morbidity in IBD.

References

1. Weedon DD, Shorter RG, Ilstrup DM *et al.* Crohn's disease and cancer. N Engl J Med. 1973;289:1099–103.
2. Gyde SN, Prior P, Macartney JC *et al.* Malignancy in Crohn's disease. Gut. 1980;21:1024–9.
3. Greenstein AJ, Sachar DB, Smith H *et al.* A comparison of cancer risk in Crohn's disease and ulcerative colitis. Cancer. 1981;48:2742–5.
4. Korelitz BI. Carcinoma of the intestinal tract in Crohn's disease: results of a survey conducted by the National Foundation for Ileitis and Colitis. Am J Gastroenterol. 1983;78:44–6.
5. Ekbom A, Helmick C, Zack M. Increased risk of large-bowel cancer in Crohn's disease with colonic involvement. Lancet. 1990;336:357–9.
6. Ekbom A, Helmick CG, Zack M *et al.* Survival and causes of death in patients with inflammatory bowel disease. Gastroenterology. 1992;103:954–60.
7. Gillen CD, Walmsley RS, Prior P *et al.* Ulcerative colitis and Crohn's disease: a comparison of the colorectal cancer risk in extensive colitis. Gut. 1994;35:1590–2.
8. Sachar DB. Cancer in Crohn's disease: dispelling the myths. Gut. 1994;35:1507–8.
9. Winawer SJ, Fletcher RH, Miller L *et al.* Colorectal cancer screening: clinical guidelines and rationale. Gastroenterology. 1997;112:594–642.
10. Itzkowitz SH. Inflammatory bowel disease and cancer. Gastroenterol Clin N Am. 1997;26:129–39.
12. Hoque AT, Hahn SA, Schurre M, Kern SE. DPC4 gene mutation in colitis associated neoplasia. Gut. 1997;40:120–2.
12. Rashid A, Hamilton SR. Genetic alterations in sporadic and Crohn's-associated adenocarcinomas of the small intestine. Gastroenterology. 1997;113:127–35.
13. Souza RF, Lei J, Yin J *et al.* A transforming growth factor $\beta1$ receptor type II mutation in ulcerative colitis-associated neoplasms. Gastroenterology. 1997;112:40–5.
14. Bernstein CN, Shanahan F, Weinstein WM. Are we telling patients the truth about surveillance colonoscopy in ulcerative colitis? Lancet. 1994;343:71–4.
15. Connell WR, Lennard-Jones JE, Williams CB *et al.* Factors affecting the outcome of endoscopic surveillance for cancer in ulcerative colitis. Gastroenterology. 1994;107:934–44.
16. Lennard-Jones JE. Colitic cancer: supervision, surveillance, or surgery. Gastroenterology. 1995;109:1388–91.
17. Langholz E, Munkholm P, Davidsen M, Binder V. Colorectal cancer risk and mortality in patients with ulcerative colitis. Gastroenterology. 1992;103:1444–51.
18. Sachar DB. Clinical and colonoscopic surveillance in ulcerative colitis: are we saving colons or saving lives? Gastroenterology. 1993;105:588–9.
19. Giardiello FM, Bayless TM. Colorectal cancer and ulcerative colitis. Radiology. 1996;199:28–30.
20. Choi PM, Nugent FW, Schoetz DJ *et al.* Colonoscopic surveillance reduces mortality from colorectal cancer in ulcerative colitis. Gastroenterology. 1993;105:418–24.

28
Role of flow cytometry in surveillance strategies in patients with ulcerative colitis*

R. PORSCHEN, K. HOLZMANN, B. KLUMP, F. BORCHARD
and the DNA PLOIDY STUDY GROUP†

INTRODUCTION

Ulcerative colitis (UC) belongs to the group of chronic inflammatory bowel diseases. Patients with UC are at a greater risk than the general population of developing colorectal carcinoma. Clinical risk factors for the development of colitis-associated carcinoma include the duration and anatomical extent of UC. The increased cancer risk has prompted a search for objective parameters allowing an individual assessment of the cancer risk.

For patients with long-standing colitis, colonoscopic surveillance is currently recommended[1]. Identification of patients with UC carrying an increased cancer risk is based on histological demonstration of dysplasia during colonoscopic surveillance. Dysplasia has been defined as an unequivocally neoplastic transformation of the colonic epithelium[2]. Although the criteria for the classification of dysplasia have been described in detail, the diagnosis is rather problematical and is often poorly reproducible. Classification of dysplasia is influenced by the degree of inflammation and is subject to inter- and intra-observer variation[3]. Because of these difficulties there is still a demand for other methods for the detection of patients prone to carcinoma development.

A rapid measurement of nuclear DNA content can be performed by flow cytometry. Abnormal DNA content (DNA aneuploidy) correlates with numerical

* Dedicated to Prof. Dr G. Strohmeyer on the occasion of his 70th birthday.
† *Members of the DNA Ploidy Study Group*: H. Bauerle, Burgfeld Hospital, Kassel; V. F. Eckardt, Gastroenterological Institute, Wiesbaden; V. Gaco, M. Weis-Klemm, University Hospital, Tübingen; H. Gordon, Red Cross Hospital, Kassel; A. Mittelstaedt, Augusta Hospital Mörsenbroich-Rath, Düsseldorf; H. E. Reis, Hospital Maria Hilf, Mönchengladbach; H. D. Schwöbel, Evangelic Hospital, Düsseldorf; M. Sporrer, Evangelic Hospital, Mettmann; H. Stockert, Evangelic Hospital Bethesda, Mönchengladbach; K. Warm, Vitalis Clinic, Bad Hersfeld.

chromosomal aberrations and may therefore reflect a neoplastic alteration. The prevalence of DNA aneuploidy and the correlation between dysplasia and DNA aneuploidy have been described by several authors in patients with ulcerative colitis[3–6]. However, the majority of these reports were restricted to patients with long-standing extensive or total colitis. To determine the correlation between the extent of UC and the prevalence of DNA aneuploidy patients with UC were included in this study independent of the extent of their disease. In addition, it was the aim of the present study to evaluate the importance of DNA ploidy measured by flow cytometry in the surveillance of patients with UC. Furthermore, the correlation between flow cytometric and molecular alterations (ras and p53 mutations) was analysed in colectomy specimen.

MATERIAL AND METHODS

Patients

A total of 368 patients with UC (147 male, 221 female) were analysed in the present study. Mean age was 44.1 years (standard deviation, 15.2 years) and mean disease duration 13.9 years (± 8.0 years). Patients with diverticulosis and irritable bowel syndrome ($n = 48$) were used as controls. All patients gave informed consent. The study was approved by the local ethical committee.

In 278 UC patients, information concerning the presence or absence of primary sclerosing cholangitis (PSC) was available. In 16 patients (15 with pancolitis, one with proctosigmoiditis, disease duration 15.6 ± 7.4 years), a definitive diagnosis of PSC was established by means of endoscopic retrograde cholangioscopy. In two other patients a suspicion of PSC existed; however, these patients refused further diagnostic work-up.

Endoscopy

At each colonoscopy the large bowel was biopsied at five different levels: the caecum/the ascending, the transverse, the descending, the sigmoid colon and the rectum. Two biopsies from each location were assessed histologically and two other biopsies taken immediately adjacent were analysed by flow cytometry. The biopsies for histology and flow cytometry were taken as close together as possible in order to facilitate a comparison between these two methods. Additional biopsies were sampled if macroscopical nodular or polypoid lesions were detected.

The biopsy specimens were fixed in formalin, embedded in paraffin and stained with haematoxylin and eosin. Dysplasia was graded by one pathologist (F.B.) in a blinded manner according to the classification proposed by Riddell et al.[2] as negative, indefinite (IND), low-grade (LGD) or high-grade (HGD).

Flow cytometry

The two biopsies from each location were pooled for flow cytometric DNA analysis. They were stored at −80°C in a dimethyl sulphoxide/citrate buffer. Before analysis the samples were rapidly thawed in a water bath. Specimens were gently ground in a 0.3 mm steel mesh with a small glass pestle[5]. After detergent/trypsin treatment of the biopsies the nuclear suspension was stained with propidium iodide according to Vindelov *et al.*[7]. In order to minimize aggregates, the nuclear suspension was constantly agitated during the incubation period. A total of 10 000 nuclei per sample were measured in a FACScan flow cytometer (Becton Dickinson, Heidelberg, Germany). The coefficient of variation of the G_1 full peak in all samples was 2.4% (standard deviation, 0.7%).

After exclusion of doublets cell cycle parameters were calculated using the RFIT software. Samples with more than one G_0/G_1 peak in the DNA histogram were judged as aneuploid. Hyperdiploid shoulders or skews that were not bimodal were not classified as aneuploid. Peaks in the tetraploid region exceeding the G_2/M value of the normal colonic mucosa by more than 3 standard deviations were classified as aneuploid. In these tetraploid samples a corresponding second peak at 8.0c was identified. For aneuploid samples a DNA index was calculated as the ratio of the abnormal G_0/G_1 mean peak channel number to the diploid G_0/G_1 mean peak channel number. If the DNA index varied no more than 10% between different parts of the large bowel, or between two examinations, it was considered to be consistent. DNA histograms were interpreted without knowledge of the histological results.

Molecular, histological and flow cytometric analysis of colectomy specimens

The colectomy specimens of seven patients with long-standing ulcerative pancolitis were analysed. Resection was performed because of dysplasia in five cases, carcinoma in one case and clinical deterioration in one case. Samples were taken from each of 30–40 positions throughout the colons. The samples were divided in order to facilitate comparison between histological, flow cytometric and molecular biological results. One part from each location was routinely fixed in formalin, embedded in paraffin, and stained with haematoxylin and eosin. Histological slides were reviewed by one experienced pathologist (F.B.), who did not know the results of the flow cytometric or molecular biological results.

After flow cytometry of the samples, high molecular weight DNA was isolated from the remaining cell nuclei according to standard methods of proteinase K/SDS digestion, phenol/chloroform extraction, and ethanol precipitation.

The highly conserved regions of the p53 gene (exon 5, 7, 8) as well as of the first exon of Ki-ras were amplified separately by polymerase chain reaction (PCR). Mutation analysis was done by the single-strand conformation polymorphism (SSCP) method. Each amplified exon was tested for optimal single-strand separation by applying different temperatures and glycerol content during electrophoresis; 15 μl of a 100 μl PCR assay were diluted with 5 μl of a formamide-dye solution (95% formamide, 20 mmol/l EDTA, 0.05% bromphenolblue, and 0.05% xylenecyanol), heated for 10 min at 90°C and subjected to gel electrophoresis in a 0.5% MDE gel (Biozym, Hessisch Oldendorf, Germany) containing 5% glycerol (p53 exon 7, 8) at room temperature or at 4°C without glycerol (p53 exon 5, Ki-ras exon 1). Bands were visualized with silver staining. Several characterized cell lines with known mutations in p53 or Ki-ras were used as controls for the SSCP reaction[8].

RESULTS

Surveillance study

The extent of UC determined by colonoscopy in the 368 patients was as follows: 22 patients with proctitis, 61 patients with proctosigmoiditis, 66 patients with left-sided colitis (involvement distal to the splenic flexure), 44 patients with extensive colitis (involvement distal to the hepatic flexure) and 175 patients with total colitis. A total of 482 colonoscopies was performed (1.3 colonoscopies per patient). In 81 patients more than one colonscopy was performed. The results refer to the last colonoscopy. A total of 5142 biopsies was analysed. In control patients no dysplasia was detected; 29 UC patients showed either dysplasia (10 indefinite, 12 low-grade, three high-grade) or carcinoma (four).

S-phase fractions and G_2/M phase fractions in control biopsies and UC biopsies are shown in Table 1. The cell proliferation values increased in biopsies showing aneuploidy. Aneuploid cell populations were detected in 32 UC patients by flow cytometry. All control patients demonstrated normal diploid DNA histograms. In 16 patients DNA aneuploidy was found at more than one location in the colorectum. In these patients aneuploid cell clones were detected dispersed throughout the whole colon in contrast to the patchy distribution of dysplasia. The percentage of aneuploid biopsies increased from 2.9% in biopsies without dysplasia to 39.5%, 35.7% and 80.0% in biopsies classified as indefinite, low-grade and high-grade dysplasia, respectively. All biopsies taken from carcinomas were aneuploid.

One important advantage of flow cytometry was the fact that aneuploid cell clones could be found again in control colonoscopies at a significantly higher percentage than dysplasias. If the calculations were restricted to the question of whether dysplastic or aneuploid samples could be re-found at the same colon segment as in the first colonoscopy the reproducibility rate amounted to only 12% and 68% for dysplasia and DNA aneuploidy, respectively. Concerning re-detection of aneuploidy or dysplasia independent of the location of the initial findings in the colon, the reproducibility rate was 38% and 79% for dysplasia and DNA aneuploidy, respectively.

The distribution of the DNA indices of aneuploid samples is shown in Figure 1. The majority of aneuploid biopsies possessed DNA indices in the near-diploid region. Two smaller peaks can be noticed in the triploid and the tetraploid regions.

Table 1 Cell proliferation measured by flow cytometry in biopsies taken from control patients and from patients with ulcerative colitis

	S phase (%)	G_2M phase (%)
Controls	6.4 ± 2.1	2.6 ± 1.0
Colitis (without aneuploidy, without dysplasia)	7.0 ± 3.3	3.0 ± 1.5
Colitis (with dysplasia)	6.6 ± 2.9	3.2 ± 1.2
Colitis (with aneuploidy)	7.8 ± 5.7	2.9 ± 1.5
Colitis (with aneuploidy, with dysplasia)	7.1 ± 5.3	3.1 ± 1.3

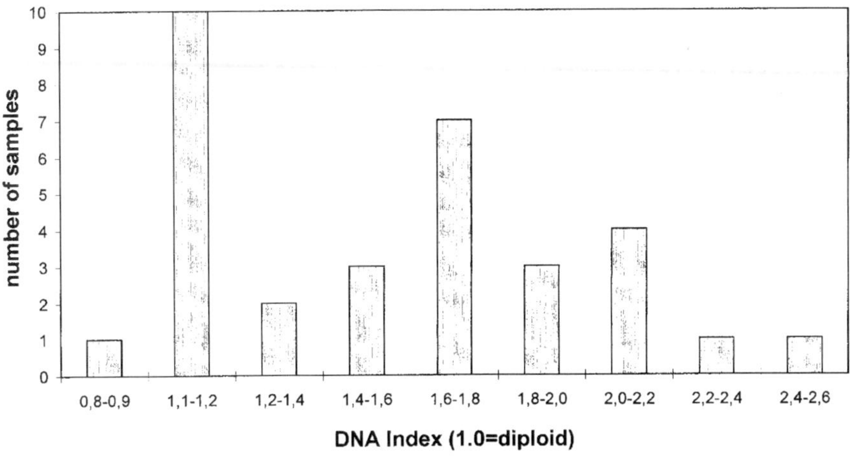

Figure 1   Distribution of the DNA indices measured by flow cytometry in patients with ulcerative colitis

The correlation between the extent of UC and DNA aneuploidy is given in Table 2. Dysplastic biopsies existed in 2.7% of the patients with proctitis, procto-sigmoiditis and left-sided colitis. This percentage increased to 7–10% in those patients with extensive or total colitis. DNA aneuploidy was almost exclusively associated with total colitis (26/32 patients). The presence of DNA aneuploidy and of dysplasia was dependent on the duration of ulcerative colitis: these percentages began to rise significantly after a disease duration of more than 10 years (Figure 2).

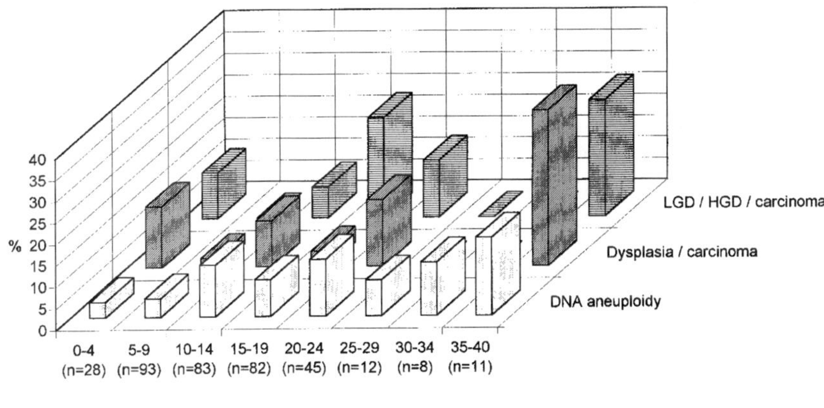

Figure 2   Relationship between the percentage of DNA aneuploidy or dysplasia and the duration of ulcerative colitis. The term 'dysplasia' refers to indefinite, low-grade and high-grade dysplasia

UC patients with PSC showed a significantly higher percentage of DNA aneuploidy than UC patients without PSC (9/16 patients versus 19/262 patients; $p < 0.000001$). The correlation between dysplasia and PSC was weaker, but still significant (4/16 patients versus 14/262 patients; $p < 0.014$).

In those patients in whom control colonoscopies have been performed (Figures 3a and 3b) 10 patients initially demonstrated DNA aneuploidy without

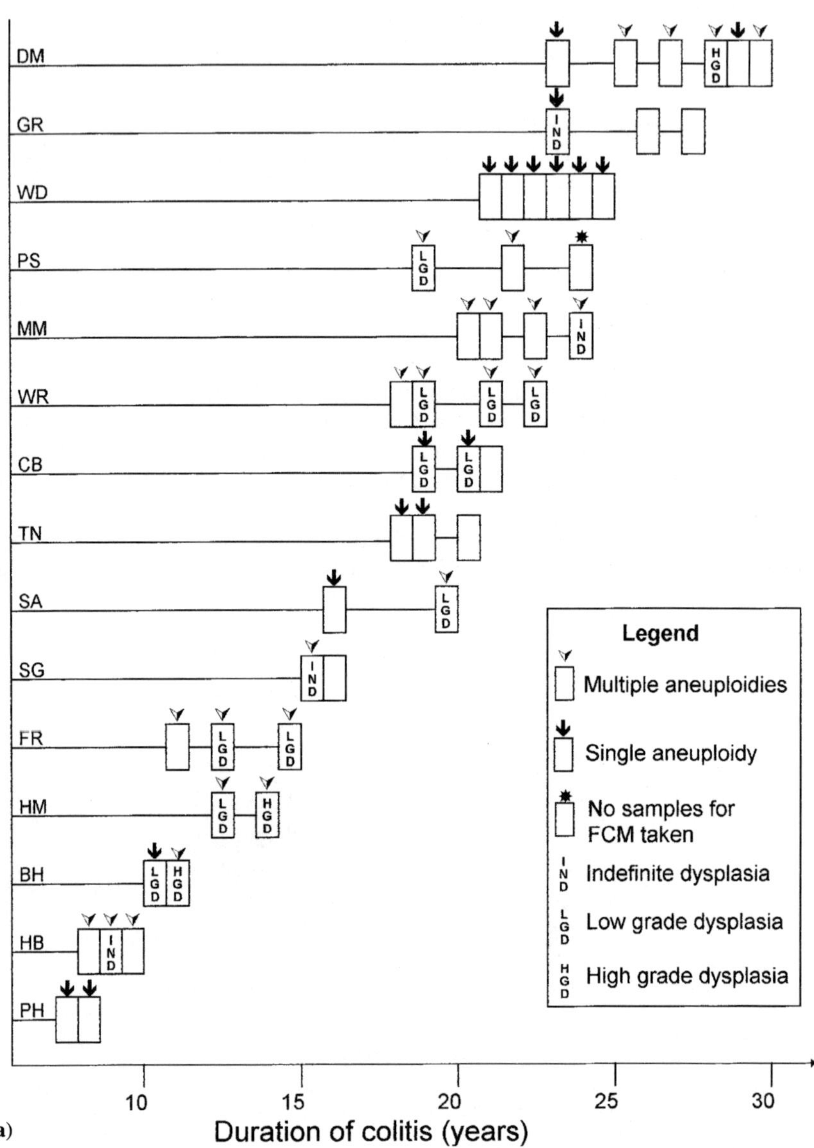

Figure 3(a) *Figure caption opposite*

Table 2 Relationship between the endoscopic extent of ulcerative colitis and the prevalence of dysplasia and of DNA aneuploidy

Extent of disease	Dysplasia* (%)	Aneuploidy (%)
Proctitis ($n = 22$)	0.0	0.0
Proctosigmoiditis ($n = 61$)	1.6	3.3
Left-sided colitis ($n = 66$)	4.5	1.5
Extensive colitis ($n = 44$)	6.8	6.8
Pancolitis ($n = 175$)	10.2	14.9

* Indefinite, low-grade, high-grade dysplasia.

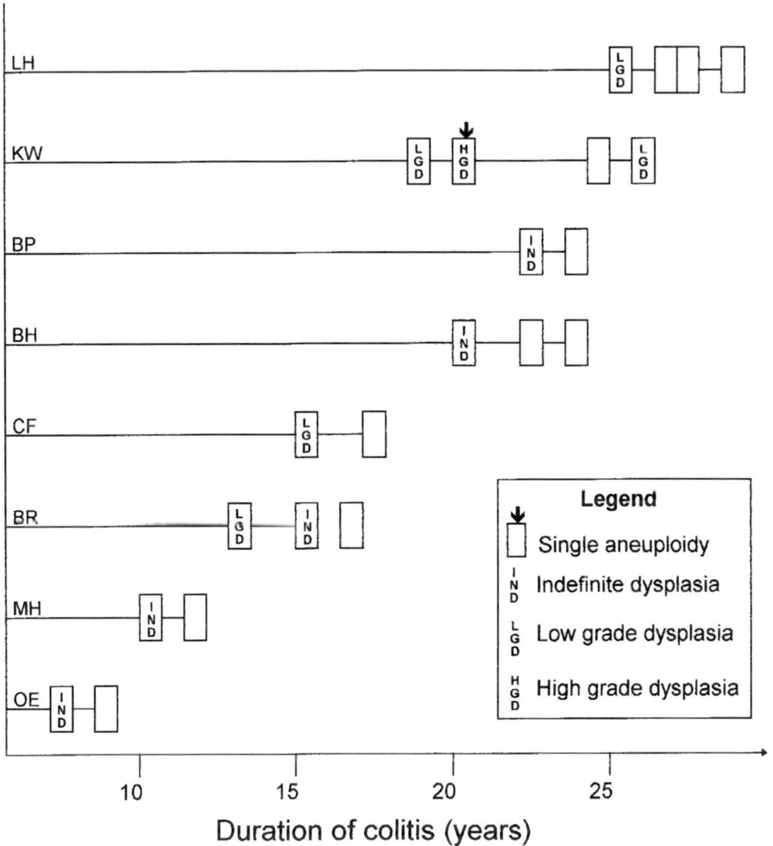

(b)

Figure 3 (a) Results of endoscopic surveillance in patients in whom control colonoscopies were performed after the initial detection of single or multiple DNA aneuploidy and/or dysplasia. Ten patients initially demonstrated DNA aneuploidy without the simultaneous detection of dysplasia. In patient D.M., single aneuploidies in the first and fifth endoscopy were detected by sigmoidoscopy. Control colonoscopies in this subgroup of patients revealed progression to dysplasia in six patients (One HGD, three LGD, two indefinite dysplasia). (b) Results of endoscopic surveillance in patients in whom control colonoscopies were performed after the initial detection of dysplasia. Only two of these eight patients showed dysplastic findings (one HGD, one indefinite dysplasia) during continued endoscopic surveillance

the simultaneous detection of dysplasia. Control colonoscopies in this subgroup of patients revealed dysplastic findings in six patients (one high-grade dysplasia (HGD), three low-grade dysplasia (LGD), two indefinite dysplasia).

In eight patients dysplasia (four LGD, four indefinite dysplasia) was present at the first colonoscopy (Figure 3b). Only two of these patients showed dysplastic findings (one HGD, one indefinite dysplasia) during continued endoscopic surveillance. In six patients, aneuploidy and dysplasia were detected simultaneously. Three patients progressed to HGD or carcinoma.

Of 55 patients without initial aneuploidy or dysplasia no-one developed aneuploidy and only two patients revealed dysplasia (one LGD, one indefinite dysplasia) during continued endoscopic surveillance.

Colectomy specimens

In this high-risk group of UC patients ($n = 7$), 44% of all the samples were aneuploid (122/278). The percentage was 35% in histologically negative samples, 45% in samples with indefinite dysplasia, 96% in samples with LGD, 75% in samples with HGD and 100% in carcinomatous samples (Figure 4).

In the SSCP analysis 25% of all the samples were positive for a p53 mutation and 3% were positive for a Ki-ras mutation. The correlation between histology, p53 mutation and Ki-ras mutation is given in Figure 4. The percentages of DNA aneuploidy and p53 mutations increase with the grade of dysplasia. However, a significant percentage of Ki-ras mutation is found only in the carcinomatous samples. Table 3 shows an overview of the correlation between aneuploidy, dysplasia and p53 mutations in the seven colectomy specimens. There is a wide range of variation in the correlation between these parameters.

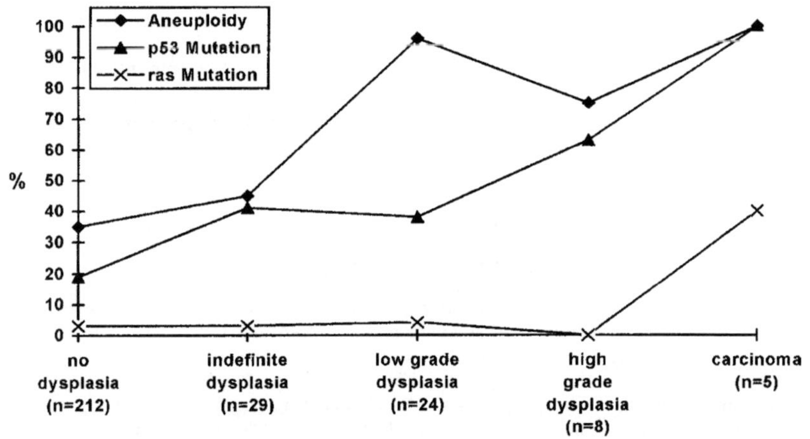

Figure 4   DNA aneuploidy, p53 and Ki-ras mutations in correlation with the grade of dysplasia in seven colectomy specimen. A total of 278 samples was analysed

Table 3 Variation of the correlation between DNA aneuploidy, p53 mutations and dysplasia in seven colectomy specimens. The patient J.G. was operated on because of clinical deterioration despite medical treatment

Patient	Percentage and numbers of aneuploid samples with a p53 mutation	Percentage and numbers of dysplastic samples with a p53 mutation	Percentage and numbers of dysplastic samples with DNA aneuploidy
M.D.	7% (2/28)	0% (0/1)	100% (1/1)
U.K.	58% (7/12)	40% (4/10)	80% (8/10)
U.G.	42% (3/7)	0% (0/6)	17% (1/6)
G.G.	70% (19/27)	74% (17/23)	87% (20/23)
M.F.	60% (3/5)	27% (3/11)	36% (4/11)
M.K.	100% (1/1)	33% (1/3)	0% (0/4)
J.G.	0% (0/0)	0% (0/0)	0% (0/0)

DISCUSSION

In surveillance studies dysplasia is used as a marker of an increased cancer risk. However, diagnosis of dysplasia may be hampered by the simultaneous presence of inflammation and classification of dysplasia by inter- and intra-individual variation[3]. Because histological interpretation is relatively subjective it would be helpful to have a more objective method to help identify those patients most likely to develop a malignant transformation in the future. The determination of DNA ploidy status by flow cytometry is emerging as a potential prognostic aid in a variety of human tumours. Alteration of DNA ploidy can also be found in pre-malignant conditions. This study demonstrates that flow cytometry is capable of detecting alterations in DNA content and cell proliferation in patients with UC.

DNA aneuploidy in our study was associated with duration of disease and almost exclusively with total colitis. This observation runs parrallel to the increased cancer risk in total UC compared to other forms of UC. Ekbom and co-workers[9] noted a significantly increased cancer risk in patients with pancolitis compared to patients with left-sided colitis or proctitis. The percentage of patients with DNA aneuploidy in the subgroup of patients with pancolitis is in agreement with other studies[10,11].

Because the appearance of dysplasia may be patchy detection of dysplasia by endoscopic biopsy may be difficult. In some of our patients widely distributed aneuploid areas were present throughout the whole colon. This wide distribution of DNA aneuploidy will naturally diminish the sampling error. This observation is supported by the high rate of reproducibility of the flow cytometric results in contrast to the low reproducibility of the histological results.

Although some studies showed a relatively good correlation between dysplasia and DNA aneuploidy this close relationship was not confirmed by some other studies[3,4,6,12]. In some patients DNA aneuploidy without the simultaneous detection of dysplasia was found. The percentage of DNA aneuploidy in non-dysplastic mucosa in other studies ranges from 2.5% to 11.6%[3,6,10,12]

The follow-up in our study is still limited. However, in some patients DNA aneuploidy was detected before the occurrence of dysplasia. These observations are supported by the data of Rubin and co-workers[13] indicating that DNA aneuploidy might precede the development of dysplasia, and that flow cytometry has the potential to reduce the cost of surveillance by identifying the subgroup of patients who require frequent follow-up and those who do not. In a prospective colonoscopic surveillance study in Sweden[14] 15 out of 59 patients with pancolitis (25.4%) had DNA aneuploidy detected at least once during the follow-up. DNA aneuploidy occurred before development of definitive dysplasia in six patients, simultaneously with development of dysplasia in six patients, and after development of dysplasia in one patient only. From these studies, and from our own results, it can be deduced that the isolated detection of DNA aneuploidy or the simultaneous detection of aneuploidy and dysplasia reflects an increased risk of the development of dysplasia or the progression of dysplastic lesions, respectively. Therefore, flow cytometry really has the potential to increase the cost–benefit ratio in surveillance of patients with UC.

Patients with PSC showed a higher percentage of DNA aneuploidy and dysplasia. This observation is in accordance with other studies showing an increased percentage of dysplastic changes in patients with PSC and UC[15]. PSC in UC has been associated with a higher risk of developing colorectal neoplasia[16].

It should be taken into consideration that flow cytometry is able to detect only numerical, but not structural, chromosomal aberrations which might be present in dysplastic and in normal mucosa. The sum of numerical chromosomal alterations is reflected by DNA aneuploidy. Vogelstein and co-workers[17] have shown that the sum of genetic alterations is crucial for colorectal carcinogenesis.

Our analysis in the colectomy specimen reveals that the occurrence of DNA aneuploidy is one of the earliest events in the development of colitis-associated carcinoma. The strong correlation of p53 mutations with the degree of dysplasia and their high percentage in histologically negative samples indicates that this genetic alteration is an important event, and occurs at an early stage of colorectal tumour development in UC. The impact of molecular genetic changes on surveillance strategies in UC has still to be defined by long-term studies, because our study in colectomy specimens showed a broad variation in the correlation of aneuploid, dysplastic and p53 mutated samples between patients.

Because DNA aneuploidy represents an early alteration during neoplastic transformation in UC, and because DNA aneuploidy can often be found widespread throughout the colorectum, thus increasing the reproducibility and the early detection of patients at risk, flow cytometry is an important tool in the surveillance of patients with UC. Flow cytometric analysis of cellular DNA content will help to improve the cost–benefit ratio in surveillance strategies because the detection of aneuploidy indicates an increased risk for the development of dysplastic changes.

Acknowledgements

This work was supported by the Deutsche Krebshilfe and Grimmke Foundation.

References

1. Porschen R, Strohmeyer G. Dysplasie und kolorektales Karzinomrisiko bei Colitis ulcerosa. Dtsch Med Wochenschr. 1991;116:1682–8.

2. Riddell RH, Goldmann H, Ransohoff DF *et al.* Dysplasia in inflammatory bowel disease: standardized classification with provisional clinical applications. Hum Pathol. 1983;14:931–68.
3. Melville DM, Jass JR, Shepherd NA *et al.* Dysplasia and deoxyribonucleic acid aneuploidy in the assessment of precancerous changes in chronic ulcerative colitis. Observer variation and correlation. Gastroenterology. 1988;95:668–75.
4. Löfberg R, Tribukait B, Öst A, Broström O, Reichard H. Flow cytometric DNA analysis in long-standing ulcerative colitis: a method of prediction of dysplasia and carcinoma development? Gut. 1987;28:1100–6.
5. Porschen R, Robin U, Schumacher A *et al.* DNA aneuploidy in Crohn's disease and ulcerative colitis: results of a comparative flow cytometric study. Gut. 1992;33:663–7.
6. Rutegard J, Ahsgren L, Stenling R, Roos G. DNA content in ulcerative colitis. Flow cytometric analysis in a patient series from a defined area. Dis Colon Rectum. 1988;31:710–15.
7. Vindelov LL, Christensen IJ, Nissen NI. A detergent–trypsin method for the preparation of nuclei for flow cytometric DNA analysis. Cytometry. 1983;3:323–7.
8. Holzmann KH, Klump B, Borchard F *et al.* Comparative analysis of histology, DNA content, p53 and Ki-ras mutations in colectomy specimens with long-standing ulcerative colitis. Int J Cancer. 1998;76:1–6.
9. Ekbom A, Helmick C, Zack M, Adami HO. Ulcerative colitis and colorectal cancer. A population-based study. N Engl J Med. 1990;323:1228–33.
10. Hammarberg G, Slezak P, Tribukait B. Early detection of malignancy in ulcerative colitis. A flow-cytometric DNA study. Cancer. 1984;53:291–5.
11. Löfberg R, Broström O, Karlén P, Tribukait B, Öst Å. Colonoscopic surveillance in long-standing total ulcerative colitis – a 15-year follow-up study. Gastroenterology. 1990;99:1021–31.
12. Fozard JBJ, Quirke P, Dixon MF, Giles GR, Bird CC. DNA aneuploidy in ulcerative colitis. Gut. 1986;27:1414–18.
13. Rubin CE, Haggitt RC, Burmer GC *et al.* DNA aneuploidy in colonic biopsies predicts future development of dysplasia in ulcerative colitis. Gastroenterology. 1992;103:1611–20.
14. Löfberg R, Broström O, Karlén P, Öst Å, Tribukait B. DNA aneuploidy in ulcerative colitis: reproducibility, topographic distribution, and relation to dysplasia. Gastroenterology. 1992;102:1149–54.
15. Brentnall TA, Haggitt RC, Rabinovitch PS *et al.* Risk and natural history of colonic neoplasia in patients with primary sclerosing cholangitis and ulcerative colitis. Gastroenterology. 1996;110:331–8.
16. Broome U, Löfberg R, Veress B, Eriksson LS. Primary sclerosing cholangitis and ulcerative colitis: evidence for increased neoplastic potential. Hepatology. 1995;22:1404–8.
17. Vogelstein B, Fearon ER, Hamilton SR *et al.* Genetic alterations during colorectal-tumour development. N Engl J Med. 1988;319:207–11.

29
K-ras and p53 mutations in colonic lavage fluid of patients with long-standing IBD

K. LOESCHKE, M. HEINZLMANN and S. M. LANG

INTRODUCTION

For the early detection of neoplastic lesions in ulcerative colitis and Crohn's disease, present surveillance strategies are not entirely satisfactory[1,2]. Among others, three fundamental problems remain unsolved. The first is that we do not know the cancer risk under present therapeutic regimens because all data stem from past decades. Improved medication may have lowered the risk, in particular 5-ASA preparations and folic acid supplementation[3–6]. If the present risk is overestimated, the clinical benefit of yearly or 2-yearly surveillance colonoscopy may be lower than presumed. A second problem is the histological assessment of dysplasia. Judgement may vary between pathologists and the clinical consequences of low-grade dysplasia are controversial. The third and probably most important issue is that even serial biopsies may fail to detect dysplasia in some spots of the large mucosal surface area not biopsied. Thus, even invasive carcinoma may remain undiscovered unless a suspicious lesion[7] is seen macroscopically. These and additional open questions have been discussed in more detail recently[2], as well as in this volume.

Therefore, means to improve cancer surveillance in inflammatory bowel disease (IBD) would be highly desirable. In this chapter we summarize our preliminary experience using methods derived from progress in the understanding of the molecular biology of colorectal carcinoma. We have investigated mutations of the K-ras and p53 genes in the colonic lavage fluid of patients with long-standing IBD.

RATIONALE FOR SEARCHING K-ras AND p53 MUTATIONS IN COLONIC LAVAGE FLUID

In sporadic colorectal carcinoma, two of the most frequent mutations are those of the K-ras oncogene and the p53 suppressor gene; they are seen in approximately 50% of these tumours. Without discussing any model of tumour progression based on molecular biology data one may state that these and other mutations may precede overt malignancy. Although data in colitis carcinoma are limited, similar mutations are found in malignant tumours developing in long-standing extensive colitis[8–15]. In this group of patients, available data suggest that the tumour risk begins after about 7 years of disease and may reach approximately 10% after 25 years[5,16–19]. Thus, we limited our studies to patients with a disease duration of at least 7 years.

Following the initial report by Sidransky *et al.*[20], several groups have shown that K-ras and p53 mutations can be detected not only in the tumour itself but also in the stool of patients with colorectal carcinoma or adenoma[21–24]. Obviously, mutated cells are shed into the stools. Instead of stool we used lavage fluid obtained at colonoscopy[25,26] which will also contain cells exfoliated from the whole intestinal tract. Such collected cells may be more representative than random biopsies of preneoplastic changes in any part of the intestine. Lavage fluid is fairly clean as compared to stools which may contain contaminants interfering with the polymerase chain reaction (PCR)[21] or causing other methodological difficulties. For these reasons we studied lavage fluid remaining in the colon before colonoscopy was performed.

PATIENTS

Our main group comprised patients with total or subtotal ulcerative colitis but patients with left-sided or distal ulcerative colitis or Crohn's disease were included later. 'Positive' controls were patients with colorectal carcinoma or adenoma, and 'negative' controls were patients without intestinal inflammation or tumour, e.g. irritable bowel syndrome or diverticulosis. Most colitis patients presented for cancer surveillance. In addition to the serial biopsies sent to the pathologist for evaluation of dysplasia, we obtained two to four biopsies to search for mutations in the tissue. So far we have found no mutations in any of the biopsies studied. Patients gave informed consent, and the protocol was approved by the local ethical committee.

ANALYSIS OF K-ras AND p53 MUTATIONS

In all patients, including the controls, the lavage fluid (50–500 ml) contained sufficient DNA for evaluation. It was washed until the supernatant became clear. DNA was extracted by lysis with guanidine thiocyanate. Codon 12 and 13 of exon 1 of the K-ras and exon 5–8 of the p53 gene were amplified by PCR. Mutations of the K-ras gene were analysed by hybridization with digoxygenin-labelled detection oligonucleotides and demonstrated by chemoluminescence on superimposed X-ray films. Mutations of the p53 gene were analysed by SSCP analysis using polyacrylamide–glycerol gel electrophoresis and visualized by silver staining. The protocol has recently been published in detail[26].

K-ras AND p53 MUTATIONS IN EXTENSIVE COLITIS

Table 1 shows our results in 32 patients with total or subtotal ulcerative colitis. In this table the patients are grouped according to disease duration, disease

Table 1   K-ras and p53 mutations in colonic lavage fluid of patients with extensive ulcerative colitis

			Mutations	
	n	*K-ras*	*p53*	*Total*
Disease duration (years)				
7–9	13	0	1	1/13
10–15	11	1	4	5/11
>15	8	1	0	1/8
Disease severity				
Mild	4	0	1	1/4
Moderate	13	2	3	5/13
Severe	15	0	1	1/15
Morphological activity				
No relevant activity	14	1	3	4/14
Moderate	15	1	2	3/15
Severe	3	0	0	0/3

severity and morphological activity at the time of colonoscopy. Disease was classified as mild when only 5-aminosalicylic acid (5-ASA) preparations had been used, as moderate when steroids had been employed, and as severe when immunosuppressive drugs – usually azathioprine – had been necessary for treatment during the course of disease. Most of the patients had moderate or severe disease but presently low morphological activity. We found K-ras mutations in two and p53 mutations in five patients. Except for one patient, all of them had the disease for 10 or more years, and up to 26 years. To evaluate a possible influence of disease severity and morphological activity, subgroups are distributed somewhat unevenly in this small series, and no clear-cut pattern emerges from these data. Taking the K-ras and p53 mutations together, seven of the 32 patients, or 22%, had a mutation of some kind in the lavage fluid. None of these seven patients had dysplasia in the serial biopsies but four patients without a mutation had mild dysplasia. There were three patients with backwash ileitis, and one of these had a K-ras mutation. There was no patient with primary sclerosing cholangitis. Both of these disease features have been described as increasing the risk of malignancy[4,27–30]. The types of mutations are shown in Table 2. One of the p53 mutations was a loss of heterozygosity[31].

Table 2   K-ras and p53 mutations in seven patients with extensive ulcerative colitis

K-ras	1× Gly → Asp 12
	1× Gly → Val 12
p53	2× exon 5
	1× exon 6
	1× exon 7
	1× exon 7 LOH

K-ras AND p53 MUTATIONS IN CONTROLS

In 27 controls without inflammation or tumour, we found one p53 mutation (3%). This 56-year-old female had a family history of pancreatic cancer, but no malignant disease was found during follow-up for 1 year. The difference in mutation frequency between extensive colitis and control patients is statistically significant ($p = 0.01$). In a small number of adenoma and carcinoma controls we found a mutation frequency of 25% and 40%, respectively. The mutations of the tumour itself have not yet been analysed, so that these figures, although somewhat low, are not unreasonable.

K-ras AND p53 MUTATIONS IN PATIENTS WITH LEFT-SIDED/DISTAL ULCERATIVE COLITIS AND CROHN'S DISEASE

In less extensive colitis, cancer risk is lower, and very low in proctitis[17], so that proctitis patients were not included. In Crohn's disease the risk is less well defined[32], but may be similar to ulcerative colitis, at least when large areas of the colon are affected[16]. In about 20 patients, each with left-sided/distal ulcerative colitis or Crohn's disease, the mutation frequency was 10% and 14%, respectively, matching the risk in these patient subgroups as derived from clinical experience.

REPEAT INVESTIGATIONS AFTER 1–3 YEARS

Some of our patients could be re-studied after an average of 2 years using the same methods. In three patients the same p53 mutation was found at the second colonoscopy. None of these three patients had developed dysplasia or carcinoma. Of two ulcerative colitis patients with mild dysplasia at the first examination, the same degree of dysplasia was still present in both, but neither carcinoma nor a mutation in the lavage was detected. One of the two other patients was colectomized without developing carcinoma, and the other could not be re-studied.

ASPECTS FOR THE FUTURE

With these initial data in mind we can now ask whether this approach is promising and should be carried further. We agree with others[33] that this should be done. One encouraging result is that, with appropriate methods, enough sediment for DNA analysis can be recovered from the lavage fluid in practically every patient, whether the disease is morphologically active or not. We also can state that mutations of the K-ras or p53 gene are present in a sizeable number of patients with IBD and liability to cancer, and that the same mutations are found in repeat studies after 1–3 years, at least in some patients. On the other hand, at present we are uncertain whether these mutations indeed indicate future cancer development, perhaps some years later as suggested by some anecdotal reports[25,34]. We also do not know which of the various mutations are clinically most important. With respect to K-ras mutations, these may also be found in non-dysplastic colorectal lesions[35,36], and in one study involving 20 patients with chronic pancreatitis and K-ras mutations in pancreatic juice, long-term follow-up did not reveal cancer development after several years[37]. With regard to p53, loss of heterozygosity may be more important than point mutations. It could also be that other gene mutations or products will prove to be more discriminative, e.g. mutations resulting in microsatellite instability[38,39] or elevated c-Src tyrosine kinase activity[40]. Therefore, for the time being we advise that our patients have a sooner follow-up when a K-ras or p53 mutation has been found, especially when it is confirmed in a repeat study.

Several approaches should be followed. First, we need a larger number of patients to discover whether the mutation frequencies found so far are representative. In particular, we need more patients with dysplasia at biopsy to see whether any correlation between mutations and dysplastic changes can be established. Second, observation periods must be extended to find out how often and which mutations are reproducible, and whether they are better predictors of malignancy as compared to random biopsies. Third, other gene mutations should be included in the analysis if practicable. If these studies substantiate the value of mutation analysis, the final goal is to simplify methods in order to improve cancer surveillance. Serum analysis of p53 antibodies or mutated DNA[41–44] may also be a perspective. A German multicentre study is in preparation to achieve some of these goals.

SUMMARY

1. Lavage fluid obtained at surveillance colonoscopy contains sufficient DNA to be analysed for gene mutations.
2. Mutations of the K-ras or p53 gene are found in 10–20% of various subgroups of patients with long-standing IBD.
3. These mutations are confirmed in some patients in repeat studies after 1–3 years.
4. This approach is promising and should be extended in longitudinal studies involving more patients with IBD and cancer risk.

Acknowledgements

Parts of this study were supported by Grant no. 82 32 11, Wilhelm Vaillant Stiftung; by Ferring GmbH, Kiel; and by the Falk Foundation, Freiburg, Germany.

References

1. Shanahan F. Discontent with dysplasia surveillance in ulcerative colitis. Inflamm Bowel Dis. 1995;1:80–3.
2. Lennard-Jones JE. Prevention of carcinoma. In: Clinical Challenges in Inflammatory Bowel Diseases. Diagnosis, prognosis and treatment. Dordrecht: Kluwer; 1998:181–93.
3. Pinczowski D, Ekbom A, Baron J, Yuen J, Adami H-O. Risk factors for colorectal cancer in patients with ulcerative colitis: a case–control study. Gastroenterology. 1994;107:117–20.
4. Bansal P, Sonnenberg A. Risk factors of colorectal cancer in inflammatory bowel disease. Am J Gastroenterol. 1996;91:44–8.

5. Moody GA, Jayanthi V, Probert CSJ, MacKay H, Mayberry JF. Long-term therapy with sulphasalzine protects against colorectal cancer in ulcerative colitis: A retrospective study of colorectal cancer risk and compliance with treatment in Leicestershire. Eur J Gastroenterol Hepatol. 1996;8:1179–83.

6. Lashner BA, Provencher KS, Seidner DL, Knesebeck A, Brzezinski A. The effect of folic acid supplementation on the risk for cancer or dysplasia in ulcerative colitis. Gastroenterology. 1997;112:29–32.

7. Blackstone MO, Riddel RH, Rogers BHG, Levin B. Dysplasia-associated lesion or mass (DALM) detected by colonoscopy in long-standing ulcerative colitis: An indication for colectomy. Gastroenterology. 1981;80:366–74.

8. Itzkowitz SH, Greenwald B, Meltzer SJ. Colon carcinogenesis in inflammatory bowel disease. Inflamm Bowel Dis. 1995;1:142–58.

9. Greenwald B, Harpaz N, Yin J et al. Loss of heterozygosity affecting the p53, Rb, and mcc/apc tumor suppressor gene loci in dysplastic and cancerous ulcerative colitis. Cancer Res. 1992;52:741–5.

10. Taylor HW, Boyle M, Smith SC, Bustin S, Williams NS. Expression of p53 in colorectal cancer and dysplasia complicating ulcerative colitis. Br J Surg. 1993;80:442–4.

11. Bell SM, Kelly SA, Hoyle JA et al. c-Ki-ras gene mutations in dysplasia and carcinomas complicating ulcerative colitis. Br J Cancer. 1991;64:174–8.

12. Benhattar J, Saraga E. Molecular genetics of dysplasia in ulcerative colitis. Eur J Cancer. 1995;31A:1171–3.

13. Redstone MS, Papadopoulos N, Caldas C, Kinzler KW, Kern SE. Common occurrence of APC and K-ras gene mutations in the spectrum of colitis-associated neoplasias. Gastroenterology. 1995;108:383–92.

14. Yin J, Harpaz N, Tong Y et al. p53 mutations in dysplastic and cancerous ulcerative colitis lesions. Gastroenterology. 1993;104:1633–9.

15. Shapiro BD, Goldblum JR, Hussain A, Lashner BA. The role of p53 mutations in colorectal cancer surveillance for ulcerative colitis. Gastroenterology. 1997;112:A1089 (abstract).

16. Gillen CD, Walmsley RS, Prior P, Andrews HA, Allan RN. Ulcerative colitis and Crohn's disease: a comparison of the colorectal cancer risk in extensive colitis. Gut. 1994;35:1590–2.

17. Ekbom A, Helmick C, Zack M, Adami H-O. Ulcerative colitis and colorectal cancer. A population-based study. N Engl J Med. 1990;323:1228–33.

18. Lennard-Jones JE, Melville DM, Morson BC, Ritchie JK, Williams CB. Precancer and cancer in extensive ulcerative colitis: findings among 401 patients over 22 years. Gut. 1990;31:800–6.

19. Katzka I, Brody RS, Morris E, Katz S. Assessment of colorectal cancer risk in patients with ulcerative colitis: experience from a private practice. Gastroenterology. 1983;85:22–9.

20. Sidransky D, Tokino T, Hamilton SR et al. Identification of ras oncogene mutations in the stool of patients with curable colorectal tumors. Science. 1992;256:102–5.

21. Smith-Ravin J, England J, Talbot IC, Bodmer W. Detection of c-Ki-ras mutations in faecal samples from sporadic colorectal cancer patients. Gut. 1995;36:81–6.

22. Eguchi S, Kohara N, Komuta K, Kanematsu T. Mutations of the p53 gene in the stool of patients with resectable colorectal cancer. Cancer. 1996;77:1707–10.

23. Villa E, Dugani A, Rebecchi AM et al. Identification of subjects at risk for colorectal carcinoma through a test based on K-ras determination in the stool. Gastroenterology. 1996;110:1346–53.

24. Hasegawa Y, Takeda S, Ichii S et al. Detection of K-ras mutations in DNAs isolated from feces of patients with colorectal tumors by mutant-allele-specific amplification (MASA). Oncogene. 1995;10:1441–5.

25. Tobi M, Luo F-C, Ronai Z. Detection of K-ras mutation in colonic effluent samples from patients without evidence of colorectal carcinoma. J Natl Cancer Inst. 1994;86:1007–10.

26. Lang SM, Heinzlmann M, Stratakis DF et al. Detection of Ki-ras mutations by PCR and differential hybridization and of p53 mutations by SSCP analysis in endoscopically obtained lavage solution from patients with long-standing ulcerative colitis. Am J Gastroenterol. 1997;92:2166–70.

27. Broomé U, Löfberg R, Veress B, Eriksson LS. Primary sclerosing cholangitis and ulcerative colitis: evidence for increased neoplastic potential. Hepatology. 1995;22:1404–8.

28. Brentnall T, Haggitt RC, Rabinovitch PS et al. Risk and natural history of colonic neoplasia in patients with primary sclerosing cholangitis and ulcerative colitis. Gastroenterology. 1996;110:331–8.

29. Marchesa P, Lashner BA, Lavery IC et al. The risk of cancer and dysplasia among ulcerative colitis patients with primary sclerosing cholangitis. Am J Gastroenterol. 1997;92:1285–8.

30. Herbay VA, Otto HF. Backwash ileitis in ulcerative colitis: a study in 302 patients. Falk Symposium 1996 Freiburg. Poster 85.

31. Lang SM, Heinzlmann M, Stratakis DF *et al.* Molecular screening of patients with long-standing extensive ulcerative colitis: detection of p53 and Ki-ras mutations by SSCP analysis and differential hybridization in colonic lavage fluid. (Submitted).

32. Bernstein D, Rogers A. Malignancy in Crohn's disease. Am J Gastroenterol. 1996;91:434–40.

33. Villa E. Molecular screening. Why haven't we started yet? Editorial. Am Gastroenterol. 1997;92:2144–6.

34. Ilyas M, Talbot IC. p53 expression in ulcerative colitis: a longitudinal study. Gut. 1995;37:802–4.

35. Jen J, Powell SM, Papadopoulos N *et al.* Molecular determinants of dysplasia in colorectal lesions. Cancer Res. 1994;54:5523–6.

36. Chaubert P, Benhattar J, Saraga E, Costa J. K-ras mutations and p53 alterations in neoplastic and nonneoplastic lesions associated with longstanding ulcerative colitis. Am J Pathol. 1994;144:767–75.

37. Furuya N, Kawa S, Akamatsu T, Furihata K. Long-term follow-up of patients with chronic pancreatitis and K-ras gene mutation detected in pancreatic juice. Gastroenterology. 1997;113:593–8.

38. Brentnall TA, Rubin CE, Crispin DA *et al.* A germline substitution in the human MSH2 gene is associated with high-grade dysplasia and cancer in ulcerative colitis. Gastroenterology. 1995;109:151–5.

39. Souza RF, Lei J, Yin J *et al.* A transforming growth factor β1 receptor type II mutation in ulcerative colitis-associated neoplasms. Gastroenterology. 1997;112:40–5.

40. Cartwright CA, Coad CA, Egbert BM. Elevated c-Src tyrosine kinase activity in premalignant epithelia of ulcerative colitis. J Clin Invest. 1994;93:509–15.

41. Shibata Y, Kotanagi H, Andoh H *et al.* Detection of circulating anti-p53 antibodies in patients with colorectal carcinoma and the antibody's relation to clinical factors. Dis Colon Rectum. 1996;39:1269–74.

42. Angelopoulou K, Stratis M, Diamandis EP. Humoral immune response against p53 protein in patients with colorectal carcinoma. Int J Cancer. 1997;70:46–51.

43. Hammel P, Boissier B, Chaumette M-T *et al.* Detection and monitoring of serum p53 antibodies in patients with colorectal cancer. Gut. 1997;40:356–61.

44. Anker P, Lefort F, Vasioukhin V *et al.* K-ras mutations are found in DNA extracted from the plasma of patients with colorectal cancer. Gastroenterology. 1997;112:1114–20.

30
The impact of therapy on colorectal cancer in ulcerative colitis

A. RAEDLER and J. HÄMLING

Spontaneous colorectal cancer is thought to be caused by genetic alterations with regard to oncogene expression, defective tumour suppression genes and insufficient DNA repair. Inherited genetic dysfunctions are supposed to be supported by environmental factors to produce malignancy. Chronic inflammation can be regarded as a factor that is definitely able to convert normal cells into cancerous cell clones. This lesson has been learned from the *Helicobacter* story. These bacteria obviously induce gastric lymphomas and possibly gastric cancer: B cell clones that show all characteristics of malignant cells can be forced to be normal mucosa-associated lymphoid tissue (MALT) cells if the antigenic stimulus is eliminated, i.e. *Helicobacter pylori* bacteria eradicated. Thus the point of no return in the development of malignancy seems to be shifted towards a more advanced lymphoma stage. This can be regarded as a change of paradigm.

It is not well understood how the inflammatory process is able to produce cell transformation. Cytokines and growth hormones are claimed to be responsible for uncontrolled cell proliferation. Moreover, free oxygen radicals, that are released by inflammatory cells, are known to produce DNA damage. It is speculated that other secondary and tertiary mediators of inflammation may partake in inducing malignancy on lymphocytes and epithelial cells.

Besides *Helicobacter*-induced MALT lymphomas there are other well-established examples for a pathophysiological relationship between inflammation and malignancy. These include Epstein–Barr virus (EBV)-induced Burkitt lymphoma, immunoproliferative small intestinal disease (IPSID) and T-cell lymphoma in coeliac disease. It is tempting to assume that, also in ulcerative colitis, development of cancer is at least partly due to chronic inflammation.

There are many arguments in favour of this hypothesis: the preferred sites of malignancy are identical with the areas of most severe inflammatory activities. One may safely assume that the agents that produce inflammation are the same as those that produce malignant transformation in patients with inflammatory bowel disease (IBD) and possibly also in patients with sporadic colorectal cancer. From experimental data, as well as epidemiological observations, these agents' effectiveness in producing malignancy also depends on bacterial flora and nutritional compounds.

Colorectal cancer in patients with ulcerative colitis is related to the extent of disease, duration of disease and age of onset: diagnosis at childhood is related to an increased risk[1]. However, a higher incidence of ulcerative colitis has been shown to be not associated with a comparable increase in IBD carcinomas[2]. This 'lower-than-expected' incidence of colorectal cancer in recent decades cannot be explained by successful surveillance programmes, increased numbers of patients with only distal colitis and proctitis (which is not a precancerous disease), or a greater proportion of patients who underwent colectomy. Thus the hypothesis was tested whether therapy of intestinal inflammation could be responsible for the decrease in cancer incidence.

The drug mainly used in medication of ulcerative colitis in recent decades is sulphasalazine. There are some hints from epidemiological studies that this drug may have a positive influence concerning prevention of malignancy. Patients in whom drug levels have been reduced, because of low compliance, drug allergy and insignificant clinical symptoms, have a higher risk of developing colorectal cancer.

There are two cohort risk factor studies that support the hypothesis that sulphasalazine is able to protect against malignancy. Pinczowski and co-workers[3] analysed 3112 patients with ulcerative colitis in a population-based cohort and compared 102 cases of colorectal cancer and 196 matched controls without cancer. They found that pharmacological therapy, especially with sulphasalazine, lasting at least 3 months, was associated with a significant protective effect (RR 0.38, 95% confidence interval 0.20–1.25). They proposed that the risk of colorectal cancer among patients with ulcerative colitis can be reduced through therapy with sulphasalazine.

Moody and co-workers[4] estimated the prognosis of a 10-year cohort as expressed by risk of colectomy and risk of colorectal cancer; moreover they assessed the impact of long-term sulphasalazine on the natural course of ulcerative colitis. They analysed 175 patients with full-blown or limited disease. The cumulative incidence of colorectal cancer 10 years after diagnosis was 2.1%, and at 20 years it was 7.4% for the total group, excluding those with a colectomy. The crude proportions developing cancer were 5/152 (= 3%) in the group who took long-term sulphasalazine but 5/16 (31%) in those who had had their treatment stopped, or who did not comply with therapy. These differences were shown to be highly significant.

Again it was claimed from these data that patients with ulcerative colitis who were not on long-term sulphasalazine or 5-aminosalicylic acid therapy independent of whether stopped by the doctor or due to lack of compliance) were significantly more likely to develop colorectal cancer.

Sulphasalazine and aminosalicylic acid have a structural configuration that resembles aspirin. This latter drug has been shown to be able to prevent cancer successfully[5]. However sulphasalazine has a different mode of action on a molecular level. It is effective in inhibiting the prostaglandin synthesis and platelet functions. 5-ASA, in contrast, is more active in reducing leukotriene action, immunoglobulin production and cytokine release. Moreover it is proposed to act as a potent scavenger for oxygen radicals, and thus inhibits the cascade of inflammation in the intestinal mucosa. On the other hand there are data showing that sulphasalazine inhibits folate acid resorption; the latter itself is known to reduce the risk of colorectal cancer[6]. Thus the protective process remains unresolved.

References

1. Ekbohm A, Helmick C, Zack M, Adami HO. Ulcerative colitis and colorectal cancer. N Engl J Med. 1990;323:1228–33.
2. Ekbohm A, Kornfeld D. Sulphasalazine use as a preventive factor for colorectal cancer in ulcerative colitis patients. Inflamm Bowel Dis. 1996;2:276–8.
3. Pinczowski D, Ekbohm A, Baron J, Yuen J, Adami HO. Risk factors for colorectal cancer in patients with ulcerative colitis: a case control study. Gastroenterology. 1994;107:117–20.
4. Moody GA, Jayanthi V, Probert CSJ, MacKay H, Mayberry JF. Long term therapy with sulphasalazine protects against colorectal cancer in ulcerative colitis: a retrospective study of colorectal risk and compliance with treatment in Leicestershire. Eur J Gastroenterol Hepatol. 1996;8:1179–83.
5. Thun MJ, Mohan M, Namboodiri BS, Heath CW. Aspirin use and reduced risk of fatal colon cancer. N Engl J Med. 1991;325:1593–6.
6. Giovannucci E, Rimm EB, Ascherio A, Stampfer MJ, Colditz GA, Willet WC. Alcohol, low-methionine–low-folate diets, and risks of colon cancer in men. J Natl Cancer Inst. 1995;87:255–73.

Section IX
Therapy in IBD

31
Therapeutic concepts in IBD

D. H. PRESENT

Much has been learned in recent years regarding the concepts of mucosal immunology in inflammatory bowel disease (IBD). This has led to an understanding of some of the mechanisms that are at work when using currently available drugs. Experimental models and basic studies have recently demonstrated a new and exciting drug, a monoclonal antibody against tumour necrosis factor (TNF) (infliximab), which has been shown to be dramatically effective in reducing Crohn's disease activity and in the healing of fistulas[1].

However, it is my opinion that current concepts of treating IBD are somewhat outdated, and as we approach the millennium we should reconsider how we manage both ulcerative colitis and Crohn's disease.

We currently understand that both these diseases are genetic disorders that are triggered by environmental factors that then produce an exaggerated immune response in the gut. However, this does not mean that each form of these diseases should be treated in the same manner. For example, there may be simple Crohn's disease involving the terminal ileum, there may be diffuse jejuno-ileitis, there may be enteroenteric fistulas or fistulas to different areas of the body, such as an enterovesical fistula. Crohn's disease is not a single entity and should at least be divided into a perforating and non-perforating pattern[2]. The perforating or fistulizing Crohn's disease is much more aggressive, shows earlier recurrence after surgery and earlier reoperation. This has been confirmed by Aeberhardt et al.[3], in which study the perforating variety recurred at a mean of 1.7 years, contrasted with the non-perforating at 13.0 years ($p = 0.005$). At the least this should make the clinician consider different types of therapy for different types of Crohn's disease.

The most common therapy for mild to moderate Crohn's disease and ulcerative colitis is either sulphasalazine or mesalamine, the latter of which is produced in various release forms. It is extremely important to look at the dose being administered in trials, as well as where the agent may be released. Unfortunately, since many of these agents are pH-dependent, we cannot be sure whether the drug is reaching the areas of bowel activity.

Four grams of 5-aminosalicylic acid (5 ASA) have been shown to be effective in the treatment of active Crohn's disease in one study[4], but not confirmed in two other similar trials, because of unexpected high placebo responses. This should not lead the clinician to conclude that 5-ASA drugs are ineffective in Crohn's disease, but rather, in a meta-analysis[5], 5-ASA drugs were shown to be approximately 15–20% better than placebo in maintaining relapse-free rates. Controlled trialists may insist that statistically significant *remission rates* are the most important criteria for judging a drug's effectiveness; however, the patient will often be quite happy if the severity of the disease can be moderately diminished. Complete remission is a desire, but not a necessity. Likewise, meta-analyses have shown that the 5-ASA drugs are statistically effective in ulcerative colitis in inducing and maintaining remission. Meta-analysis has failed to show any benefit, dose-for-dose, of the newer 5-ASA drugs compared to the older sulphasalazine, and my personal preference, especially for distal ulcerative proctosigmoiditis, is to start with sulphasalazine. In my experience toxicity occurs in about 10%, and can be avoided if the drug is introduced gradually and taken with food. For those who develop upper gastrointestinal symptoms, the coated tablet should be prescribed. Relapse-free rates are increased as the dosage is increased. Likewise, topical 5-ASA enemas and suppositories are prophylactic in ulcerative colitis. They have never been shown effective in distal Crohn's proctosigmoiditis. In the latter situation I recommend that immunosuppressives be instituted earlier, since Crohn's proctosigmoiditis is often a refractory form of the disorder.

In summary, our current concepts as regards 5-ASA drugs in IBD management are that both ulcerative colitis and Crohn's disease respond, but doses of at least 3 g or higher should be used to induce remission. The clinician should not be afraid to treat with doses up to 4–4.8 g daily and short-term studies using even higher doses of 5-ASA are probably warranted in Crohn's disease. Use the same induction dose as the maintenance dose in both ulcerative colitis and Crohn's disease.

5-ASA drugs are effective as postoperative prevention in doses of 3 g or higher. Several controlled and uncontrolled trials have shown the efficacy of several 5-ASA agents when used in adequate doses. Metronidazole has shown prevention lasting up to 1 year when used in high doses[6]. Trials are currently under way to discover whether lower doses for longer periods can keep the patient disease-free. A recent placebo-controlled trial has shown that 3 g of mesalamine is superior to placebo, and that 50 mg of 6-mercaptopurine (6-MP) is superior to placebo[7]. 6-MP appeared in several parameters to be more effective than the mesalamine. Current concepts should be changed so that all patients with Crohn's disease are considered for treatment with 6-MP postoperatively to prevent recurrence. Compliance should be excellent, since patients will only have to take a single pill of 6-MP daily.

Whether higher-dose 6-MP would be more effective, or whether the combination of 6-MP and 5-ASA and metronidazole would be the most effective regimen, remains to be determined.

Corticosteroids have been the mainstay as the initial therapy in moderate to severe Crohn's disease and ulcerative colitis. Unfortunately, many physicians also use it for mild ulcerative colitis and mild Crohn's disease, and I believe that this is inappropriate.

Steroids have been shown to be effective in a large controlled trial in active ulcerative colitis at each stage of severity[8]. However, two subsequent controlled trials have failed to show that corticosteroids are more effective than placebo in maintaining remission[9]. Therefore, steroids should not be used long term in the treatment of ulcerative colitis. Steroids are often used inappropriately in ulcerative colitis even when clinically indicated. For example, physicians should use higher doses (40–60 mg daily) rather than starting with lower doses and increasing gradually. Intravenous administration is more effective than oral administration. In addition, my experience has been that continuous infusions are more effective than pulse infusions. Most important, let me clearly state once again that steroids do not maintain remission in ulcerative colitis.

As regards Crohn's disease, the same is true. Steroids have been shown to be effective in the National Cooperative Crohn's Disease Study[10], which was of 17 weeks duration, and effective in the European Cooperative Study, which was a 6-week trial[11]. It must be clearly reinforced to clinicians that Crohn's disease is not a disease of 6 or 17 weeks, but rather a disease of a lifetime. There were four subsequent controlled trials, all of which failed to show that steroids could maintain remission in Crohn's disease. The toxic side-effects of steroids are well known to everybody, and therefore are little discussed. However, if a pharmaceutical company tried to bring a new drug on to the market, which produced cushingoid features, psychological side-effects (including psychosis), glaucoma, peptic disease, hypertension, diabetes, myopathy, avascular necrosis, osteoporosis and profound hypokalaemia, my guess is that it would never pass through the regulatory agencies. Nevertheless, physicians continue to use steroids for prolonged periods, despite this disastrous toxicity profile.

Gastroenterologists are currently using colonoscopy to diagnose Crohn's disease. I would recommend that barium studies are much more rewarding in that one can usually see fistula or fissuring in the bowel wall, which antedates the fistulization. In having my patients undergo barium studies I have seen that steroids will often 'worsen' the inflammatory process when fistulization is present. Until recently no controlled trial in Crohn's disease has randomized for patients with internal and external fistula. For example, budesonide has recently shown efficacy in two controlled trials[12,13]. All patients with fistula were excluded from the trials. However, in a prevention trial[14] there was no difference between budesonide and placebo at 1 year. Therefore this new effective agent, which appears to have less toxicity than standard corticosteroids, has not demonstrated any preventative ability. Since all patients with fistula were excluded from the budesonide studies we do not know the effect of this drug on fistulas. The final limitation on the use of steroids comes from both the National Cooperative Crohn's Disease Study and a study by Munkholm *et al.*, showing that almost 40% of patients who are started on prednisone will become steroid-dependent[10,15].

I therefore feel that we should adopt new concepts in IBD management as regards steroids in ulcerative colitis and Crohn's disease. First, start with the higher dose when treating, and use multiple dosing rather than a single dose. Remember that, if the patient is very sick, intravenous administration is more effective than oral administration, and that continuous infusions may be more effective than pulse therapy. However, remember that steroids do not have a role in the long-term prevention of either ulcerative colitis or Crohn's disease, and possibly may worsen Crohn's fistulas. The extensive toxicity of steroids precludes their use for longer than 3 months without a strong consideration for a change in therapy.

If I am advocating less use of steroids, what do clinicians have as alternatives? These would include high-dose 5-ASA, antibiotics, combinations of the above two, as well as immunomodulators and newer agents.

As regards antibiotics there are no 'large' controlled trials demonstrating efficacy with either broad-spectrum antibiotics or with antimycobacterial therapy. An initial uncontrolled study by Moss et al.[16] showed there was a clinical response of almost 90% and a radiological improvement in about two-thirds of patients when broad-spectrum antibiotics were used for 6 or more months. Recently a study by Prantera[17] has shown than metronidazole, in combination with ciprofloxacin, was effective in about 46% of active Crohn's patients. Another study by Colombel[18] has shown a 56% response to 1 g of ciprofloxacin daily. Consider that these response rates are only about 10% less than that seen with corticosteroids.

Finally, metronidazole in several controlled trials[19] has shown efficacy in both low and high doses. Because of the lack of extensive controlled data there are many conflicting opinions regarding the use of antibiotics in IBD management. In my clinical opinion it is clear that antibiotics are effective therapy. I believe they should always be used in fistulizing Crohn's disease and especially when steroids are introduced in patients with fistula. If there is no response to a single antibiotic, use combinations. There have been suggestions in uncontrolled trials that there may be a long-term role for broad-spectrum antibiotics in maintenance.

In summing up this section, in the treatment of mild to moderate Crohn's disease use high-dose 5-ASA and double antibiotic therapy in preference to oral steroids. The efficacy is almost equal to steroids and the toxicity is significantly lower.

We now turn to immunosuppressive therapy for IBD. As noted above, it has been shown that there is an exaggerated inflammatory process in the bowel. Cytokines such as interleukin 2 (IL-2), interferon-γ and TNFα are elevated. Strategies include trying to suppress these cytokines or, alternatively, to increase the anti-inflammatory cytokines, such as IL-10, IL-4 and TGFβ. For many years the strategy has been to use steroids and 5-ASA compounds to try to clear up the inflammatory process that has already occurred, whereas current strategy should be focused on trying to quiet the immunological process before excessive cytokines are released.

The most effective drugs in treating chronic Crohn's disease and chronic ulcerative colitis are 6-MP and azathioprine. An initial controlled trial from Mount Sinai Medical Center[20] showed overall clinical improvement, significant steroid sparing as well as fistula healing in chronic Crohn's disease. The National Cooperative Study failed to confirm these results, but the design of the trial was poor, in that it was completed in 17 weeks. Data have shown that the mean time to respond is approximately 3.1 months. Therefore, the study missed about 20% of the potential responders. Both barium studies and endoscopy have shown significant healing with 6-MP/azathioprine; however, its greatest efficacy has been with fistulization, where approximately 30% of fistulas close, and another 30% are clinically improved. Neither steroids nor 5-ASA products have ever shown closure of major fistulas (gastrocolic, ileovesical, perianal) as has been observed with 6-MP/azathioprine. Several uncontrolled studies, as well as one controlled trial[21], demonstrated that if the patient remains on 6-MP/azathioprine, the relapse rate over the next 1–2 years occurs in only 5%, whereas if the drug is discontinued the relapse rate ranges from 40% to 70%.

Although the controlled data are less clear, there are several large uncontrolled studies[22] showing that 6-MP is equally effective in steroid-refractory ulcerative colitis. In the largest study[23], 105 chronic patients who had failed steroids as well as oral and topical 5-ASA were treated with 6-MP. Responses noted include complete clinical remission in 65% and partial remission in 24%. Only 11% of patients failed. The longer the drug was continued the more likely the patient was to enter remission. In this large series it was shown that after initiation of 6-MP only 12% of this refractory group of patients required colectomy. A similar placebo-controlled trial using azathioprine has been carried out in ulcerative colitis[24], and showed maintenance of remission, in almost twice as many patients who were maintained on azathioprine as compared to those who discontinued it. The conclusion is quite clear: azathioprine and 6-MP prevent relapse both in Crohn's disease and ulcerative colitis.

Toxicity with 6-MP/azathioprine is significantly less than is observed with steroids[25]. An acute allergic reaction, with rash, fever and joint pain, is seen in approximately 2%. Self-limiting pancreatitis (which occurs in approximately 2–3 weeks) was observed in another 3–4%. If the drug is withdrawn the patient improves, and chronic pancreatitis has not been observed. Bone marrow depression rarely occurs, and can be prevented if complete blood counts are drawn weekly during the first month.

As regards long-term toxicity, super-infections are almost never observed and mortality from infection is rare. It had been feared that an increased risk of neoplasms would occur with the use of these agents; however, in the large series by Connell *et al.*[26] there has been no significant excess of colon cancers in azathioprine-treated patients. The same study observed no lymphomas, and although several lymphomas have been reported in a scattered form in the literature, the Greenstein *et al.* study[27] has shown that there is an increased risk of lymphoma in ulcerative colitis and Crohn's disease independent of azathioprine. A recent study has demonstrated that 6-MP is safe in pregnancy when used before conception, at conception and during pregnancy[28]. There is no increased association with prematurity, spontaneous abortions, congenital abnormalities, neonatal or childhood infections and neoplasia.

The current concept in IBD management should be that 6-MP and azathioprine are the most effective and safest long term therapeutic agents in the treatment of both ulcerative colitis and Crohn's disease. They should be used earlier in the course. If patients are unable to wean off steroids by 3 months, 6-MP or azathioprine should be started in both ulcerative colitis and Crohn's disease. If there is no improvement in 4 months after the introduction of 6-MP/azathioprine, then leukopenia should be induced. The drug is safe in pregnancy and does not pose any long-term neoplastic risk.

Turning to methotrexate, there have been several uncontrolled and one controlled trial in the treatment of active Crohn's disease. The controlled trial[29] showed a 39% success rate with the active drug compared to 19% with the placebo. In addition, several moderate-sized uncontrolled studies[30–32] have shown a clinical short-term response rate ranging from 65% to 83% in active Crohn's disease. Long-term responses range from 16% up to 44%, depending upon the definition of long-term response (that is, complete or incomplete discontinuation of steroids). In many of the studies, steroids have had to be maintained at low doses in order to maintain a clinical response and methotrexate does not appear to be as effective as 6-MP/azathioprine as regards steroid sparing.

In summary, concepts in using methotrexate should be that it is an effective short-term drug in Crohn's disease, that it is effective in 6-MP/azathioprine failures, that steroid sparing is not as effective as 6-MP/azathioprine, and that parenteral administration appears to be more effective than oral administration. The drug is not as effective in ulcerative colitis. Long-term toxicity is uncertain, since in my small series 3% of patients have developed cirrhosis and there has not been a very long-term follow-up.

As regards cyclosporine, the medical community appears to have written off this drug as ineffective in Crohn's disease. This is certainly not true, in that in the initial Brynskov *et al.* study[33] a dose up to 7.5 mg/kg daily was statistically effective as compared to placebo. Several subsequent studies, looking at both induction and maintenance of disease activity, report that cyclosporine is not effective in Crohn's disease. However, it must be noted that in these subsequent trials the drug was administered in a lower dose, 5 mg/kg daily. When administered intravenously in a dose of 4 mg/kg daily by continuous infusion, cyclosporine is very effective in the management of perianal fistula[34]. Closure of these chronic fistulas can be seen in as little as 6 days. Another small study[35] has been reported, and both were similar, showing a combined response rate of 86% with closure of fistulas in slightly over 60%. The mean response time was 4–7 days; however, relapse occurred in 42% of patients. In several small studies using intravenous cyclosporine for activity of disease, a 70–75% response rate to the high-dose intravenous cyclosporine has been observed[36]. Maintenance with cyclosporine alone has been poor unless 6-MP/azathioprine are added to the regimen.

In summary, as regards concepts in IBD management in using cyclosporine in Crohn's disease, it is definitely effective in Crohn's disease when administered intravenously in both fistulous disease and active disease. The response rate is approximately 70%; however, the drug is not effective when used orally for maintenance. Therefore, patients who respond to cyclosporine should be placed on 6-MP or azathioprine for maintenance therapy.

As regards ulcerative colitis, fulminant disease has been noted in about 10–15% of all ulcerative colitis patients. Approximately one-third of these patients will lose their colon at the initial episode and another third will lose their colon to chronic activity in the next year. It has been shown that if steroids are used for 7–10 days with no response, then further use of this agent will not be effective. Therefore, in a pilot study intravenous cyclosporine was used in severe ulcerative colitis patients who had failed at least 10 days of steroids. If the patient responded, he/she was transferred to oral cyclosporine with a goal of steroid discontinuation, endoscopic healing and alleviation of clinical symptoms. In this pilot study the short-term response was 81% and the long-term response rate was 56%. A double-blind placebo-controlled trial was initiated[37], with the intention of treating 42 patients. The study was terminated after only 20 patients were entered because the results showed a dramatic efficacy with cyclosporine

(82% response) and no response with placebo ($p < 0.001$). If one looks at the overall response rate in the controlled and uncontrolled trials, the acute response was 83% and the long-term success was 59%. This 59% figure must be compared to long-term response using steroids alone for more than 10 days, which is less than 1%. Finally, we have shown in a smaller series that when 6-MP is added to the regimen of responders, remission is maintained in 77% of all patients[38].

Therefore, our concepts using cyclosporine in ulcerative colitis are that cyclosporine is effective when given intravenously in acutely ill steroid-refractory patients. Long-term maintenance with this drug is good but not ideal; therefore 6-MP/azathioprine should be added to the regimen. Use of intravenous cyclosporine requires expertise, since the toxicity rate may be high, ranging up to 10%.

Recently, a new agent has been used in clinical trials in the treatment of Crohn's disease. This is a chimeric monoclonal antibody against TNF[1]. When administered acutely to patients with active Crohn's disease, clinical response was seen in 65%, compared to 17% with placebo. When looking at clinical remission at 4 weeks the result was 43% compared to 4%. In patients who were re-treated every 8 weeks, maintenance of remission was seen in the group receiving the active drug, and there was a gradual fall-off of response in those receiving placebo. A recent study has been completed, looking at fistulization in Crohn's disease[39]. In this protocol the drug was given at week 0, 2 and 6, with a primary goal of closing more than 50% of fistulas on two consecutive visits. Secondary goals included complete healing of all fistulas, decrease in Crohn's Disease Activity Index, improvement in quality of life and a decreased perianal disease activity index. The primary endpoint was reached in 62% of patients compared to 26% with placebo. If one looks at complete closure of fistulas, this was observed in 46% of patients compared to 12% with placebo. This was statistically significant ($p = 0.001$). Both perianal fistulas and abdominal wall fistulas have shown response to this agent. Although some patients have relapsed with discontinuation after the initial three infusions, some patients have maintained their response for over 1 year without any further infusions.

Finally, how do we summarize our approaches to IBD management? First, one should use combination therapy, that is, 5-ASA plus antibiotics in Crohn's disease and immunomodulators in both Crohn's and ulcerative colitis. The treating physician should use higher doses of 5-ASA and avoid the acute use of steroids in mild Crohn's disease and ulcerative colitis, and should avoid chronic steroids in both diseases. Let me again emphasize that immunomodulators should be instituted much earlier in the course of management. The use of anti-inflammatory agents alone for chronic disease is outdated. The author would like to make the prediction that in the future newer immunobiological therapies (for example infliximab, the antibody against TNF-α) will be used earlier in the course of Crohn's disease and will lower the over-activated immune 'thermostat'. Once this has been accomplished then 6-MP/azathioprine and/or 5-ASA drugs can be used as maintenance. Because of toxicity I further predict that steroids will become a third-line agent in the treatment of active Crohn's disease.

References

1. Targan SR, Hanauer SD, van Deventer SJH *et al.* A short term study of chimeric monoclonal antibody cA2 to tumor necrosis factor alpha for Crohn's disese. N Engl J Med. 1997;337:1029–35.
2. Greenstein AJ, Lachman P, Sachar DB *et al.* Perforating and nonperforating indications for surgery in Crohn's disease. Evidence for two clinical forms. Gut. 1986;29:588–92.
3. Aeberhardt P, Berchtold W, Riedtmann HJ *et al.* Surgical recurrence of perforating and non-perforating Crohn's disease. Dis Colon Rectum. 1996;39:80–7.
4. Singleton JW, Hanauer SB, Gitnick GL *et al.* Mesalamine capsules for the treatment of active Crohn's disease. Results of a 16-week trial. Gastroenterology. 1993;104:1293–301.
5. Messori A, Brignola C, Trallori G *et al.* Effectiveness of 5-aminosalicylic acid for maintaining remission in patients with Crohn's disease. A meta analysis. Am J Gastroenterol. 1994;89:692–8.
6. Rutgeerts T, Hiele M, Gedoes K *et al.* Controlled trial of metronidazole treatment for prevention of Crohn's recurrence after ileal resection. Gastroenterology. 1995;108:1617–21.
7. Korelitz D, Hanauer S, Rutgeerts T *et al.* Postoperative prophylaxis of 6-MP/5-ASA or placebo in Crohn's disease: a two year multicenter trial. Gastroenterology. 1998;114:A1011.
8. Truelove SC, Witts LJ. Cortisone in ulcerative colitis: final report on a therapeutic trial. Br Med J. 1955;2:1041.
9. Lennard-Jones JE, Misiewicz JJ, Connell AM *et al.* Prednisone as maintenance treatment for ulcerative colitis in remission. Lancet. 1965;1:188.
10. Summers RW, Switz DM, Sessions JT *et al.* National Cooperative Crohn's Disease Study. Results of drug treatment. Gastroenterology. 1979;77:847–69.
11. Malchow H, Ewe K, Brandes JW *et al.* European Cooperative Crohn's Disease Study. Results of drug treatment. Gastroenterology. 1984;86:249–66.
12. Greenberg GR, Feagan BG, Martin F *et al.* Oral budesonide for active Crohn's disease. N Engl J Med. 1994;331:836–41.
13. Rutgeerts P, Lofberg R, Malchow H *et al.* A comparison of budesonide with prednisolone for active Crohn's disease. N Engl J Med. 1994;331:842–5.
14. Greenberg GR, Feagan BG, Martin F *et al.* Oral budesonide as maintenance treatment for Crohn's disease. A placebo-controlled dose ranging study. Gastroenterology. 1996;110:45–51.
15. Munkholm P, Langholz E, Davidsen M *et al.* Frequency of glucocorticoid resistance and dependency in Crohn's disease. Gut. 1994;35:360–2.
16. Moss AA, Carbone JV, Kressel HY. Radiological and clinical assessment of broad spectrum antibiotic therapy in Crohn's disease. Am J Roentgenol. 1978;131:787–90.
17. Prantera C, Zannoni F, Scribano ML *et al.* An antibiotic regimen for the treatment of active Crohn's disease. A randomized controlled clinical trial with metronidazole versus ciprofloxacin. Am J Gastroenterol. 1996;91:328–32.
18. Colombel JF. A controlled trial comparing ciprofloxacin with mesalazine for the treatment of active Crohn's disease. Gastroenterology. 1997;112:A951.
19. Sutherland L, Singleton J, Sessions J *et al.* Double blind placebo controlled trial of metronidazole in Crohn's disease. Gut. 1991;32:1071–5.
20. Present DH, Korelitz BI, Wisch N *et al.* Treatment of Crohn's disease with 6-mercaptopurine in a long term, randomized, double blind study. N Engl J Med. 1983;2:981–7.
21. O'Donoghue VP, Dawson AM, Powell-Tuck J *et al.* Double blind withdrawal trial of Azathioprine as maintenance treatment for Crohn's disease. Lancet. 1978;2:955–7.
22. Present DH. 6-Mercaptopurine and other immunosuppressive agents in the treatment of Crohn's disease and ulcerative colitis. Gastroenterol Clin N Am. 1989;18:57–71.
23. George J, Present DH, Pou R *et al.* The long term outcome of ulcerative colitis treated with 6-mercaptopurine. Am J Gastroenterol. 1996;91:1711–14.
24. Hawthorne AB, Logan RFA, Hawkey CJ *et al.* Randomized controlled trial of Azathioprine withdrawal in ulcerative colitis. Br Med J. 1992;305:20–2.
25. Present DH, Meltzer SJ, Krumholz MD *et al.* 6-Mercaptopurine in the management of inflammatory bowel disease: short and long term toxicity. Ann Intern Med. 1989;111:641–9.
26. Connell WR, Kamm MA, Dickson M *et al.* Long term neoplasia risk after azathioprine treatment in inflammatory bowel disease. Lancet. 1994;343:1249–52.
27. Greenstein AJ, Mullin GE, Heimann T *et al.* Lymphoma in inflammatory bowel disease. Cancer. 1992;69:1119–23.

28. Francella A, Dayan A, Rubin P *et al.* 6-Mercaptopurine is safe therapy for childbearing patients with inflammatory bowel disease: a case controlled study. Gastroenterology. 1996;110A:909 (abstract).
29. Feagan BG, Rochon J, Fedorak RN *et al.* Methotrexate for the treatment of Crohn's disease. N Engl J Med. 1995;332:292–7.
30. Kozarek PA, Patterson DJ, Gelfand MD *et al.* Methotrexate induces clinical and histologic remission in patients with refractory inflammatory bowel disease. Ann Intern Med. 1989;110:353–6.
31. Lemann M, Chamiot-Prieur C, Mesnard B *et al.* Methotrexate for the treatment of refractory Crohn's disease. Aliment Pharmacol Ther. 1996;10:309–14.
32. Muhadevan U, Marion J, Present DH. The place for methotrexate in the treatment of refractory Crohn's disease. Gastroenterology. 1997;112:A1031.
33. Brynskov V, Freund L, Rasmussen SN *et al.* Placebo controlled double blind randomized trial of cyclosporine therapy in active Crohn's disease. N Engl J Med. 1989;321:845–50.
34. Present DH, Lichtiger S. Efficacy of cyclosporine in treatment of fistula of Crohn's disease. Dig Dis Sci. 1994;39:374–80.
35. Hanauer SB, Smith MB. Rapid closure of Crohn's disease fistula with continuous intravenous cyclosporine A. Am J Gastroenterol. 1993;88:646–9.
36. Lemann M, de la Valussiere F, Vouhnik Y *et al.* Intravenous cyclosporine for refractory attacks of Crohn's disease: long term follow-up of patients. Gastroenterology. 1998;114:A1020.
37. Lichtiger S, Present DH, Kornbluth A *et al.* Cyclosporine in severe ulcerative colitis refractory to steroid therapy. N Engl J Med. 1994;330:1841–5.
38. Marion JF, Present DH. 6-MP maintains cyclosporine induced response in patients with severe ulcerative colitis. Am J Gastroenterol. 1996;91:A1975.
39. Present DH, Mayer L, Van Deventer SJH *et al.* Anti TNF-alpha chimeric antibody (cA2) is effective in the treatment of the fistula of Crohn's disease: a multicenter randomized double blind placebo controlled study. Am J Gastroenterol. 1997;92:A1746.

32
Salicylates

J. KELLER, A. DIGNASS and P. LAYER

INTRODUCTION

Standard therapy of inflammatory bowel disease (IBD) includes application of salicylates such as mesalazine (5-aminosalicylic acid, 5-ASA) and its derivatives. These substances have been shown to be effective both in treatment of active disease and in maintaining remission in Crohn's disease and ulcerative colitis[1–19]. Even long-term application for maintenance therapy is usually well tolerated, which is an important advantage over corticosteroids and immunosuppressive agents.

The precise mechanism of action of mesalazine is obscured by the failure to understand the aetiopathogenesis of IBD. However, several mediators identified in the inflammatory cascades activated in IBD are obviously modulated by mesalazine. Possible mechanisms of action include inhibition of leukotrienes (e.g. LTB4), prostaglandins and platelet-activating factor[20–22], modulation of production, binding and action of several cytokines (interleukin 1 (IL-1), IL-2, tumour necrosis factor alpha (TNF-α), interferon gamma (IFN-α))[23,24] and inhibition of chemotactic activity of formylated bacterial peptides. Other studies have demonstrated that mesalazine is a potent scavenger of oxygen free radicals[25–27] and modulates immune functions of the intestinal mucosa[28,29]. Virtually all anti-inflammatory effects of mesalazine are mediated *topically*.

A recent meta-analysis which compared the efficacy of rectal corticosteroids and rectal mesalazine preparations revealed that mesalazine is superior to corticosteroids in the management of distal ulcerative colitis[30]. These data stress that mesalazine may be one of the most efficacious drugs available for treatment of IBD, provided that appropriate delivery systems induce sufficient concentrations within inflamed regions of the gut.

In left-sided colitis this can be achieved by *topical* application. However, orally administered plain aminosalicylic acid is rapidly and completely absorbed within the upper gastrointestinal tract. Therefore, appropriate pharmacological and pharmaceutical *oral* formulations are of critical importance to achieve liberation of mesalazine at the site of inflammation in IBD patients with small intestinal and/or extensive colonic disease. Sulphasalazine (SASP) was the first salicylate which was introduced into treatment of IBD in the 1930s[31]. SASP allows delivery of large amounts of 5-ASA to the colon by linkage of the therapeutically active 5-ASA moiety to sulphapyridine[32]. 5-ASA is set free predominantly within the colonic lumen after cleavage of the azo-bond by colonic bacteria. However, transport of 5-ASA to the distal gut has to be paid for by considerable side-effects caused by sulphapyridine. In order to overcome preterm absorption of pure mesalazine and to avoid sulphapyridine-related side-effects of SASP, several new oral mesalazine preparations have been developed during recent years with different release patterns.

This chapter will review therapeutic use of salicylates in IBD with special respect to the pharmacokinetic properties of different preparations.

ORAL MESALAZINE PREPARATIONS

Sulphasalazine (SASP)

SASP is a composite of 5-aminosalicylic acid (5-ASA, mesalazine), an aspirin analogue, and sulphapyridine, a sulphonamide. Both residues are covalently linked by a diazo bond. In humans, less than 10% of intact SASP is absorbed during small intestinal transit and most of the compound is delivered into the colon. Cleavage of SASP by the bacterial enzyme azoreductase starts in the distal ileum but is predominantly achieved in the colon[33]. This leads to the delivery of large quantities of sulphapyridine and mesalazine into the proximal colonic lumen. Sulphapyridine, the sulphonamide moiety, is absorbed quantitatively by the colonic mucosa and undergoes hepatic metabolism (acetylation, glucuronidation, hydroxylation) with subsequent renal excretion. Luminal mesalazine is acetylated and thereby inactivated to a small extent by colonic bacteria. The major proportion of acetyl–5-ASA is produced by the intestinal epithelium which requires mucosal absorption of mesalazine[34]. Apparently, re-secretion of the inactive acetylated 5-ASA (ac-5-ASA) into the intestinal lumen occurs, whereas luminal ac-5-ASA does not appear to cross back into the epithelium[34]. The pioneering studies by Azad Khan and colleagues[32] have revealed that the therapeutic effect of suphasalazine in IBD is achieved by the 5-ASA moiety, while the sulphapyridine residue has no significant anti-inflammatory activity on gut mucosa. On the other hand, most of the side-effects of SASP, such as rush, arthritis, pericarditis, pancreatitis, pleuritis, reversible infertility in man, pancytopenia because of folate deficiency and other reactions are caused by sulphapyridine. These side-effects occur dose-dependently in 13–60% of patients taking SASP[35,36]. However, the sulphapyridine residue prevents preterm absorption and metabolism of mesalazine which would make it unavailable to the most commonly inflamed distal regions of the gut. Therefore, in this formulation, sulphapyridine is necessary for therapeutic efficacy.

Uncoated 5-ASA

Following oral administration, uncoated mesalazine is rapidly and completely absorbed by the upper gastrointestinal mucosa. Mesalazine is subsequently inactivated by acetylation[37–39]. Consequently, the major portion (> 80%) of the absorbed amount is present in the plasma as ac-5-ASA[39]. Acetylation of mesalazine also takes place in the liver. Systemic elimination of mesalazine occurs almost exclusively in the acetylated form by renal excretion[38]. The half-life of mesalazine and its acetylated metabolite is dose-dependent. For mesalazine the half-life varies between 40 and 90 min; the half-life of ac-5-ASA is 6–10 h[40]. Approximately half of the absorbed mesalazine is bound to plasma proteins. In the colon the absorption rate of 5-ASA is lower than in the proximal gastrointestinal tract. Only 20–30% of the dose administered is absorbed when mesalazine is administered directly into the colon by oral delayed-release preparations, enema or suppositories, whereas the major proportion is eliminated by faecal excretion[40,41].

Modern delayed-release mesalazine preparations

In order to overcome rapid absorption and inactivation of pure mesalazine in the proximal gastrointestinal tract, and to avoid the sulphapyridine-related side-effects of SASP, several oral mesalazine preparations have been developed during recent years. There are two basic principles which have been employed to ensure delivery of therapeutic amounts of mesalazine to the distal small intestine and the colon: on the one hand a pharmacological approach was undertaken by coupling of mesalazine to a carrier molecule other than sulphapyridine. Probably the most elegant approach is the coupling of two 5-ASA molecules as in olsalazine (Dipentum®) which are released in the colon by cleavage of the diazo bond by bacterial enzymes. On the other hand, a pharmaceutical approach employing encapsulation of mesalazine in special matrices also allows delayed release in the distal intestine. One example for this is coating of mesalazine with pH-sensitive acrylic resins (Asacol®, Salofalk®, Claversal®). This leads to disintegration of mesalazine tablets and release of increasing amounts of 5-ASA due to increasing pH during gastrointestinal transit. Alternatively, mesalazine can be encapsulated with a semipermeable ethylcellulose membrane (as in Pentasa®). This preparation is supposed to release more constant rates of 5-ASA into the intestinal lumen by osmotic mechanisms.

Coupling of mesalazine to carrier molecules

SASP is the prototype of this group of mesalazine derivatives and is still used to compare effectiveness of other mesalazine preparations in clinical studies. However, alternative carrier molecules have been developed in order to avoid the sulphapyridine-related side-effects. One of the most interesting pharmacological approaches is the synthesis of a 5-ASA dimer by coupling of two molecules of 5-ASA (olsalazine; Dipentum®). This 5-ASA dimer is stable and is not absorbed within the proximal gastrointestinal tract. Similar to SASP, it is cleaved by the bacterial enzyme azoreductase. This leads to the release of two molecules of free 5-ASA in the colon[42]. Only small amounts of mesalazine are absorbed from olsalazine[43]. Other carrier molecules which have been used to ensure delivery of mesalazine to the distal gut include inert carriers such as para-aminobenzoic acid (benzalazine), 4-aminobenzoyl-alanine (balsalazide) and 4-aminobenzoyl-glycine (ipsalazide). These new preparations currently play no significant role in the treatment of IBD and are not available in most European countries or the United States. Interestingly, a recent study has shown that balsalazide may be more effective in treatment of acute ulcerative colitis than conventional delayed-release preparations[44].

Encapsulation of mesalazine in a delayed-release matrix

Protection of mesalazine from absorption and inactivation within the upper gastrointestinal tract, and delivery of sufficient amounts to the distal small intestine and the colon, can also be achieved by encapsulation of 5-ASA with acrylic resins or ethylcellulose. Commercially available oral mesalazine preparations use the acrylic resins Eudragit S (Asacol®) or Eudragit L in combination with sodium bicarbonate/glycine buffering (Salofalk®, Claversal®). Preparations with Eudragit S permit disintegration at pH > 7, those with Eudragit L at about pH 6[45]. Alternatively, mesalazine can be packed in microgranules and separately coated with a semipermeable ethylcellulose membrane. This preparation is available as a tablet (Pentasa®) which releases acid-stable microgranules of mesalazine within the stomach. Throughout intestinal transit, active 5-ASA diffuses through the ethylcellulose membrane with a velocity that is pH-dependent (time to 50% release at pH 2: 15 h, at pH 7: 4–5 h)[46].

Release of orally administered mesalazine during gastrointestinal transit

Therapeutic efficacy of mesalazine in IBD requires sufficient luminal concentrations at the site of inflammation. However, the release patterns of mesalazine from delayed-release preparations differ substantially. Because of varying sites of inflammation in patients with IBD, the choice of an adequate mesalazine preparation may be critical for effective treatment. There are several indirect methods which give limited information about luminal availability of mesalazine. These methods include measuring of urinary or faecal excretion as well as plasma appearance and disappearance rates of 5-ASA and its main metabolite acetyl-5-ASA[47–50]. In addition, radiographic tracings of a barium sulphate marker, scintigraphic tracings of radioactive isotopes released from coated tablets in Crohn's disease patients or healthy volunteers[51–53] or the recovery of mesalazine from the ileostomy effluent of patients are utilized in order to study the luminal liberation of 5-ASA[51,54]. These approaches provide rather indirect methods to study the global delivery of 5-ASA into the colon, whereas its availability within individual levels of the small bowel cannot be characterized. This information is necessary, however, because of the potential value of mesalazine in the treatment of small intestinal Crohn's disease.

In order to determine the luminal release and fate of different oral slow-release mesalazine preparations, we recently studied two different galenic preparations (Salofalk® and Pentasa®) by direct luminal measurement in volunteers[55–57]. Healthy volunteers were intubated with an integrated multilumen oro-ileal tube which allowed marker perfusion; aspiration of chyme from the duodenum, mid-jejunum and terminal ileum; and intestinal manometry[56–59]. Our studies demonstrated significantly different release patterns of these oral delayed-release formulations. While both preparations predominantly release mesalazine into the colon, significantly different patterns of small intestinal transit and bioavailability within the small intestinal lumen were observed (Figure 1), which reflect the interaction between specific pharmacokinetic properties and physiological gastric emptying mechanisms in humans.

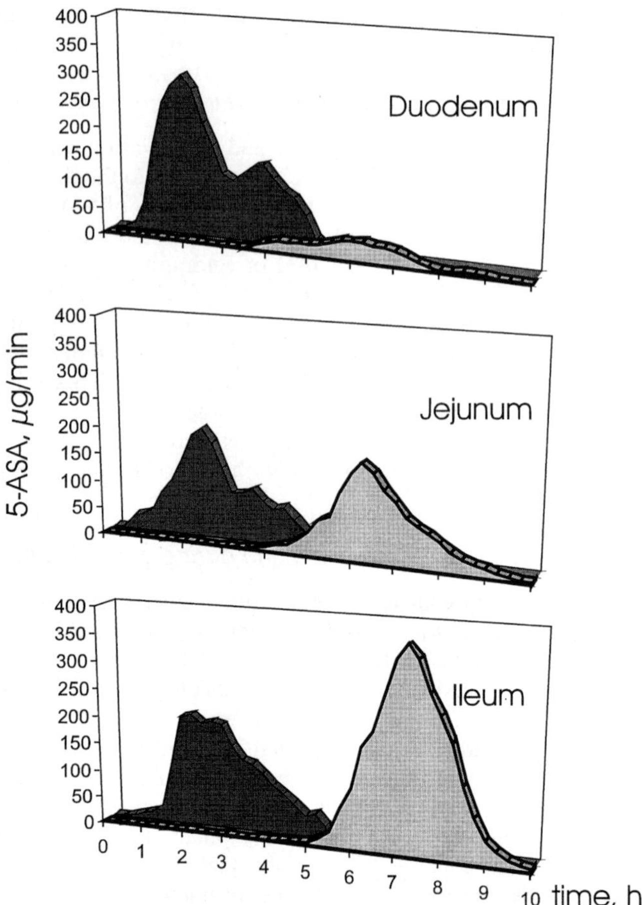

Figure 1 Mean delivery rates to the duodenum, jejunum and ileum following oral administration of 500 mg 5-ASA together with a test meal from two different delayed-release preparations: light areas: 5-ASA coated with Eudragit L (Salofalk®, n = 6); dark areas: 5-ASA microspheres coated with a semipermeable membrane (Pentasa®, n = 6). Data are presented as three-term moving average

Eudragit L-coated mesalazine preparations. 5-ASA coated with a pH-sensitive release matrix (Eudragit L, Salofalk®) coadministered with a test meal is emptied from the stomach about 3 h postprandially together with the first phase III of recurring interdigestive motility. This is in accordance with physiological gastric emptying mechanisms which do not allow gastric emptying of solid particles in the digestive period if their diameter exceeds 1–2 mm. The quantity of 5-ASA released increases during small intestinal transit. Less than 2% of the total dose of free 5-ASA is cumulatively delivered to the duodenum, approximately 6% is released in the jejunum and about 13% in the ileum. In parallel, increasing amounts of ac-5-ASA are detected in the small intestine, averaging about 1.5% in the duodenum, 12% in the jejunum and 18% in the ileum. Consequently, once the tablet has left the stomach, concentrations of 5-ASA and ac-5-ASA increase continuously from the duodenum to the distal ileum over 3 h and decrease over the next 3 h. Overall, about 10% of the dose administered is excreted in urine within 10 h after ingestion, whereas about 90% reaches the colon either in solution (30%) or still unreleased from tablets (60%). Since a major proportion of mesalazine released during small bowel transit is inactivated by acetylation before it reaches the colon, about 70% of the total dose enters the colon as active drug[56].

Ethylcellulose-coated mesalazine microspheres. In contrast, due to the small diameter of individual microspheres, 5-ASA in an ethylcellulose-coated microsphere preparation (Pentasa®) is emptied from the stomach during the digestive period, simultaneously with a meal[57]. Although small intestinal transit times are similar to those of Salofalk®, cumulative delivery of free 5-ASA from Pentasa® to the duodenum, jejunum and ileum is in each case approximately 10% of the total dose, reflecting significant pharmacokinetic differences between these two preparations. Cumulative amounts of ac-5-ASA tend to be slightly greater at distal intestinal sites. Following oral administration of identical doses of 5-ASA, systemic bioavailability of both 5-ASA and its acetylated metabolite are considerably lower with Pentasa® than with Salofalk®. Only traces of 5-ASA are present in urine; the cumulative excretion of ac-5-ASA amounts to approximately 5% of the total dose. Overall analysis suggests that 70% of the total dose reaches the colon unreleased from microspheres. During small intestinal transit about 20% is released and enters the colon dissolved in luminal juice; half of this as active drug. Taken together, similar to Salofalk® about 80% of the dose administered reaches the colon as active drug.

TOPICAL MESALAZINE PREPARATIONS

There are several different galenic preparations for topical application of mesalazine in left-sided colitis such as enemas, suppositories or foams. Enemas have been shown to spread retrogradely to the sigmoid region in all, and to reach the splenic flexure in most patients, whereas spreading to the transverse colon is observed in only a small minority of patients[60]. Scintigraphic evaluations revealed that distribution of mesalazine foam is similar to that of enemas, but foam appeared to have a more uniform distribution and a longer persistence in the descending and sigmoid colon[61]. These advantages were reflected by prompter remission of symptoms in patients using foam compared with liquid enema in a multicentre, randomized and prospective study[62] performed on 233 patients with ulcerative colitis.

In patients with a temporary or permanent (ileal) stoma, high concentrations of active drug can be achieved within the intestinal lumen by instillation of mesalazine foam or enema via the stoma.

Treatment with mesalazine suppositories is a therapeutic alternative in patients with mild to moderate proctitis who cannot tolerate or retain enemas sufficiently. Effective treatment may be achieved by application of mesalazine suppositories containing 500 mg 5-ASA only twice per day[63].

Similar to oral preparations, topical mesalazine preparations are available for uncoupled 5-ASA (Salofalk®, Claversal®, Pentasa®), 5-ASA coupled with sulphapyridine (Azulfidine®) and 5-ASA dimers (Dipentum®).

ADVERSE EFFECTS OF MESALAZINE

In general, mesalazine preparations are well tolerated even in long-term therapy. The rate of side-effects is significantly higher in patients treated with sulphasalazine, mainly due to the sulphapyridine moiety which causes substantial dose-related intolerance in addition to allergic and toxic reactions (compare above). The most common adverse effects of mesalazine itself are headache (up to 13%) nausea (up to 8%) and epigastric discomfort (up to 8%)[64,65]. Itching, dizziness, indigestion, muscular ache and fever occur in less than 5% of patients and were seen with a similar frequency in patients who received placebo[64]. Allergic reactions to mesalazine occurred in 0.5% of patients treated with 1.5 g oral mesalazine per day in a large general-practice study[65]. Rare adverse effects of mesalazine include acute pancreatitis, perimyocarditis, bronchospasm, retrosternal chest pain, neutropenia, lupus-like syndrome, accelerated hair loss, acute alveolitis and interstitial lung fibrosis[64,66–69].

Because mesalazine shares structural similarities with acetylsalicylic acid and phenacetin, both drugs with known nephrotoxicity, a nephrotoxic potential has also been suspected for mesalazine. There are conflicting data as to whether (long-term) application of mesalazine may induce renal damage or not. No clinically significant nephrotoxicity has been reported by two large studies[70,71]. However, increasing dosages may enhance the risk of chronic nephrotoxicity. Recent studies have shown that in IBD patients treated with mesalazine proteinuria can be detected by sensitive methods. Since in these studies proteinuria was also associated with markers of disease activity, it remained unclear whether disturbance of renal function was a consequence of mesalazine treatment or of increased disease activity[72–75]. Another study suggests that renal impairment of any severity may occur in 1 in 100 patients treated with Asacol® (mesalazine preparation which employs a pH-dependent release mechanism) and that clinically significant interstitial nephritis is seen in less than 1 in 500 patients. Impairment of renal function may become irreversible if diagnosis of nephrotoxicity is delayed for more than 18 months and is most reliably detected by elevated serum creatinine concentrations[76]. Meanwhile it has been accepted that serum creatinine concentrations should be monitored at baseline, within the first 3 months after introduction of mesalazine therapy and annually thereafter[77].

The most frequent and disturbing side-effect of olsalazine is secretory watery diarrhoea, which occurs dose-dependently in 15–35% of patients[78] and necessitates discontinuation of the drug in 5–10%[79]. The underlying mechanism appears to be stimulation of ileal secretion. Lowering the dose of olsalazine may attenuate or eliminate diarrhoea. Indeed, a recent study suggests that maintenance therapy with 1 g per day of olsalazine is well tolerated and induces diarrhoea in less than 5% of patients[80].

Apart from this, there are rare case reports of paradoxical effects of sulphasalazine and mesalazine therapy leading to exacerbation of ulcerative colitis with increased stool frequency, rectal bleeding and fever[81–83].

Due to the overall small risk of side-effects and missing evidence for teratogenic potential, therapeutic use of mesalazine is considered to be safe in pregnancy. A recent study has supported the notion that pregnant women suffering from IBD should be encouraged to continue mesalazine medication to prevent relapses which are associated with increased perinatal risk[84].

CLINICAL APPLICATION OF MESALAZINE IN IBD

Oral and topical mesalazine preparations have been studied in the treatment of active chronic IBD of mild to moderate severity and as maintenance therapy. There is convincing evidence that these preparations are effective in acute-phase and maintenance therapy both in ulcerative colitis and in Crohn's disease[1-19].

Ulcerative colitis

Topical mesalazine preparations have been firmly established as therapy for acute disease and maintenance of remission in left-sided ulcerative colitis and ulcerative proctitis[1].

A recent meta-analysis has shown that mesalazine enemas are even superior to topical corticosteroids in the management of distal ulcerative colitits[30]. Typically, response rates of 80% are achieved by use of mesalazine enemas in such patients. The onset of action may take 3–21 days and the treatment time for an acute, uncomplicated flare of ulcerative colitis requires 3–6 weeks[1].

Oral mesalazine preparations are as effective as sulphasalazine in the treatment of mild to moderately active ulcerative colitis if equimolar doses of 5-ASA are applied[2,19]. The beneficial effect of mesalazine is dose-dependent[19]. Therefore, larger doses (3–4.8 g per day) seem to be warranted, though smaller doses (0.8–1.5 g per day) have also been effective in treatment of acute inflammation[2-6]. Interestingly, a recent study has shown that balsalazide may be more effective and is better tolerated than conventional delayed-release preparations[44].

Both oral mesalazine preparations coated with pH-sensitive acrylic resins (Asacol®, Salofalk®, Claversal®) and mesalazine microgranules coated with a semipermeable ethylcellulose membrane (Pentasa®) deliver 70–80% of the dose administered into the colon as active drug (compare p. 281). Therefore, these preparations may be equally effective in treatment of ulcerative colitis. Possibly olsalazine might be used preferentially since with this preparation almost all 5-ASA is delivered to the colon[85]. Besides, systemic absorption of 5-ASA from olsalazine is low, which may reduce the risk of systemic side-effects[43].

Mesalazine preparations are of special importance for maintenance therapy of ulcerative colitis[7-9,19]. Maintenance therapy should be initiated if the frequency of active phases exceeds one per year and/or if disease activity impairs quality of life[10]. Therapy should be continued for 2 years if patients remain in remission. In most cases doses between 750 and 1500 mg mesalazine per day or 1000 mg diazo-bonded 5-ASA (olsalazine) significantly reduce relapse rates. A recent study showed that a combination treatment with oral mesalazine and topical application twice per week may be more effective in maintaining remission than oral application alone[86]. This form of treatment might be appropriate for patients at high risk of relapse.

Crohn's disease

In contrast to earlier studies using low doses of mesalazine[17], there is now increasing evidence that mesalazine is also effective in the treatment of active Crohn's disease, provided that sufficient doses (up to 4.5 g oral mesalazine per day) are applied[11–13,18]. In patients with inflammation restricted to the distal colon, topical mesalazine preparations induce high intraluminal 5-ASA concentrations at the site of inflammation and may be of value as in ulcerative colitis. However, most patients have ileal and/or proximal colonic involvement, and therefore benefit from oral mesalazine. Delayed-release preparations have been shown to induce and maintain remission, reduce postoperative relapse rates and spare steroids if combined with conventional steroid therapy[11–13,18,87–91]. Theoretically, compound-specific release patterns suggest that preparations coated with acrylic resins (Salofalk®, Claversal®) may be favourably utilized in predominantly terminal ileal disease, while Pentasa® is probably particularly effective in extensive small intestinal disease which includes proximal involvement (compare pp. 280, 281). In colonic disease, both types of galenic preparations may be equally effective. It has to be kept in mind, however, that these assumptions have not yet been confirmed in clinical trials.

There are conflicting data as to whether mesalazine is effective as maintenance monotherapy in Crohn's disease patients[91]. Several studies suggest that mesalazine preparations are safe and effective drugs for maintenance therapy[12–16,84], at least if higher doses are employed (> 2 g per day) and maintenance therapy is started shortly after achieving remission. However, these promising results are questioned by a more recent study which showed no significant difference between relapse rates in Crohn's disease patients receiving mesalazine 3 g/day or placebo followed up for 1 year[92].

SUMMARY

The beneficial effects of mesalazine on inflammatory processes and clinical outcome in IBD depend on delivery of sufficient amounts of active 5-ASA at the site of inflammation. Against the background of the different characteristics of gastrointestinal transit and bioavailability within the lumen of the small and large bowel of specific 5-ASA preparations described above, it appears to be of importance to adapt the choice of a particular preparation to the specific pattern of inflammation in individual patients.

References

1. Lichtenstein GR. Medical therapies for inflammatory bowel disease. Curr Opin Gastroenterol. 1994;10:390–403.
2. Rachmilewitz D, on behalf of an international study group. Coated mesalazine (5-aminosalicylic acid) vs. sulphasalazine in the treatment of active ulcerative colitis: a randomized trial. Br Med J. 1989;298:82–6.
3. Schröder KW, Tremaine WJ. Oral 5-aminosalicylic acid (Asacol®) for treatment of symptomatic chronic ulcerative colitis. Gastroenterology. 1986;90:A1620.
4. Schröder KW, Tremaine WJ, Ilstrup DM. Coated oral 5-aminosalicylic acid therapy for mildly to moderately active ulcerative colitis. N Engl J Med. 1987;317:1625–9.
5. Sninski CA, Cort DH, Shanahan F *et al.* Oral mesalamine (Asacol) for mildly to moderately active ulcerative colitis. Ann Intern Med. 1991;115:350–5.

6. Hanauer S, Schwartz J, Robinson M *et al.* and the Pentasa® Study Group. Mesalamine capsules for treatment of active ulcerative colitis: results of a controlled trial. Am J Gastroenterol. 1993;88:1188–97.

7. Azad Khan AK, Howes DT, Piris J, Truelove SC. Optimum dose of sulphasalazine for maintenance treatment in ulcerative colitis. Gut. 1980;21:232–40.

8. Riley SA, Mani V, Goodman MJ, Herd ME, Dutt S, Turnberg LA. Comparison of delayed release 5-aminosalicylic acid (Mesalazine) and sulfasalazine as maintenance treatment for patients with ulcerative colitis. Gastroenterology. 1988;94:1383–9.

9. Travis SPL, Tysk C, de Silva HJ, Sandberg-Gertzén H, Jewell DP, Järnerot G. Optimum dose of olsalazine for maintaining remission in ulcerative colitis. Gut. 1994;35:1282–6.

10. Robinson M, Hanauer S, Hoop R, Zbrozek A, Wilkinson C. Mesalamine capsules enhance the quality of life for patients with ulcerative colitis. Aliment Pharmacol Ther. 1994;8:27–34.

11. Singleton JW, Hanauer SB, Gitnick GL *et al.* and the Pentasa Crohn's Disease Study Group. Mesalamine capsules for the treatment of active Crohn's disease: results of a 16 week trial. Gastroenterology. 1993;104:1293–301.

12. Hanauer SB, Krawitt EL, Robinson M, Rick GG, Safdi MA and the Pentasa Crohn's Disease Compassionate Use Study Group. Long term management of Crohn's disease with mesalamine capsules (Pentasa®). Am J Gastroenterol. 1993;88:1343–51.

13. Gross V, Schölmerich J, Roth M *et al.* Vergleich zwischen hoch dosierter 5-Aminosalizylsäure (5-ASA) und 6-Methylprednisolon (6-MP) bei aktiver Ileocolitis Crohn. Med Klin. 1994;89(Suppl. 1):158.

14. Brignola C, Iannone P, Pasquali S *et al.* Placebo-controlled trial of oral 5-ASA in relapse prevention of Crohn's disease. Dig Dis Sci. 1992;37:29–32.

15. Gendre J-P, Mary J-Y, Florent C *et al.* and the Groupe d'Etudes Thérapeutiques des affections inflammatoires digestives. Oral masalamine (Pentasa) as maintenance treatment in Crohn's disease: a multicenter placebo-controlled study. Gastroenterology. 1993;104:435–9.

16. Messori A, Brignola C, Trallori G *et al.* Effectiveness of 5-aminosalicylic acid for maintaining remission in patients with Crohn's disease: a metaanalysis. Am J Gastroenterol. 1994;89:692–8.

17. Rasmussen SN, Lauritsen K, Tage-Jensen U *et al.* 5-Aminosalicylic acid in the treatment of Crohn's disease. Scand J Gastroenterol. 1987;22:877–88.

18. Brynskov J, Norby Rasmussen S. Clinical pharmacology: development of new forms of treatment of inflammatory bowel disease. Scand J Gastroenterol. 1996;31(Suppl. 216):175–80.

19. Sutherland LR *et al.* Alternatives to sulphasalazine: a meta-analysis of 5-ASA in the treatment of ulcerative colitis. Inflam Bowel Dis. 1997;3:65–78.

20. Nielsen OH, Bukhave K, Elmgreen J, Ahnfelt-Ronne I. Inhibition of 5-lipoxygenase pathway of arachidonic acid metabolism in human neutrophils by sulphasalazine and 5-aminosalicylic acid. Dig Dis Sci. 1987;32:577–82.

21. Lauritsen K, Hansen J, Bytzer P, Bukhave K, Rask-Madsen J. Effects of sulphasalazine and disodium azodisalicylate on colonic PGE_2 concentrations determined by equilibrium *in vivo* dialysis of faeces in patients with ulcerative colitis and healthy controls. Gut. 1984;25:1271–8.

22. Greenfield SM, Punchard NA, Teare JP, Thompson RPH. Review article: The mode of action of the aminosalicylates in inflammatory bowel disease. Aliment Pharmacol Ther. 1993;7:369–83.

23. Barve S, Joshi-Barve S, Talwalker R, McClain CJ, Varilek GW. Mesalamine (5-ASA) and the anti-oxidant, vitamin E inhibit interleukin-1 (IL-1) mediated activation of nuclear factor (B (NF(B)) in CACO-2 cells. Gastroenterology. 1995;108:A777.

24. Stevens C, Lipman M, Fabry S *et al.* 5-Aminosalicylic acid abrogates T-cell proliferation by blocking interleukin-2 production in peripheral blood mononuclear cells. J Pharmacol Exp Ther. 1995;272:399–406.

25. Miyachi Y, Yoshioka A, Imamura S, Niwa Y. Effect of sulphasalazine and its metabolites on the generation of reactive oxygen species. Gut. 1987;28:190–5.

26. Liu ZC, McClelland RA, Uetrecht JP. Oxidation of 5-aminosalicylic acid by hypochlorus acid to a reactive iminoquinone. Drug Metab Dispos. 1995;23:246–50.

27. Hiller KO, Willson RL. Hydroxyl free radicals and anti-inflammatory drugs: biological inactivation studies and reaction rate constants. Biochem Pharmacol. 1973;13:2109–11.

28. Mahida YR, Lamming CED, Gallagher A *et al.* 5-Aminosalicylic acid is a potent inhibitor of interleukin 1 beta production in organ culture of colonic biopsy specimens from patients with inflammatory bowel disease. Gut. 1991;32:50.

29. MacDermott RP, Schloemann SR, Bertovich MJ *et al.* Inhibition of antibody secretion by 5-aminosalicylic acid. Gastroenterology. 1989;96:442–8.

30. Marshall JK, Irvine EJ. Rectal corticosteroids versus alternative treatments in ulcerative colitis: a meta-analysis. Gut. 1997;40:775–81.
31. Svartz N. Salazopyrin, a new sulfonilamide preparation. Acta Med Scand. 1942;110:577–98.
32. Azad Khan AK, Piris J, Truelove SC. An experiment to determine the active therapeutic moiety of sulphasalazine. Lancet. 1977;1:892–5.
33. Azad Khan AK, Truelove SC, Aronson R. The disposition and metabolism of sulphasalazine (salicylazosulphapyridine) in man. Br J Pharmacol. 1982;3:523.
34. Allgayer H, Ahnfefelt NO, Kruis W *et al.* Colonic *N*-acetylation of 5-aminosalicylic acid in inflammatory bowel disease. Gastroenterology. 1989;97:38–41.
35. Hanauer SB. Evolving medical therapies for inflammatory bowel disease. Prog Inflam Bowel Dis. 1994;15:1–6.
36. Bachrach WH. Sulphasalazine. An historical perspective. Am J Gastroenterol. 1988;83:487–96.
37. Peppercorn MA, Goldman P. Distribution studies of salicylazosulphapyridine and its metabolites. Gastroenterology. 1973;64:240–5.
38. Shafi A, Chowdhury JR, Das KM. Absorption, enterohepatic circulation and excretion of 5-aminosalicylic acid in rats. Am J Gastroenterol. 1982;77:297–9.
39. Nielson OH, Bondesen S. Kinetics of 5-aminosalicylic acid after jejunal instillation in man. Br J Clin Pharmacol. 1983;16:738–40.
40. Klotz U, Maier KE, Fischer C, Bauer KH. A new slow-release form of 5-aminosalicylic acid for the oral treatment of inflammatory bowel disease. Biopharmaceutic and clinical pharmacokinetic characteristics. Arzneimittel Forschung/Drug Res. 1985;35:636–9.
41. Bondesen F, Bronn-Schou J, Pedersen V, Rafiolsadat Z, Hansen S, Huidberg EF. Absorption of 5-aminosalicylic acid from colon and rectum. Br J Clin Pharmacol. 1988;25:269.
42. Ewe K. Differentialtherapie von chronisch entzündlichen Darmerkrankungen mit oralen Aminosalizylaten. Dtsch Ärztebl. 1994;91:B2223–5.
43. Ewe K, Becker K, Ueberschaer B. Systemic uptake of 5-aminosalicylic acid from olsalazine and eudragit L coated mesalazine in patients with ulcerative colitis in remission. Z Gastroenterol. 1996;34:225–9.
44. Green JRB, Lobo AJ, Holdsworth CD *et al.* and the ABACUS investigator group. Balsalazide is more effective and better tolerated than mesalamine in the treatment of acute ulcerative colitis. Gastroenterology. 1998;114:15–22.
45. Brogden RN, Sorkin EM. Mesalazine. A review of its pharmacodynamic and pharmacokinetic properties, and therapeutic potential in chronic inflammatory bowel disease. Drugs. 1989;38:500–23.
46. Brynskov J, Norby Rasmussen S. Clinical pharmacology: development of new forms of treatment of inflammatory bowel disease. Scand J Gastroenterol. 1996;31(Suppl. 216):175–80.
47. Klotz U, Maier KE, Fischer C, Bauer KH. A new slow-release form of 5-aminosalicylic acid for the oral treatment of inflammatory bowel disease. Biopharmaceutic and clinical pharmacokinetic characteristics. Arzneimittel Forschung/Drug Res. 1985;35:636–9.
48. Myers B, Evans DNW, Rhodes J *et al.* Metabolism and urinary excretion of 5-aminosalicylic acid in healthy volunteers when given intravenously or released for absorption at different sites in the gastrointestinal tract. Gut. 1987;28:196–200.
49. Rasmussen SN, Bondesen S, Huidberg EF *et al.* 5-Aminosalicylic acid in a slow release preparation: bioavailability, plasma level and excretion in humans. Gastroenterology. 1982;83:1062–70.
50. Rijk MCM, van Schaik A, van Tongeren JHM. Disposition of 5-aminosalicylic acid by 5-aminosalicylic acid-delivering compounds. Scand J Gastroenterol. 1988;23:107–12.
51. Christensen LA, Fallingborg J, Jacobsen BA, Abildgaard K, Rasmussen HH, Hansen SH, Rasmussen SN. Comparative bioavailability of 5-aminosalicylic acid from a controlled release preparation and an azo-bond preparation. Aliment Pharmacol Ther. 1994;8:289–94.
52. Christensen LA, Fallingborg J, Jacobsen BA *et al.* Comparative bioavailability of 5-aminosalicylic acid from a controlled release preparation and an azo-bond preparation. Aliment Pharmacol Ther. 1994;8:289–94.
53. Hardy JG, Harvey WJ, Sparrow RA *et al.* Localization of drug release sites from an oral sustained-release formulation of 5-ASA (Pentasa) in the gastrointestinal tract using gamma scintigraphy. J Clin Pharmacol. 1993;33:712–18.
54. Christensen LA, Fallingborg J, Jacobsen BA, Rasmussen SN. Pharmakokinetik der oral verabreichten 5-Aminosalizylsäure (Mesalazin)-Präparate: Unterschiede und mögliche klinische Auswirkungen. Chirurg Gastroenterol. 1993;9(Suppl. 1):38–43.

55. Keller J, Goebell H, Klotz U, Layer P. Release patterns of 5-aminosalicylic acid in human small intestine. Importance of galenic preparation. Med Klin. 1998 (In press).

56. Goebell H, Klotz U, Nehleen B, Layer P. Oro-ileal transit of slow release 5-aminosalicylic acid. Gut. 1993;34:669–75.

57. Layer PH, Goebell H, Keller J, Dignass A, Klotz U. Delivery and fate of oral mesalamine microgranules within the human small intestine. Gastroenterology. 1995;108:1427–33.

58. Layer P, Chan ATH, Go VLW, DiMagno EP. Human pancreatic secretion during phase II antral motility of the interdigestive cycle. Am J Physiol. 1988;254:G249–53.

59. Layer P, Peschel S, Schlesinger T, Goebell H. Human pancreatic secretion and intestinal motility: effects of ileal nutrient perfusion. Am J Physiol. 1990;258:G196–201.

60. Chapman NJ, Brown NL, Phillips SF et al. Distribution of mesalamine enemas in patients with active distal ulcerative colitis. Mayo Clin Proc. 1992;67:245–8.

61. Campieri M, Corbelli C, Gionchetti P et al. Spread and distribution of 5-ASA colonic foam and 5-ASA enemas in patients with ulcerative colitis. Dig Dis Sci. 1992;37:1890–7.

62. Campieri M, Paoluzzi P, D'Albasio G, Brunetti G, Pera A, Barbara L. Better quality of therapy with 5-ASA colonic foam in active ulcerative colitis: a multicenter comparative trial with 5-ASA enema. Dig Dis Sci. 1993;38:1843–50.

63. Campieri M et al. Mesalazine (5-aminosalicylic acid) suppositories in the treatment of ulcerative proctitis or distal proctosigmoiditis. A randomized controlled trial. Scand J Gastroenterol. 1990;25:663–8.

64. Brogden RN, Sorkin EM. Mesalazine. A review of its pharmacodynamic and pharmacokinetic properties, and therapeutic potential in chronic inflammatory bowel disease. Drugs. 1989;38:500–23.

65. May B. Behandlung chronisch entzündlicher Darmerkrankungen. Studie über Mesalazin (5-Aminosalizylsäure) an mehr als 1700 Patienten unter Praxisbedingungen. Münchener Med Wochenschr. 1987;129:786–9.

66. Rünzi M, Layer P. Drug-associated pancreatitis – facts and fiction. Pancreas. 1996;13:100–9.

67. Dent MT, Ganapathy S, Holdsworth CD, Channer KC. Mesalazine induced lupus-like syndrome. Br Med J. 1992;305:159.

68. Largler U, Schulthess HK, Kuhn M. Akute Alveolitis unter Mesalazin. Schweiz Med Wochenschr. 1992;122:1332–4.

69. Sviri S, Gafanovich I, Kramer MR, Tsvang E, Ben-Chetrit E. Mesalamine-induced hypersensitivity pneumonitis. J Clin Gastroenterol. 1997;24:34–6.

70. Riley SA, Lloyd DR, Mani V. Tests of renal function in patients with quiescent colitis: effects of drug treatment. Gut. 1992;33:1348–52.

71. Walker AM, Szneke P, Bianchi LA, Field LG, Sutherland LR, Dreyer NA. 5-Aminosalicylates, sulphasalazine, steroid use and complications in patients with ulcerative colitis. Am J Gastroenterol. 1997;92:816–20.

72. Schreiber S, Hämling J, Zehnter E et al. Renal tubular dysfunction in patients with inflammatory bowel disease treated with aminosalicylate. Gut. 1997;40:761–6.

73. Mahmud N, O'Connell MA, Stinson J, Goggins MG, Weir DG, Kelleher D. Tumour necrosis factor-α and microalbuminuria in patients with inflammatory bowel disease. Eur J Gastroenterol Hepatol. 1995;7:215–19.

74. Mahmud N, Stinson J, O'Connell MA et al. Microalbuminuria in inflammatory bowel disease. Gut. 1994;35:1599–604.

75. Kreisel W, Wolf LM, Grotz W, Grieshaber M. Renal tubular damage: an extraintestinal manifestation of chronic inflammatory bowel disease. Eur J Gastroenterol Hepatol. 1996;8:461–8.

76. World MJ, Stevens PE, Ashton MA, Rainford DJ. Mesalazine-associated interstitial nephritis. Nephrol Dial Transplant. 1996;11:614–21.

77. De Broe ME, Stlear JC, Nouwen ET, Elseviers MM. Mesalazine and chronic interstitial nephritis: is there a role for urinary markers to detect early changes? In: Pharmacokinetics and Safety Profile of Mesalazine. Adis International; 1997:42–52.

78. Meyers S, Sachar DB, Present DH, Janowitz HD. Olsalazine sodium in the treatment of ulcerative colitis among patients intolerant of sulfasalazine. A prospective, randomized, placebo-controlled, double-blind, dose-ranging clinical trial. Gastroenterology. 1987;93:1255–62.

79. Jarnerot G. Clinical tolerance of olsalazine. Scand J Gastroenterol. 1988;23(Suppl.):21–3.

80. Courtney MG, Nunes DP, Bergin CF et al. Randomised comparison of olsalazine and mesalazine in prevention of relapse in ulcerative colitis. Lancet. 1992;339:1279–81

81. Werlin S, Grand R. Bloody diarrhea – a new complication of sulphasalazine. J Pediatr. 1978;92:450–1.
82. Ruppin H, Domschke S. Acute ulcerative colitis – a rare complication of sulphasalazine therapy. Hepatogastroenterology. 1984;31:192–3.
83. Kapur KC, Williams GT, Allison MC. Mesalazine induced exacerbation of ulcerative colitis. Gut. 1995;37:838–9.
84. Orna DC, Park YH, Veerasuntharam G *et al.* The safety of mesalamine in human pregnancy: a prospective controlled cohort study. Gastroenterology. 1998;114:23–8.
85. Christensen LA, Fallingborg J, Jacobsen BA *et al.* Comparative bioavailability of 5-aminosalicylic acid from a controlled release preparation and an azo-bond preparation. Aliment Pharmacol Ther. 1994;8:289–94.
86. D'Albasio G, Pacini F, Camarri E *et al.* Combined therapy with 5-aminosalicylic acid tablets and enemas for maintaining remission in ulcerative colitis. A randomized double-blind study. Am J Gastroenterol. 1997;92:1143–7.
87. Bayless TM. Maintenance therapy for Crohn's disease. Gastroenterology. 1996;110:299–302.
88. McLeod RS, Wolff BG, Steinhart AH *et al.* Prophylactic mesalamine treatment decreases postoperative recurrence of Crohn's disease. Gastroenterology. 1995;109:404–13.
89. Peppercorn MA. A critical evaluation of the therapeutic benefits and side effects of aminosalicylate analogues in the treatment of inflammatory bowel disease. Inflammopharmacology. 1993;2:263–76.
90. Modigliani R. Colombel JF, Dupas J-L *et al.* Mesalamine in Crohn's disease with steroid-induced remission: effect on steroid withdrawal and remission maintenance. Gastroenterology. 1996;110:688–93.
91. Sahmoud T, Mary JY. Mesalazine as a maintenance treatment in Crohn's disease: is it the long-awaited solution? Gut. 1997;40:284–5.
92. De Franchis R *et al.* Controlled trial of oral 5-aminosalicylic acid for the prevention of early relapse in Crohn's disease. Aliment Pharmacol Ther. 1997;11:845–52.

33
Glucocorticosteroids in the treatment of IBD

J. SCHÖLMERICH

INTRODUCTION

Since the aetiology of chronic inflammatory bowel diseases (IBD) has not yet been elucidated, and pathogenesis is only partly understood, no causal treatment exists. Glucocorticosteroids (GCS) have been successfully used in the treatment of symptoms and inflammation in several disorders[1,2]. Since an excessive acute and chronic inflammation is an essential part of the mucosal tissue injury, GCS have been a mainstay of treatment for both ulcerative colitis (UC) and Crohn's disease (CD), for over 30 years.

PHARMACOLOGY

The ubiquitous distribution of glucocorticoid receptors in the body explains the large number of unwanted effects of GCS. Receptors are present in practically every cell of the human organism in a concentration between 2000 and 30 000 binding sites per cell, corresponding to about 5×10^{13}/mg cytosolic protein (in leukocytes). Plasma concentrations of glucocorticoids vary considerably after oral ingestion of the same dose by normal subjects or patients with IBD[3]. In some studies an impaired absorption of prednisolone in IBD patients, in particular in patients with extensive small bowel CD, is found[3–5] while others described a normal absorption compared to healthy controls[6–8]. Biological half-life is 16–38 h while plasma half-life is only 2–4 h[9]. The rectal administration, bioavailability and maximal plasma concentrations are lower in patients with UC as compared to controls[10]. In particular with foam preparations the bioavailability is only 2% and peak plasma concentrations are even further decreased to about 5% of values achieved with enemas[11]. Steroid receptors seem to be downregulated in patients with IBD, at least in the mucosa[12] (Table 1).

Synthetic steroids, mainly substituted in C17 position, have been developed for treatment of pulmonary disorders. Due to a high first-pass elimination in the liver or in the mucosa these substances have a lower bioavailability. In particular

Table 1 Glucocorticoid receptors in IBD and other immune-mediated diseases[12]: receptors (10^{12}/mg cytosolic protein) in leukocytes or mucosal homogenate

	Treated	*Untreated*	*Control*
IBD, mucosa	1.5 ± 3.2	2.5 ± 4.2	27 ± 22
IBD, leukocytes	14 ± 13 ($n = 24$)	41 ± 39 ($n = 29$)	51 ± 20 ($n = 31$)
Collagen disorders, leukocytes	17 ± 17 ($n = 47$)	23 ± 15 ($n = 12$)	51 ± 20 ($n = 31$)

budesonide, when given rectally or orally in time- or pH-dependent release preparations, has a systemic bioavailability of only 10%. Accordingly systemic effects are much less pronounced, as shown in a number of studies.

In the following clinical applications of steroids and the newer 'non systemic' steroids in IBD will be discussed.

ULCERATIVE COLITIS

Distal UC treatment with steroid enemas is superior to placebo[13]. However, 5-aminosalicylic acid (5-ASA) seems to be somewhat superior to steroid treatment[14]. Patients prefer suppositories versus foams, and foams compared to enemas, and rectal treatment is more effective when compared to oral treatment.

Budesonide enemas have been used in a number of trials for distal UC and were found to be better than placebo and comparable to conventional steroids[15,16]. However, they were not better than 5-ASA enemas[17,18]. A dose of 2 mg was found to be optimal. Interestingly a combination of another non-systemic steroid (beclomethasone dipropionate) with 5-ASA as enemas had better therapeutic effects than either of the drugs alone[19] (Table 2).

Patients with more extensive colitis and with severe colitis are treated with oral or intravenous steroids. However, in severe cases only about 50% of patients achieve remission and 42% need colectomy, while in moderate colitis 80%, and in mild colitis 84%, reach remission[20]. Only one study has assessed divided doses compared to a single dose, and this did not find a difference[21]. Oral budesonide in a time-dependent release form did not show better efficacy when compared to prednisolone[22].

Steroids have been used for maintenance treatment in some earlier trials[23], showing that alternate-day use is better than no treatment. However, the success

Table 2 Beclomethasone dipropionate (BDP) vs 5-ASA enemas vs combination in distal ulcerative colitis[19] (percentages)

4 weeks	*BDP (3 mg)* *(n = 20)*	*5-ASA (1 g)* *(n = 21)*	*Combination* *(n = 19)*
Endoscopic remission	30	10	37
Clinical improvement	70	76	100
Endoscopic improvement	75	71	100

rates of surgical treatment indicate that all long-term medical treatments have to be weighed against surgical treatment which is able to cure disease.

In summary, in UC most patients do not need steroids. Distal disease can be treated with hydrocortisone foam, betamethasone enemas or budesonide enemas. 5-ASA is in most cases sufficient. Severe colitis needs systemic steroids in high doses given orally or intravenously. Steroids are probably not of much use in maintenance treatment and should not be given long term.

CROHN'S DISEASE

In active CD steroids are still the mainstay of treatment. However, a recent study[24] showed that only 44% of patients reached a long-term remission with their first steroid treatment, 36% become steroid-dependent and 20% were initially steroid-resistant. In patients with responding disease activity normally declined rapidly during the first 2 weeks and overall 70–80% responded initially[25–28]. Steroids are superior to 5-ASA[27]; a comparison with higher doses (4.5 g/day) of 5-ASA decreases this difference[28]. The effect of steroids is limited to clinically symptomatic patients, as evidenced in a recent study[29].

A number of trials have been performed using time-dependent or pH-dependent oral budesonide release preparations (Table 3). All studies showed very similar effects, indicating that remission rates were somewhat lower when compared to systemic steroids, although statistical significance was never achieved. However, side-effects were always statistically less frequent than with systemic steroids, when a dose of 9 mg/day of budesonide was used. No major difference between divided and single doses has been demonstrated up to now, although one trial indicated that a single dose may be better[33]. Our own studies have shown that patients with a longer disease duration (> 8 years), and with initially highly active disease (CDAI > 300), show less response when compared to patients with shorter disease duration and lower activity at the start of treatment[34]. A dose-finding study demonstrated that for the time-dependent release form 9 mg/day was the optimal dose, and 15 mg/day did not add more benefit[31]. In contrast, the pH-dependent release form improved remission rates in patients who were not pretreated, from 55% with 9 mg/day to 66% with 18 mg/day. This was particularly due to an effect in those patients having initially higher activity[35]. Slightly more systemic side-effects were observed with the highest dose; their incidence remained, however, still much lower than with systemic steroids[35].

A switch from conventional steroids to budesonide is possible in active and already inactive disease. While 79% of patients who have already been brought into remission maintain this state for 8 weeks, in patients in whom systemic steroids have not yet been effective, about 39% achieve remission during subsequent weeks. The total number of side-effects, and the percentage of patients having side-effects, decreased after switching during the next 6 weeks from 269 to 90 and from 65% to 43%, respectively[36]. However, lower doses of 3 or 6 mg/day do not achieve these success rates[37].

Several attempts have been made to maintain remission in CD using glucocorticosteroids. While one trial did not find a difference between 4 weeks and 12 weeks treatment[38], the European multicentre trial[26] demonstrated that in

Table 3 Randomized controlled studies with oral budesonide in active Crohn's disease (percentages)

| | Remission (%) | | | | | | | Steroid side-effects (%) | | | | | | |
| | | Budesonide | | | | | | | Budesonide | | | | | |
Study	Placebo	3 mg	6 mg	9 mg	15 mg	18 mg	Prednisolone	Placebo	3 mg	6 mg	9 mg	15 mg	18 mg	Prednisolone
Rutgeerts et al.[30]				53			66				33			55
Greenberg et al.[31]	20	33		51	43			26	15	26	38			
Gross et al.[32‡]				56			73				29			70
Campieri et al.[33]				60*			60				14			38 §
				42†							11			
Gross et al[35‡]			36	55		66					20	21		31	

* 1 × 9 mg.
† 2 × 4.5 mg.
‡ pH-modified release budesonide.
§ Moon face only.

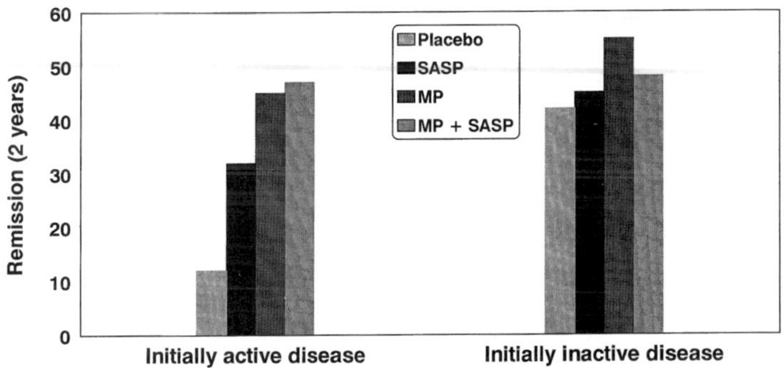

Figure 1 Relapse prevention with low-dose (8 mg) methylprednisolone (MP) or sulphasalazine (SASP) in Crohn's disease[26]. There is an effect of drugs in patients with initially active disease treated with the respective drug, but not in those with initially inactive disease

Table 4 Budesonide-pH-dependent release for active Crohn's disease – dose finding[35]

	Remission 6 weeks (%)		
	2 × 2 mg *(n = 104)*	*3 × 3 mg* *(n = 99)*	*3 × 6 mg* *(n = 106)*
Not pretreated, CDAI > 150 (n = 104)	**36**	**55**	**66**
Pretreated, CDAI > 150 (n = 80)	40	32	47
Pretreated, CDAI < 150 (n = 125)	63	71	73
Side-effects (n)	81	79	88

Bold figures indicate significant effects.

patients being brought into remission using steroids there is an effect in maintenance of such remission using low-dose steroids (10 mg prednisolone equivalent) while this is not the case for patients treated for 2 years being in remission at the start of treatment (Figure 1)[26].

A dose of 3 mg/day pH-dependent-release budesonide slightly prolongs time to relapse but does not maintain remission in patients who have been brought into remission using conventional steroids[39] (Figure 2). Two trials using the time-dependent release form indicated that 6 mg/day budesonide leads to a delay of relapse. However after 1 year relapse rates were identical regardless of treatment with placebo, 3 mg, or 6 mg/day of this preparation (Table 5)[39–41]. A dose of 6 mg led to somewhat decreased side-effects and more suppression of basal cortisol, as shown in a recent meta-analysis from three trials using time-dependent-release budesonide[42]. In this analysis, including one as-yet-unpublished trial, a significant shift of the time to relapse was found only for 6 mg/day budesonide. An initially high CDAI and female gender were indicating a higher relapse rate.

Budesonide was also not very useful in postoperative relapse prevention, where again a shift in time to relapse, but no difference after 1 year treatment, was found[43,44]. Only in the subgroup of patients operated for initially highly active disease was there some benefit after 1 year (30% versus 65% relapse rate).

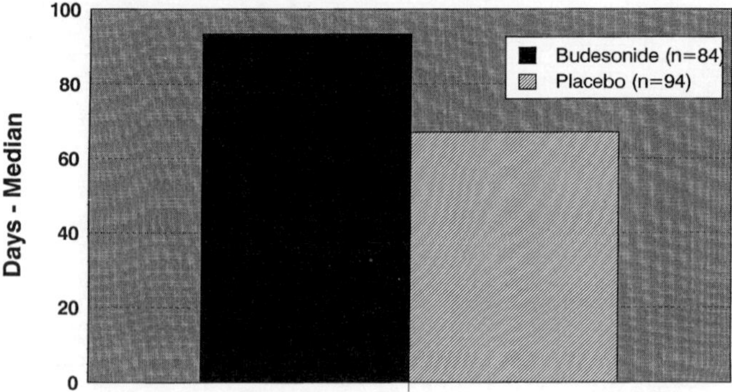

Figure 2   Time to relapse in patients with Crohn's disease brought into remission using conventional steroids and thereafter treated with budesonide (3 × 1 mg/day) or placebo[39]

Table 5   Maintenance of glucocorticosteroid-induced remission of Crohn's disease

| | *Median time to failure (days)* | | | *One-year failure rate (%)* | | |
| | | *Budesonide* | | | *Budesonide* | |
	Placebo	*3 mg*	*6 mg*	*Placebo*	*3 mg*	*6 mg*
Greenberg *et al.*[40]	39	124	178[†]	64	58	58
Loefberg *et al.*[41]	92	139	258[†]	63	74	59
Gross *et al.*[39]*	67	91	–	65	67	–

* pH-modified release budesonide.
[†] $p < 0.05$.

Table 6   Remission maintenance in Crohn's disease with budesonide (time-dependent release) – pooled trials data[42]

	6 mg (n = 90)	*3 mg (n = 90)*	*Placebo (n = 90)*
Prior prednisolone (%)	34	18	28
Time to relapse (days)	**263**	170	150
Side-effects			
Percentage	**48**	31	24
No. per day	0.24	0.20	0.34
Δ Cortisol (basal, ng/ml)	**+11**	+60	+42
Normal HPA function (%)			
Baseline	67	78	92
After treatment	55	73	84

Bold figures indicate significant effects versus placebo.

In summary, steroids are still a mainstay of treatment in active CD. In patients with mild and modest activity oral budesonide can be used to decrease side-effects. Steroids have no place in maintenance treatment at present. A prolonged course of low-dose steroids may be useful in patients brought into remission with systemic steroids. Steroid-dependent patients should receive alternative treatment, i.e. azathioprine. Further developments are needed to improve the remission rate in active CD and the effect of maintenance treatment.

References

1. Schölmerich J, Andus T. Old and new steroids. In: Fleig WE, editor. Inflammatory Bowel Disease. Lancaster: Kluwer; 1995:193–224.
2. Andus T, Targan SR. Corticosteroids. In: Targan S, Shanahan F, editors. Inflammatory Bowel Disease: From Bench to Bedside. Baltimore, MD: Williams & Wilkins; 1993:487–502.
3. Pickup ME. Clinical pharmacokinetics of prednisone and prednisolone. Clin Pharmacokinet. 1979;4:111–28.
4. Elliot PR, Powell-Tuck J, Gillespie PE et al. Prednisolone absorption in acute colitis. Gut. 1980;21:49–51.
5. Rodrigues CA, Nabi EM, Spiliadis C et al. Prednisolone absorption in inflammatory bowel disease, including cases with proximal to distal small bowel involvement. Gastroenterol Clin Biol. 1985;9:564–71.
6. Tanner AR, Halliday JW, Powell L. Serum prednisolone levels in Crohn's disease and celiac disease following oral prednisolone administration. Digestion. 1981;21:310–15.
7. Olivesi A. Normal absorption of oral prednisolone in children with active inflammatory bowel disease, including cases with proximal to distal small bowel involvement. Gastroenterol Clin Biol. 1985;9:564–71.
8. Milsap RL, George DE, Szefler SJ, Murray KA, Lebenthal E, Jusko WJ. Effect of inflammatory bowel disease on absorption and disposition of prednisolone. Dig Dis Sci. 1983;28:161–8.
9. Swartz S, Dluhy R. Corticosteroids: clinical pharmacology and therapeutic use. Drugs. 1978;16:238–55.
10. Petitjean O, Wendling JL, Tod M et al. Pharmacokinetics and absolute rectal bioavailability of hydrocortisone acetate in distal colitis. Aliment Pharmacol Ther. 1992;6:351–7.
11. Möllmann H, Barth J, Möllmann C, Tunn S, Krieg M, Derendorf H. Pharmacokinetics and rectal bioavailability of hydrocortisone acetate. J Pharmacol Sci. 1991;80:835–6.
12. Rogler G, Meinel A, Lingauer A et al. Glucocorticoid-receptors are downregulated in inflamed colonic mucosa of patients with inflammatory bowel disease. Eur J Clin Invest. 1999;(in press).
13. Marshall JK, Irvine EJ. Rectal corticosteroids versus alternative treatments in ulcerative colitis: a meta-analysis. Gut. 1997;40:775–81.
14. Farup PG, Hovde O, Halvorsen FA, Raknerud N, Brodin U. Mesalazine suppositories versus hydrocortisone foam in patients with distal ulcerative colitis. Scand J Gastroenterol. 1995;39:164–70.
15. Bianchi-Porro G, Campieri M, Bianchi P et al. Comparative trial of budesonide and methylprednisolone enemas in the treatment of ulcerative colitis. Eur J Gastroenterol Hepatol. 1994;6:125–30.
16. Danielsson A, Hellers G, Lyrenäs E et al. A controlled randomized trial of budesonide versus prednisolone retention enemas in active distal ulcerative colitis. Scand J Gastroenterol. 1987;22:987–92.
17. Lamers C, Meijer J, Engels L et al. Comparative study of the topically acting glucocorticosteroid budesonide and 5-aminosalicylic acid enema therapy of proctitis and proctosigmoiditis. Gastroenterology. 1991;101:A223.
18. Leman M, Rutgeerts P, van Heuverzwijn R et al. Comparison of budesonide enema and 5-ASA enema in the treatment of active distal ulcerative colitis. Hellenic J Gastroenterol. 1995;5:194.
19. Mulder CJ, Fockens P, Meijer JW et al. Beclomethasone dipropionate (3 mg) versus 5-aminosalicylic (2 g) versus the combination of both (3 mg/2 g) as retention enemas in active ulcerative proctitis. Eur J Gastroenterol Hepatol. 1997;8:549–52.
20. Kjeldsen J. Treatment of ulcerative colitis with high doses of oral prednisolone: the rate of remission, the need for surgery, and the effect of prolonging the treatment. Scand J Gastroenterol. 1993;28:821 6.
21. Powell-Tuck J, Brown, R, Lennard-Jones JE. A comparison of oral prednisolone as single or multiple daily doses for active proctocolitis. Scand J Gastroenterol 1987;13:883–7.

22. Löfberg R, Danielsson A, Suhr O *et al.* Oral budesonide versus prednisolone in patients with active extensive and left-sided ulcerative colitis. Gastroenterology. 1996;110:1713–18.
23. Powell-Tuck J, Brown RL, Chambers TJ, Lennard-Jones JE. A controlled trial of alternate day prednisolone as a maintenance treatment of ulcerative colitis in remission. Digestion. 1981;22:263–70.
24. Munkholm P, Langholz E, Davidsen M, Binder V. Frequency of glucocorticoid resistance and dependency in Crohn's disease. Gut. 1994;35:360–2.
25. Summers RW, Switz DM, Sessoins Jr JT *et al.* National Cooperative Crohn's Disease Study: results of drug treatment. Gastroenterology. 1979;77:847–69.
26. Malchow H, Ewe K, Brandes JW *et al.* European Cooperative Crohn's Disease Study (ECCDS): results of drug treatment. Gastroenterology. 1984;86:249–66.
27. Schölmerich J, Jenss H, Hartmann F and the German 5-ASA Study Group. Oral 5-aminosalicylic acid versus 6-methylprednisolone in active Crohn's disease. Can J Gastroenterol. 1990;4:446–51.
28. Gross V, Andus T, Fischbach W and the German 5-ASA Study Group. Comparison between high dose 5-aminosalicylic acid and 6-methylprednisolone in active Crohn's ileocolitis. A multicenter randomized double-blind study. Z Gastroenterol. 1995;33:582–4.
29. Landi B, Anh TN, Cortot A *et al.* Endoscopic monitoring of Crohn's disease treatment: a prospective, randomized clinical trial. Gastroenterology. 1992;102:1647–53.
30. Rutgeerts P, Löfberg R, Malchow H *et al.* A comparison of budesonide with prednisolone for active Crohn's disease. N Engl J Med. 1994;33:842–5.
31. Greenberg GR, Feagan BG, Martin F and the Canadian Inflammatory Bowel Disease Study Group. Oral budesonide for active Crohn's disease. N Engl J Med. 1994;331:836–41.
32. Gross V, Andus T, Caesar I *et al.* and the German/Austrian Budesonide Study Group. Oral pH-modified release budesonide versus 6-methylprednisolone in active Crohn's disease. Eur J Gastroenterol Hepatol. 1996;8:905–9.
33. Campieri M, Ferguson A, Doe W and the International Budesonide Study Group. Oral budesonide competes favorably with prednisolone in active Crohn's disease. Gut. 1997;41:209–14.
34. Caesar I, Gross V, Roth M *et al.* Treatment of active Crohn's ileocolitis with an oral slow release Eudragit-coated budesonide formulation. Z Gastroenterol. 1995;33:247–50.
35. Gross V, Caesar I, Andus T *et al.* and the German/Austrian Budesonide Study Group. Dose-finding study with oral budesonide in patients with active Crohn's ileocolitis. Gastroenterology. 1997;112:A986 (abstract).
36. Caesar I, Gross V, Andus T *et al.* and the German/Austrian Budesonide Study Group. Replacement of conventional steroids by oral pH-modified release budesonide in active and inactive Crohn's disease. Dig Dis Sci. 1998 (In press).
37. Novacek G, Kleinberger M, Vogelsand H, Moser G, Lochs H. Budesonide in glucocorticoid dependent chronic active Crohn's disease; a pilot study. Z Gastroenterol. 1995;33:251–4.
38. Brignola C, De Simone G, Belloli C *et al.* Steroid treatment in active Crohn's disease: a comparison between two regimens of different duration. Aliment Pharmacol Ther. 1994;8:465–8.
39. Gross V, Andus T, Ecker KW *et al.* and the Budesonide Study Group. Low-dose oral pH-modified release budesonide for maintenance of steroid induced remission in Crohn's disease. Gut. 1998;42:493–6.
40. Greenberg GR, Feagan BG, Marin F *et al.* and the Canadian Inflammatory Bowel Disease Study Group. Oral budesonide as maintenance treatment for Crohn's disease: a placebo-controlled dose-ranging study. Gastroenterology. 1996;110:45–51.
41. Loefberg R, Rutgeerts P, Malchow H *et al.* Budesonide prolongs time to relapse in ileal and in ileocaecal Crohn's disease. A placebo controlled one year study. Gut. 1996;39:82–6.
42. Feagan B, Greenberg GR, Löfberg R, Ferguson A, Persson T. Budesonide controlled ileal release prolonged remission in Crohn's disease: meta-analysis. Gut. 1997:41(Suppl. 3)A17.
43. Ewe K. Non-systemic steroids for relapse prevention in Crohn's disease. In: Tytgat GNJ, Bartelsman JFWM, van Deventer SJH, editors. Inflammatory Bowel Disease. Lancaster: Kluwer;1995:666–71.
44. Hellers G, Löfberg R, Rutgeerts P *et al.* Oral budesonide for prevention of recurrence following ileocecal resection of Crohn's disease. A one year placebo-controlled study. Gastroenterology. 1996;110:A923.

34
Immunosuppressive therapy

E. F. STANGE

INTRODUCTION

The standard immunosuppressive agents in inflammatory bowel disease (IBD) are azathioprine and 6-mercaptopurine. More recently, methotrexate, cyclosporine A, tacrolimus and mycophenolate have been introduced in steroid-dependent or refractory disease. The rationale for the use of these drugs lies in the multiple immunological abnormalities described in both types of disease[1]. The role of these treatment alternatives will be reviewed in this chapter.

AZATHIOPRINE AND 6-MERCAPTOPURINE

The precise mechanism of action of both azathioprine and 6-mercaptopurine remains enigmatic, although some progress has been made in this regard. Azathioprine has been demonstrated to be converted to 6-mercaptopurine *in vivo*, suggesting that there is no principal difference in action between the two agents. 6-Mercaptopurine is subsequently metabolized to 6-thioinosinic acid, the presumed active metabolite which becomes incorporated into developing strands of DNA. In lymphocytes this substitution blocks critical gene activation of effector lymphocyte clones, thus inhibiting their proliferation.

In Crohn's disease nine reports on controlled trials of azathioprine or 6-mercaptopurine in either active or quiescent disease[2-10] have been fully published. An overview of these studies is given in Table 1. The two initial small trials[2,3] failed to show a significant benefit, probably due to insufficient statistical power (β-error) and the short treatment course. In the milestone study by Present *et al.*[6] 83 chronically ill patients were entered into a 2-year double-blind study comparing 6-mercaptopurine with placebo. Crossover data showed that improvement occurred in 26 of 39 courses of the drug (67%) as compared with three of 39 courses of placebo (8%, $p < 0.0001$). Non-crossover data likewise confirmed the superiority of 6-mercaptopurine. The drug was more effective in closing fistulas (31% versus 6%) and in permitting discontinuation or reduction of steroid dosage (75% versus 36%). It is important to note that the onset of response was often delayed, with 32% of the patients taking longer than

Table 1 Azathioprine and 6-mercaptopurine: controlled trials

	Dose (mg/kg per day)	Duration (months)	n	Response Plac/Aza (%)
Crohn's disease				
Active disease				
Rhodes et al.[2]	2–4	2 + 2	16	0/0
Klein et al.[3]	3	4 + 4	26	46/46
Willoughby et al.[4]	2–4	6	22	17/100 ($p < 0.01$)
Summers et al.[5*]	2.5	4	136	26/36
Present et al.[6†]	1.5	12 + 12	83	14/72 ($p < 0.001$)
Ewe et al.[7]	2.5	4	42	38/76 ($p = 0.03$)
Candy et al.[8]	2.5	3	63	67/76
Quiescent disease				
Rosenberg et al.[9]	2	6.5	20	40/70 ($p < 0.05$)
O'Donoghue et al.[10]	2	12	51	30/57 ($p < 0.01$)
Summers et al.[5*]	1	12–24	155	64/69
Candy et al.[8]	2.5	12	45	7/42 ($p < 0.001$)
Ulcerative colitis				
Acute active disease				
Caprilli et al.[15*]	2.5	3	20	80/60
Jewell et al.[16]	2.5	1	80	68/78
Chronic active disease				
Kirk et al.[17]	2–2.5	6	44	Pred dose reduced ($p < 0.001$)
Rosenberg et al.[18]	1.5	6	30	7/44 ($p < 0.05$)
Maintenance				
Jewell et al.[16]	1.5–2.5	12	80	23/40
Hawthorne et al.[19]	Variable	12	79	31/61 ($p < 0.01$)

Plac: placebo; Aza: azathioprine; pred: prednisolone.

* No concomitant steroids.

† 6-Mercaptopurine.

3 months to respond, and 19% taking longer than 4 months. The National Cooperative Crohn's Disease Study[5] gave a negative result but was biased against azathioprine for several reasons. First, corticosteroids were withdrawn in a significant proportion of the patients immediately before the start of the trial so that many patients experienced an early relapse. Since azathioprine requires several months for its action this design probably doomed the azathioprine arm of the trial. Also for this reason the treatment period of 4 months may simply have been too short and the data actually indicate an improved action after 7 weeks of treatment[5]. A large uncontrolled study also supports a corticoid-sparing effect in 76% of patients, control of refractory disease in 73%, lessening of fistulization in 63% and overall achievement of treatment goals in 72%[11].

A recent small study examined whether azathioprine combined with standard prednisolone therapy improved the therapeutic outcome compared with monotherapy with prednisolone in active Crohn's disease[7]. At the end of the 4-month trial, 16 of 21 patients (76%) with combined therapy versus eight of 21 patients treated with corticosteroids alone (38%) were in remission ($p = 0.03$). The differences in activity indices became significant after 8 weeks. In addition, the average steroid dose was significantly lower in the combined-treatment group. However, in the initial period of 3 months in the trial of Candy *et al.* the minimal difference between the placebo and azathioprine was not significant[8], confirming the slower onset of its action. Thus, an early synergistic effect of azathioprine and corticosteroids is unproven, but the combination of the two agents in chronic active disease is probably wise. A recent meta-analysis of the controlled trials, by Pearson *et al.*, supports the significant advantage of azathioprine/6-mercaptopurine in active disease[12]. It was also found that the response rate was dependent on treatment time and dose, in particular cumulative dose. An interesting new approach to speed up the slow onset of action is the use of high-dose intravenous therapy during an initial 36-h treatment phase, as suggested by Sandborn *et al.*[13] However, this may be detrimental to patients with a defect in 6-mercaptopurine metabolism, and the results of an ongoing trial supporting this approach are eagerly awaited. Finally, the combined studies of the meta-analysis[12] demonstrated a steroid-sparing effect both in active and quiescent disease with an odds ratio of 3.7 and 4.6, respectively. In addition, fistulas improved with azathioprine therapy with an odds ratio of 4.4.

Azathioprine in this meta-analysis was found to exert a more limited but still statistically significant effect in Crohn's disease patients with quiescent disease. Again, in the large negative study by Summers *et al.*[5] the patients did not receive a comedication with steroids and the dose of azathioprine at 1 mg/kg body weight per day was lower than in most other treatment regimes (2–4 mg/kg body weight per day). Interestingly, in the trial by Candy *et al.* steroids could be successfully weaned following the initial phase of combined therapy with steroids plus azathioprine[8]. The French trial by Bouhnik *et al.*[14], although uncontrolled, suggests that azathioprine therapy should be maintained for at least 4 years, because during this period the relapse rate is unacceptably high. After 4 years the relapse rates of those continued on the drug and those weaned from azathioprine were comparably low.

The trials using azathioprine in ulcerative colitis are fewer and less conclusive. Conspicuously, both studies in patients with acute relapse failed to detect a significant benefit[15,16], whereas two trials focusing on patients with chronic active disease reported significant improvement[17,18]. In an early report azathioprine was ineffective in both achieving and maintaining a remission[16]. In contrast, patients who had been taking azathioprine for 6 months prior to another trial, and who were in remission for at least 2 months, displayed a significantly higher relapse rate when withdrawn from the drug (59%) as compared to the group continued on the medication (36%)[19].

The benefit of these immunosuppressive agents, which is now generally accepted, has to be weighed against eventual toxicity. In the large experience of Present *et al.*[20] in 396 patients treated with 6-mercaptopurine, based on a mean period of follow-up of 5 years, toxicity included pancreatitis (3.3%), bone marrow depression (2%), allergic reactions (2%) and drug hepatitis (0.3%). All complications were reversible, with no mortality. Infectious complications were seen in 7.4% of the patients, of which 1.8% were severe. Again, all infections were cured with no deaths; 3.1% of the cohort developed neoplasms but only one (0.3%), a diffuse histiocytic lymphoma of the brain, had a probable association with the drug.

It may be concluded that azathioprine and 6-mercaptopurine represent a reasonable and reasonably safe medication in otherwise intractable IBD, provided that surgery is not indicated. Most importantly, all patients have to be carefully monitored to detect potential side-effects early.

METHOTREXATE

Use of methotrexate, another cytotoxic immunosuppressant, in refractory Crohn's disease has been introduced by Kozarek et al.[21] in an uncontrolled trial of limited size. Nevertheless, this study, reporting an improvement in the majority of patients with chronic active disease, formed the basis for a series of ongoing controlled trials. Methotrexate is usually administered as weekly intramuscular injections of 25 mg during a 12-week treatment period. Thereafter the dosing may be switched to oral medication in tapered fashion if remission is achieved. The single fully published controlled trial on this drug in Crohn's disease, by Feagan et al., reported a limited therapeutic benefit of approximately 20%[22]. The uncontrolled French study by Lémann et al.[23] confirmed an initial response to methotrexate but the relapse rate amounted to 60% after 10 months. Thus, methotrexate is a second-line drug in this indication, particularly reserved for those not responding or intolerant to azathioprine/6-mercaptopurine. Finally, a trial[24] using a low dose (12.5 mg orally per week) in ulcerative colitis was negative. Since published experience with the drug is limited, a final evaluation of the role of methotrexate in chronic active IBD clearly awaits full publication of further controlled trials.

CYCLOSPORINE A

Despite its revolutionary role in transplantation medicine and its well-known mechanism of action, cyclosporine A has only recently been introduced in the field of IBD. This hydrophobic undecapeptide is obtained by extraction of the soil fungus *Tolypocladium infatum gams*. After entering the target cell the drug binds to cyclophilin, inactivates calcineurin and prevents the nuclear factor of activated T cells (NFAT)-induced transcription of messenger-RNA encoding for interleukin-2 and its receptor[25]. In addition, cyclosporine interferes with B cell

Table 2 Methotrexate: controlled trials

	Dose per week	Duration (months)	n	Response Plac/Mtx
Crohn's disease				
Chronic active disease				
Feagan et al.[22]	25 mg intramuscular	4	141	19/39 ($p < 0.025$)
Ulcerative colitis				
Chronic active disease				
Oren et al.[24]	12.5 mg oral	9	67	47/49

Plac: placebo; Mtx: methotrexate.

activation indirectly by suppressing the formation of activating factors by helper
T cells. These molecular mechanisms are responsible for the unique selectivity
of cyclosporine which acts only on lymphocytes but not on granulocytes, monocytes or macrophages. Since the T cell is currently believed to play a pivotal role
in the mucosal inflammatory process[1] the rationale for the use of the drug in
these diseases is obvious.

As reviewed recently by Tremaine and Sandborn[25], cyclosporine has been
used extensively in uncontrolled trials in both Crohn's disease and ulcerative
colitis. The number of patients studied ranged from one to 32, the dose from 1 to
15 mg/kg body weight per day and the duration of therapy from 2 to 56 weeks.
Overall, the impression of rapid clinical response within 1–3 weeks prevailed in
the majority of patients and studies, but many patients relapsed rapidly after discontinuation of treatment[25]. Our own early encouraging results on fistulation[26]
are in agreement with several other trials reporting on a rapid closure of fistulas
in Crohn's disease[25] but, again, the success often was not maintained. Of particular interest is the intravenous route which excludes problems arising in some
patients because of inconsistent or poor absorption in those with rapid intestinal
transit[27].

The first fully reported controlled trial on cyclosporine A was that of
Brynskov et al. in active chronic Crohn's disease[28]. Following a 3-month study
period 59% of cyclosporine-treated patients, but only 32% of placebo patients,
showed improvement ($p = 0.032$). The effect became evident after 2 weeks.
However, during the subsequent 3 months, when the drug was gradually withdrawn, the proportion of patients with improvement dropped to 38%[28] and the
benefit was essentially lost after 1 year[29]. The study was criticized because
response was measured by a somewhat subjective grading score rather than the
standard Crohn's disease activity index. Unfortunately, none of the following
three large controlled trials[30–32] confirmed these findings. Therefore it seems that
there is little long-term benefit of oral cyclosporine even if the medication is
continued for a full year or more.

In ulcerative colitis a small controlled trial supports use of intravenous
cyclosporine in severe, fulminant disease[33]. It appears from the experience in

Table 3 Cyclosporine A: controlled trials

	Dose (mg/kg per day)	Duration (months)	n	Response Plac/CyA
Crohn's disease				
Chronic active disease				
Brynskov et al.[28]	5–7.5 (oral)	3	71	32/59 ($p = 0.032$)
Feagan et al.[30]	5–15	18	305	48/40
Jewell et al.[31]	5	3	147	43/36
Stange et al.[32]	5	12	182	20/20
Ulcerative colitis				
Severe disease				
Lichtiger et al.[33]	4 (intravenous)	Variable	20	0/82 ($p < 0.001$)

Plac: placebo; CyA: cyclosporine A.

several centres that this aggressive therapy indeed may avert colectomy in approximately 40–50% of the patients[34,35]. Although it is difficult to predict outcome, such simple data as stool frequency and C-reactive proteins may be helpful[35]. However, cyclosporine should not be overused simply to postpone and possibly delay an unavoidable operation. It is critically important in this situation to integrate both the internist and the surgeon in decision finding. Side-effects are frequent but rarely serious[25,32]. Paraesthesias (30%) and hypertrichosis (14%) are common, followed by tremor, hyertension and nausea. Renal insufficiency may occur (7%) but is usually reversible. Taken together, the data support the use of cyclosporine in very severe disease as a last resort, particularly in fistulating Crohn's disease and severe ulcerative colitis. However, patient monitoring has to be very close, indicating that the drug should be given only in centres with particular experience in its prudent use.

Possibly newer drug developments such as tacrolimus (FK506) may further improve therapeutic options[36]. This drug is well absorbed, more potent than cyclosporine A and, at least in the transplant field, is associated with less infections. In our hands, using 1–2 weeks of intravenous therapy followed by a switch to the oral route, nine out of 11 patients responded. In contrast to cyclosporine, it also seems possible to maintain remission during the oral phase. It should be emphasized that this represents only preliminary and uncontrolled experience, and needs to be confirmed by formal controlled trials. Most importantly, the caveat holds that the potential benefit of all immunosuppressive agents should be considered in the light of known, and possibly unknown, untoward effects of these aggressive and often long-term treatments. Particularly in the case of chronic active ulcerative colitis many patients may prefer to have a definite operation such as a colectomy with ileoanal pouch.

References

1. Podolski DK. Inflammatory bowel disease (first of two parts). N Engl J Med. 1991;324:928–37.
2. Rhodes J, Beck P, Bainton D, Campbell H. Controlled trial of azathioprine in Crohn's disease. Lancet. 1971;2:1273–6.
3. Klein M, Binder HJ, Mitchell M, Aaronson R, Spiro H. Treatment of Crohn's disease with azathioprine: a controlled evaluation. Gastroenterology. 1974;66:916–22.
4. Willoughby JMT, Beckett J, Kumar P, Dawson AM. Controlled trial of azathioprine in Crohn's disease. Lancet. 1971;2:944–6.
5. Summers RW, Switz DM, Sessions JT *et al.* National Cooperative Crohn's Disease Study: results of drug treatment. Gastroenterology. 1979;77:847–69.
6. Present DH, Korelitz BI, Wisch N, Glass JL, Sachar DB, Pasternack BS. Treatment of Crohn's disease with 6-mercaptopurine. A long-term, randomized, double-blind study. N Engl J Med. 1980;302:981–7.
7. Ewe K, Press AG, Singe CC *et al.* Azathioprine combined with prednisolone or monotherapy with prednisolone in active Crohn's disease. Gastroenterology. 1993;105:367–72.
8. Candy S, Wright J, Gerber M *et al.* A controlled double blind study of azathioprine in the management of Crohn's disease. Gut. 1995;37:674–8.
9. Rosenberg JL, Levin B, Wall AJ, Kirsner JB. A controlled trial of azathioprine in Crohn's disease. Am J Dig Dis. 1975;20:721–6.
10. O'Donoghue DP, Dawson AM, Powell-Tuck J, Bown RL, Lennard-Jones JL. Double-blind withdrawal trial of azathioprine as maintenance treatment for Crohn's disease. Lancet. 1978;2:955–7.
11. O'Brien JJ, Bayless TM, Bayless JA. Use of azathioprine or 6-mercaptopurine in the treatment of Crohn's disease. Gastroenterology. 1991;101:39–46.
12. Pearson DC, May GR, Fick GH, Sutherland LR. Azathioprine and 6-mercaptopurine in Crohn's disease. A meta-analysis. Ann Intern Med. 1995;2:132–42.

13. Sandborn WJ, Van OEC, Zins BJ *et al*. An intravenous loading dose of azathioprine decreases the time to response in patients with Crohn's disease. Gastroenterology. 1995;109:1806–17.
14. Bouhnik Y, Lémann M, Mary JY *et al*. Long-term follow-up of patients with Crohn's disease treated with azathioprine or 6-mercaptopurine. Lancet. 1996;27:215–19.
15. Caprilli R, Carratu R, Babbini M. A double-blind comparison of the effectiveness of azathioprine and sulphasalazine in idiopathic proctocolitis. Am J Dig Dis. 1975;20:115–20.
16. Jewell DP, Truelove SC. Azathioprine in ulcerative colitis: final report on a controlled therapeutic trial. Br Med. J. 1974;4:627–30.
17. Kirk AP, Lennard-Jones JE. Controlled trial of azathioprine in chronic ulcerative colitis. Br Med J. 1982;284:1291–2.
18. Rosenberg JL, Wall AJ, Levin B, Binder HJ, Kirsner JB. A controlled trial of azathioprine in the management of chronic ulcerative colitis. Gastroenterology. 1975;69:96–9.
19. Hawthorne AB, Logan RFA, Hawkey CJ *et al*. Randomized controlled trial of azathioprine withdrawal in ulcerative colitis. Br Med J. 1992;305:20–2.
20. Present DH, Meltzer STJ, Krumholz MP, Wolke A, Korelitz BI. 6-Mercaptopurine in the management of inflammatory bowel disease: short- and long-term toxicity. Ann Intern Med. 1989;111:641–9.
21. Kozarek RA, Patterson DJ, Gelfand MD, Botoman VA, Ball TJ, Wilske KR. Methotrexate induces clinical and histologic remission in patients with refractory inflammatory bowel disease. Ann Intern Med. 1989;110:353- 6.
22. Feagan BG, Rochon J, Fedorak RN *et al*. Methotrexate for the treatment of Crohn's disease. N Engl J Med. 1995;2:292–7.
23. Lémann M, Chamiot-Prieur C, Mesnard B *et al*. Methotrexate for the treatment of refractory Crohn's disease. Aliment Pharmacol Ther. 1996;10:309–14.
24. Oren R, Arber N, Odes S *et al*. Methotrexate in chronic ulcerative colitis; a double-blind, randomized, Israeli multicenter trial. Gastroenterology. 1996;110:1416–21.
25. Tremaine WJ, Sandborn WJ. Cyclosporine treatment of inflammatory bowel disease. Mayo Clin Proc. 1992;67:981–90.
26. Stange EF, Fleig W, Rehklau E, Ditschuneit H. Ciclosporin A treatment in inflammatory bowel disease. Dig Dis Sci. 1089;34:1387–92.
27. Brynskov J. Cyclosporin for inflammatory bowel disease: mechanisms and possible actions. Scand J Gastroenterol. 1993;28.849–57.
28. Brynskov J, Freund L, Rasmussen SN *et al*. A placebo-controlled, double-blind, randomized trial of cyclosporine therapy in active chronic Crohn's disease. N Engl J Med. 1989;321:845–50.
29. Brynskov J, Freund L, Norby R *et al*. Final report on a placebo-controlled, double-blind, randomized, multicentre trial of cyclosporin treatment in active chronic Crohn's disease. Scand J Gastroenterol. 1991;26:689–95.
30. Feagan BG, McDonald JWD, Rochon J *et al*. For the Canadian Crohn's relapse prevention trial investigators. Low-dose cyclosporine for the treatment of Crohn's disease. N Engl J Med. 1994;330:1846–51.
31. Jewell DP, Lennard-Jones JE and the Cyclosporin Study Group of Great Britain and Ireland. Oral cyclosporin for chronic active Crohn's disease: a multicentre controlled trial. Eur J Gastroenterol Hepatol. 1994;6:499–505.
32. Stange EF, Modigliani R, Peña A, Wood AJ, Feutren PD, Smith PR and the European Study Group. European trial of ciclosporin in chronic active Crohn's disease: A 12 month study. Gastroenterology. 1995;107:774–82.
33. Lichtiger S, Present D, Kornbluth A *et al*. Cyclosporin in severe ulcerative colitis refractory to steroid therapy. N Engl J Med. 1994;330:1841–5.
34. Carbonnel F, Boruchowicz A, Duclos B *et al*. Intravenous cyclosporine in attacks of ulcerative colitis. Dig Dis Sci. 1996;41:2471–6.
35. Travis SPL, Farrant JM, Ricketts C *et al*. Predicting outcome in severe ulcerative colitis. Gut. 1996;38:905–10.
36. Fellermann K, Ludwig D, Stahl M, David-Walek T, Stange EF. Steroid-unresponsive acute attacks of inflammatory bowel disease: immunomodulation by tacrolimus. Am J Gastroenterol. 1998;93:1860–6.

35
Monoclonal antibodies and interleukins

J. EMMRICH and S. LIEBE

INTRODUCTION

Immunological reactions and immunoregulatory abnormalities play a central role in the pathogenesis of inflammatory bowel diseases[1-5]. Different initial factors induce local mucosal inflammatory reactions which can be down-regulated in normal individuals. These inflammatory reactions are followed by tissue repair and healing. In patients with chronic inflammatory bowel diseases the mucosal immune system is activated showing an over-reaction directed against micro-organisms and other luminal antigens. Therefore, the local inflammation cannot be down-regulated. This mucosal inflammation is mediated mainly by immunocompetent cells and cytokines. Cytokines are small proteins mediating interactions among cells in a paracrine fashion. They interact in complex cascades in which production of one cytokine can influence target cells to produce other cytokines or to reduce cytokine production, which in turn triggers yet other cytokines. Standard medical therapy for inflammatory bowel disease uses drugs with a variety of anti-inflammatory effects and poorly defined targets. Advances in the understanding of the mechanisms of mucosal inflammation have provided a means for the development of specific immunomodulatory treatment[6]. Interactions of leukocytes and inflammatory mediators as targets of immunomodulatory therapies are shown in Figure 1. T-cell activation, interactions between antigen-presenting cells and CD4 T cells, cytokine expression, leukocyte recruitment, and cell injury are different levels of the immune reaction[4-6]. The aim of our therapy is to modulate this immune reaction using monoclonal antibodies and cytokines.

MONOCLONAL ANTIBODIES AGAINST T CELLS

There is increasing evidence for activation of mucosal T cells indicated by the expanded mucosal T-cell population, elevated expression of activation markers on the surface of mucosal T cells, increased cytotoxic T-cell function, and

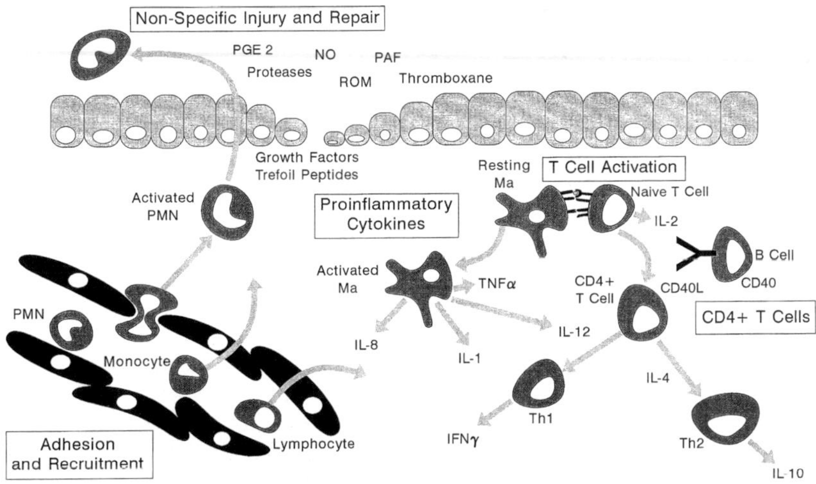

Figure 1 Targets of immunomodulatory therapy (modified from Reference 6)

increased production of cytokines[1–5]. Recent studies using a variety of animal models of inflammatory bowel disease have also shown an important role for CD4+ T cells in the pathogenesis of chronic intestinal inflammation[7]. There are different strategies to treat patients with inflammatory bowel diseases using T-cell-directed therapies: T-cell apheresis, blocking of T-cell activation, inhibition of CD4, immunomodulatory cytokines and blocking of costimulatory signals, arc the principal approaches to decrease inflammatory activity by influencing T cells[6].

Beneficial therapeutic effects of monoclonal antibodies directed against CD4 surface molecules have been demonstrated in clinical trials of autoimmune diseases[8–10] . However, there were differences in the clinical efficacy using different anti-CD4 antibody preparations. In human pilot studies, three antibodies have been administered to patients with therapy-refractory inflammatory bowel diseases, including the monoclonal mouse antibodies, MAX16H5 and B5, as well as the chimeric antibody cM-T412.

Six patients with Crohn's disease and four patients with ulcerative colitis were treated in an open-label fashion using cM-T412[11]. All patients achieved clinical as well as endoscopic remission with a mean duration of 11 months in Crohn's disease and 12 months in ulcerative colitis. However, application of this antibody resulted in a marked depletion of CD4+ T cells. The antibody cM-T412 was used in another study as a daily infusion of 10 mg, 30 mg or 100 mg for a week to treat three groups of four patients with active therapy-resistant Crohn's disease[12]. The authors reported a moderate potential efficacy of the antibody cM-T412, indicated by a mean reduction in Crohn's disease activity index (CDAI)[13] of 25%, 24% and 36%, respectively, in the three groups of patients at 4 weeks, and 24% and 52% at 10 weeks in the 30-mg and 100-mg groups. CD4+ cell counts were reduced to nearly 25% of baseline.

Twelve patients with severe refractory Crohn's disease were treated in an open-label clinical trial using intravenous application of the murine monoclonal antibody B-F5[14]. Eight patients received 0.5 mg kg^{-1} day^{-1} for 7 consecutive days. Four patients were treated with 0.5 mg kg^{-1} on the first day and 1 mg kg^{-1} day^{-1} for the next 6 days. CD4+ T cell numbers were not affected by this treatment. Only two patients experienced clinical improvement and two other patients responded with partial improvement. The authors concluded that this antibody was not successful in treating inflammatory bowel disease.

In an open-label clinical trial, we treated 7 patients with ulcerative colitis and 5 patients with Crohn's disease using the monoclonal mouse IgG$_1$ antibody MAX16H5[15,16]. The antibody was infused daily at a concentration of 0.3 mg/kg for 7 days. Four of the treated patients received a second therapy cycle 4 weeks later in the same manner. Clinical response was evaluated using the CDAI for patients with Crohn's disease and the clinical activity index CAI[17] for patients with ulcerative colitis. We were able to induce remission of the disease in ten of the twelve treated patients with chronic active inflammatory bowel disease. All four patients treated with a second therapy cycle achieved remission for 5–15 months which was longer than in patients treated with a single therapy cycle. Clinical remission was also indicated by decreased CRP levels. CD4+ T cells were reduced only immediately after antibody infusion followed by nearly normal values after the therapy cycle. The other lymphocyte subpopulations were not affected by this antibody.

We can conclude that anti-CD4 antibody treatment using antibody MAX16H5 induced reduction of disease activity as well as decreased laboratory parameters in patients refractory to conventional treatment regimens. Additional controlled studies with prolonged or repeated courses of antibody therapy or in combination with immunosuppressive drugs should be considered.

CYTOKINES

Interleukin-10

The cytokine interleukin-10 is produced by T cells, B cells and monocytes. IL-10 inhibits a wide variety of leukocyte functions, including the production of inflammatory cytokines and the expression of co-stimulatory molecules[18,19]. A phase I trial of recombinant human IL-10 in patients with chronic active Crohn's disease was the first application of this cytokine in the treatment of human disease[20]. This study was a multicentre randomized double-blind, placebo-controlled trial which tested different dose levels of IL-10 from 0.5 μg/kg to 25 μg/kg per day. Patients with a CDAI between 200 and 350 were given a once-daily intravenous bolus dose over 7 consecutive days. Results showed that IL-10 was safe and well tolerated. Patients in all groups receiving IL-10 had a 50% rate of remission during the study compared with 23% in the placebo group (Figure 2). Patients with remission after interleukin-10 therapy seemed to maintain the response through the 4 weeks. However, in a subsequent larger study of patients with chronic active Crohn's disease, the use of IL-10 has not been as successful[21]. There appears to be a small group of Crohn's disease patients who responded to IL-10 but this represents only about 30%. This difference may be

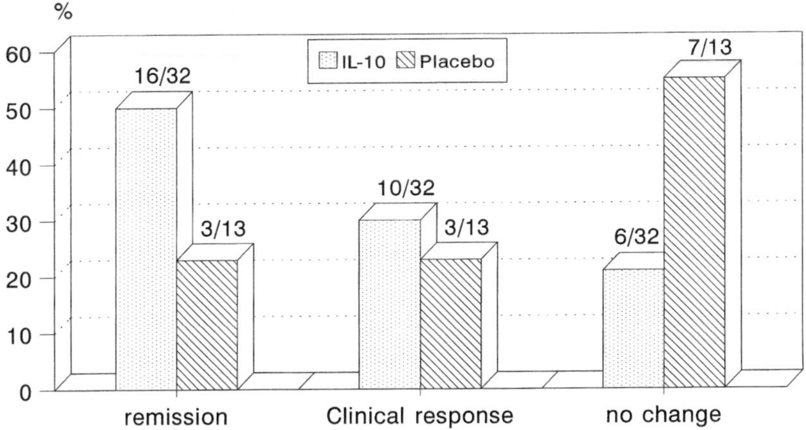

Figure 2 Results of IL-10 application in patients with Crohn's disease[20]

related to the differences in inflammation patterns that exist in the responding patients in comparison with those who did not.

Interleukin-11

In animal models, beneficial effects of the multifunctional cytokine interleukin-11 have been shown[22]. It was reported that IL-11 accelerates recovery of the intestine after injury. In a controlled multicentre trial, patients with active Crohn's disease were treated either twice or five times per week for 3 weeks at 5, 16 and 40 μg/kg of rhIL-11[23]. At the 16 μg/kg dose, 33–41% of patients went into remission. In the placebo group, only 7.6% of patients had a remission.

Anti-TNF-α antibody

The immunomodulatory therapy best explored up to the present is anti-TNF-α treatment. The cytokine TNF-α is produced mainly by macrophages and has multiple effects, including activation of macrophages, neutrophils and lymphocytes. It could be shown that TNF-α is one of the earliest cytokines produced in the inflammatory cascade, activating the production of other cytokines such as IL-1β, IL-6, and IL-8[24]. Therefore, inhibition of TNF-α should reduce the production of those other cytokines. Clinical trials using antibodies against TNF-α have already been shown to be effective in the treatment of patients with rheumatoid arthritis[25].

First, the anti-TNF-α antibody cA2 was used to treat patients with inflammatory bowel disease. An open-label trial of this humanized chimeric antibody resulted in remission of steroid-unresponsive Crohn's disease in 8 of 10 patients after one infusion, with no side-effects[26]. In this study, the average duration of response after a single infusion was 4 months. A 12-week double-blind placebo-controlled trial studied 108 patients with moderate to severe refractory Crohn's disease of least 6 months duration, with CDAI scores between 220 and 400[27]. All patients received a single 2-h intravenous infusion of placebo or cA2 at

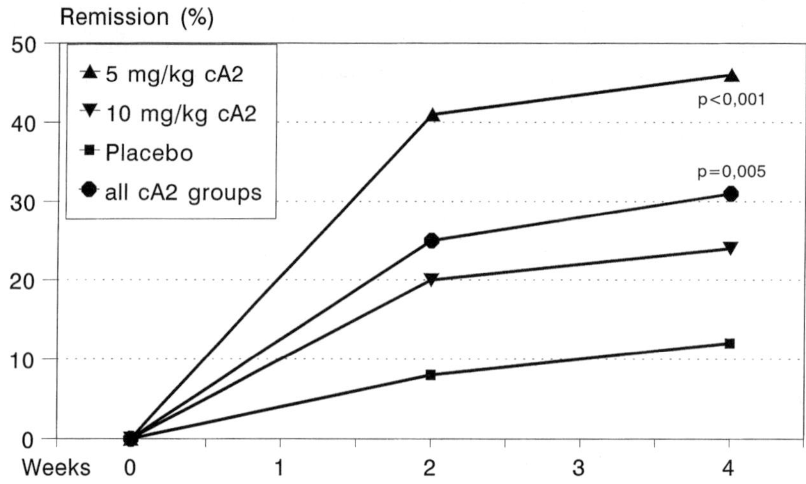

Figure 3 Results of anti-TNF-α antibody therapy in Crohn's disease[27]

doses of 5, 10 or 20 mg/kg (Figure 3). At 4 weeks, there was a significant clinical response in 81% of the patients who received the 5-mg/kg dose (22 of 27), 50% of those who received the 10-mg/kg dose (14 of 28) and 64% of those who received the 20-mg/kg dose (18 of 28), when compared with placebo. The effect of antibody therapy was sustained at 12 weeks. There were similar side-effects in cA2 and placebo groups. Anti-TNF-α antibodies reduced mucosal cell infiltrates producing inflammatory mediators[28] and induced mucosal healing[29].

However, four cases of lymphoma have been reported after treatment with cA2 (one in a patient with Crohn's disease, two in patients with rheumatoid arthritis, and one in a patient with AIDS)[30]. It is not known whether they are attributable to the inhibition of TNF-α or to the underlying disease. Therefore, the long-term benefits and risks of cA2 therapy need further investigation.

A second humanized monoclonal antibody (CDP571) has also been tested in patients with Crohn's disease[31]. This IgG$_4$ humanized chimeric monoclonal antibody was given in a double-blind placebo-controlled study to patients with mild-to-moderate active disease. Twenty-one patients received CDP571 and 10 received placebo. The median CDAI fell significantly at 2 weeks in the antibody-treated patients but not in the placebo group. Six of the 21 patients treated with the antibody achieved remission, whereas none of the placebo patients did. However, there was no difference between antibody-infused and placebo patients at 4, 6 or 8 weeks.

OTHER IMMUNOMODULATORY PRINCIPLES

New data suggest that interleukin-12 may be involved in mediating the immune response in inflammatory bowel disease. Blocking of IL-12 may be a promising way of controlling the mucosal inflammatory process.

In inflammatory bowel disease, several adhesion molecules, such as ICAM-1, are expressed followed by leukocyte infiltration in the mucosa. Preliminary data are available for the application of ICAM-1 antisense oligonucleotide[32] to inhibit the expression of this adhesion molecule at RNA level. Results of larger trials are awaited at present.

Cytokine genes can be specifically targeted using specific carriers, including liposomes, adeno- and retroviral vectors. These approaches are now being tested in animal models[33]. Instead of targeting cytokines directly, it is possible to interfere with the signal transduction proteins regulating cytokine production. Agents that specifically target these proteins are currently being developed.

SUMMARY

Taken together, we can say that molecules of the immune system are beginning to be used to treat human diseases. T cells and cytokines are targets for immunomodulatory therapy because they mediate disease manifestations and tissue injury. Many of our current therapies probably work by inhibition of immunocompetent cells and cytokines. However, our current agents are non-specific in their effects. Targeted therapy is now possible with specific monoclonal antibodies as well as cytokines. Anti-TNF-α monoclonal antibodies effectively down-regulated inflammation in steroid-refractory Crohn's disease in a multicentre trial, and remissions in patients who responded to treatment could be maintained by repeated administration of the antibody. The preliminary results with other immunomodulatory agents also appear promising. These agents not only represent important new therapeutic principles for patients suffering from inflammatory bowel diseases, but should give us new insights into the pathogenesis of the disease.

References

1. Zeitz M. Immunoregulatory abnormalities in inflammatory bowel disease. Eur J Gastroenterol Hepatol. 1990;2:246–50.
2. Podolsky DK. Inflammatory bowel disease. N Engl J Med. 1991;325:928–37.
3. Sartor RB. Cytokines in intestinal inflammation: Pathophysiological and clinical considerations. Gastroenterology. 1994;106:533–9.
4. Elson CO, McCabe RP. The immunology of inflammatory bowel disease: In: Kirsner JB, Shorter RG, editors. Inflammatory Bowel Disease. Baltimore: Williams & Wilkins; 1995:203–51.
5. Powrie F. T cells in inflammatory bowel disease: protective and pathogenetic roles. Immunity. 1995;3:171–4.
6. Sands BE. Biologic therapy for inflammatory bowel disease. Inflam Bowel Dis. 1997;3:95–113.
7. Strober W, Ehrhardt RO. Chronic intestinal inflammation: an unexpected outcome in cytokine or T cell receptor mutant-mice. Cell. 1993;75:203–5.
8. Emmrich F, Schulze-Koops H, Burmester G. Anti-CD4 and other antibodies to cell surface antigens for therapy. In: Davies ME, Dingle JT, editors. Immunopharmacology of Joints and Connective Tissue. London: Academic Press; 1994:87–117.
9. Horneff G, Burmester G, Emmrich F, Kalden JR. Treatment of rheumatoid arthritis with an anti-CD4 monoclonal antibody. Arthritis Rheum. 1991;34:129–40.
10. Olive D, Mawas C. Therapeutic applications of anti-CD4 antibodies. Crit Rev Ther Drug Carrier Sys. 1993;10:29–63.
11. Deusch K, Manthe B, Reiter C, Riethmüller G, Classen M. CD4-antibody treatment of inflammatory bowel disease: One year follow up. Gastroenterology. 1993;104:A691.

12. Stronkhorst A, Radema S, Yong SL, *et al*. CD4 antibody treatment in patients with active Crohn's disease: a phase I dose finding study. Gut. 1997,40:320–7.
13. Best WR, Becktel JM, Singleton JW, Kern F. Development of a Crohn's disease activity index. Gastroenterology. 1976;70:439–44.
14. Canva-Delcambre V, Jacquot S, Robinet E, *et al*. Treatment of severe Crohns disease with anti-CD4 monoclonal antibody. Aliment Pharmacol Ther. 1996;10:721–7.
15. Emmrich J, Seyfarth M, Fleig WE, Emmrich F. Treatment of inflammatory bowel disease with anti-CD4 monoclonal antibody. Lancet. 1991;338:570–1.
16. Emmrich J, Seyfarth M, Liebe S, Emmrich F. Anti-CD4 antibody treatment in inflammatory bowel disease without a long CD4+-cell depletion. Gastroenterology. 1995;108:A815.
17. Rachmilewitz D. Coated mesalazine (5-aminosalicylic acid) versus sulphasalazine in the treatment of active ulcerative colitis: A randomized trial. Br Med J. 1989;298:82–6.
18. Moore KW, O'Garra A, de Waal Malefyt R, *et al*. Interleukin-10. Annu Rev Immunol. 1993;11:165–90.
19. de Vries JE. Immunosuppressive and anti-inflammatory properties of interleukin-10. Ann Med. 1995;27:537–41.
20. van Deventer SJ, Elson CO, Fedorak RN and the Crohn´s Disease Study Group. Multiple doses of intravenous interleukin-10 in steroid-refractory Crohn's disease. Gastroenterology. 1997;113:383–9.
21. Schreiber S, Fedorak RN, Nielsen OH, *et al*. A safety and efficacy study of recombinant human interleukin-10 (rhuIL-10) treatment in 329 patients with chronic active Crohn's disease. Gastroenterology. 1998;114:A1080.
22. Qiu BS, Pfeiffer CJ, Keith JC. Protection by recombinant human interleukin-11 against experimental TNB-induced colitis in rats. Dig Dis Sci. 1996;41:1625–30.
23. Bank S, Sninsky C, Robinson M, *et al*. Safety and activity evaluation of rhIL-11 in subjects with active Crohn's disease. Gastroenterology. 1997;112:A927.
24. Maini RN, Elliott M, Brennan FM, *et al*. Targeting TNFα for the therapy of rheumatoid arthritis. Clin Exp Rheumatol. 1994;12(Suppl. 11):S63–6.
25. Elliott M, Maini RN, Feldmann M, *et al*. Randomized double-blind comparison of chimeric monoclonal antibody to tumor necrosis factor alpha (cA2) versus placebo in rheumatoid arthritis. Lancet. 1994;344:1105–10.
26. van Dullemen HM, van Deventer SJ, Hommes DW, *et al*. Treatment of Crohn's disease with anti-tumor necrosis factor chimeric monoclonal antibody (cA2). Gastroenterology. 1995;109:129–35.
27. Targan SR, Hanauer SB, van Deventer SJ, *et al*. A short-term study of chimeric monoclonal antibody cA2 to tumor necrosis factor alpha for Crohn's disease. N Engl J Med. 1997;337:1029–35.
28. Baert F, D'Haens G, Geboes K, *et al*. TNFα antibody therapy causes a fast and dramatic decrease of histologic colonic inflammation in Crohn's disease but not in ulcerative colitis. Gastroenterology. 1996;110:A859.
29. D'Haens GR, van Deventer SJH, van Hogezand R, *et al*. Anti-TNFα monoclonal antibody (cA2) produces endoscopic healing in patients with treatment-resistant, active Crohn's disease. Gastroenterology. 1998;114:A964.
30. Bickston SJ, Cominelli F. Treatment of Crohn's disease at the turn of the century. N Engl J Med. 1998;339:401–2.
31. Stack WA, Mann SD, Roy AJ, *et al*. Randomised controlled trial of CDP571 antibody to tumor necrosis factor-α in Crohn's disease. Lancet. 1997;349:521–4.
32. Yacyshin B, Woloschuk B, Yacyshyn MB, *et al*. Efficacy and safety of ISIS 2302 (ICAM-1 antisense oligonucleotide) treatment of steroid-dependent Crohn's disease. Gastroenterology. 1997;112:A1123.
33. Hogaboam CM, Vallance BA, Kumar A, *et al*. Therapeutic effects of interleukin-4 gene transfer in experimental inflammatory bowel disease. J Clin Invest. 1997;100:2766–76.

36
Antibiotic therapy in Crohn's disease

C. PRANTERA, M. L. SCRIBANO, G. FALASCO and
F. ZANNONI

Crohn's disease (CD) is a chronic inflammatory bowel disease of uncertain origin, which is usually treated with anti-inflammatory drugs, steroids and/or immunosuppressive agents. Many gastroenterologists use antibiotics in their clinical practice to improve symptoms and to induce remission of active CD phases.

RATIONALE FOR ANTIBIOTIC THERAPY IN CROHN'S DISEASE

- CD lesions are usually located on upstrain valves where the flow of bowel content slows down[1] and bacteria may overgrow.
- The diversion of faecal stream usually heals CD lesions[2].
  In operated patients, CD post-surgical recurrence does not appear in the pre-anastomotic ileum if a terminal ileostomy is performed proximal to the ileocolonic anastomosis; CD lesions usually reappear in the neoterminal ileum after the closure of the ileostomy[3].
- In the jejunum, 'fistulizing CD' is less frequent than in the terminal ileum and in the colon where the bacteria concentration is higher[4].
- Antibiotics are used successfully in the treatment of perianal fistulae and in the management of entero-enteric and entero-cutaneous fistulae[5,6].
- Some mycobacterial diseases, such as intestinal tuberculosis and Johne's disease of ruminants, show pathological aspects similar to those of CD[7].
- Some chronic intestinal diseases characterized by diarrhoea, such as Whipple's disease and tropical sprue, are successfully treated with antibiotics.

Rather than a specific bacterium being the aetiological agent of CD, it seems that commensal bacteria with their products may amplify and perpetuate the inflammatory activity, although the primary mechanism of CD lesions is still unknown.

INFECTIVE CAUSE OF CROHN'S DISEASE: SUPPORTING DATA

Results of epidemiological studies from France and England seem to point to an infective factor being one of the possible causes of CD[8,9]. *Mycobacterium*

"

paratuberculosis has been the most investigated infectious agent, mainly because of certain results collected over the last fifteen years[10,11], and also because it is the cause of Johne's disease in ruminants. However, an equal number of proofs argue against the supposition that CD is caused by *Mycobacterium paratuberculosis* or other mycobacterial species[12,13]. Thus, the hypothesis that mycobacteria are responsible for CD has not so far been adequately proved.

THE ROLE OF INTESTINAL MICROFLORA

As in the case of an infected wound, the intestinal flora might perpetuate intestinal inflammation by colonizing the initial bowel lesion induced by an unknown aetiological agent which has broken through the epithelial barrier. A recent study has demonstrated that an increased intestinal permeability may cause the absorption of bacteria and toxic bacterial products from the lumen[14]. In fact, an increased intestinal permeability predicted relapse of symptoms in 76% of 72 CD patients followed-up for one year[14]. Moreover, bacterial overgrowth over the lesions accounts for bacterial penetration of the bowel wall. Several different factors could justify bacterial overgrowth in CD bowel, such as faecal stasis, bowel wall lesions impairing gut motility, intestinal narrowing and strictures. Elevated antibody levels directed against the normal intestinal bacteria such as *E. coli*, *Bacterioides* and other species, have been found in the serum of CD patients; this could support the hypothesis of intraluminal bacteria translocation across the intestinal wall[15]. Furthermore, various products from the gut flora have inflammatory properties and might have an impact on the local immune system. In conclusion, there seems to be substantial evidence that intestinal microflora and bacterial products amplify and perpetuate the inflammatory response of CD[16], and are responsible for the frequently found septic state of these patients.

ANTIMYCOBACTERIAL THERAPY

Different antibiotics active against mycobacteria, in single or multiple regimen, have been used in CD. Anecdotal reports have reported positive results in treating CD patients with different antimycobacterial drugs. Open and controlled trials have given contrasting results. The trials of Shaffer *et al.*[17] and Swift *et al.*[18] which employed classic antitubercular therapy obtained completely negative results, whereas a trial employing clarithromycin reported positive results[19]. In between these two results, two trials from Ireland and Italy demonstrated a certain efficacy of clofazimine alone vs. placebo[20], and of a combination of rifampicin, ethambutol, clofazimine and dapsone in acute-phase CD[21].

The heterogeneity of CD, as well as the differences in the drugs used, the length of treatment and the evaluation of results, make any conclusion impossible.

ANTIBIOTIC THERAPY IN CROHN'S DISEASE

Although antibiotics do not have a definite role as a primary therapy of CD, they are usually employed in the treatment of CD complications, such as abscesses and toxic state, in order to reduce bacterial overgrowth in the bowel lumen, and to improve abdominal symptoms, such as diarrhoea, pain and meteorism. Nevertheless, the results are sometimes conflicting.

Metronidazole

Metronidazole is the antibiotic most frequently employed for CD treatment. This imidazole compound is particularly active against parasites and most anaerobic bacteria, and its use is now widely accepted in perianal CD therapy. In a randomized crossover trial from Sweden, the Cooperative CD Study, metronidazole was compared with sulphasalazine; both the drugs were equally effective but only when the colon was involved. It is interesting to note that metronidazole was effective in patients who failed on sulphasalazine, but the reverse was not observed[22]. In a randomized trial from Birmingham, metronidazole alone or in combination with co-trimoxazole, had little therapeutic value in active CD[23]. In a double-blind placebo-controlled trial from Canada, remission rates at 16 weeks were 36% with 10 mg kg^{-1} day^{-1} of metronidazole and 27% with double dosage[24]. This is similar to previous results[22] and this trial also confirmed that metronidazole seems to be more effective when the colon is involved. These studies suggest that metronidazole is efficacious in Crohn's colitis and ileocolitis but not in small bowel disease. In the trial from Birmingham, the small number of patients with colitis who were included in the 'metronidazole arm' could be the reason for the negative results[23]. Recently, a trial of metronidazole vs. placebo for recurrence prevention of Crohn's ileitis after operation was performed[25]; the antibiotic, started on the seventh day after surgery for a 3-month period, decreased the severity of early endoscopic recurrent lesions in the neoterminal ileum and also seemed to delay clinical recurrence at one year follow-up.

Side-effects

Metronidazole is usually well tolerated, even at a dosage of 1.5 g/day. The side-effects rate varies between 10 and 20% according to the dosage and duration of treatment. The most frequent adverse events are gastrointestinal intolerance, neurotoxicity and metallic taste. Peripheral neuropathy occurs in 50–85% of long-term metronidazole-treated patients[5].

Ciprofloxacin

Ciprofloxacin is a quinolone derivative with a selective suppressive effect on the intestinal microflora. *Escherichia coli* and aerobic Enterobacteriaceae are especially sensitive to this antibiotic which, by contrast, does not particularly affect *Bacterioides* and *Clostridium* spp.

Ciprofloxacin has been reported to be effective in the long-term treatment of ten cases of active perianal CD[6] and in four cases of Crohn's ileitis[26]. Two open studies on ciprofloxacin and metronidazole in the treatment of active CD have been performed recently. In the first, from Italy, 52% of patients with active refractory CD reached complete remission (CDAI<150), 19% had no clinical remission, and 13% withdrew because of side-effects[27]; more than 65% of patients with Crohn's colitis had a positive clinical response. The second study, from Canada, was a retrospective analysis of 72 patients, 29 of whom were concurrently receiving steroids[28]; in the non-steroid group, 67% of patients had a clinical response.

Three controlled trials on ciprofloxacin in active CD have been published. The first double-blind placebo-controlled study enrolled 89 patients concomitantly treated with steroids and metronidazole who were randomized to be treated with placebo or ciprofloxacin[29]. Eleven patients on ciprofloxacin and 12 of the control group did not achieve clinical and endoscopic remission. The high rate of success normally achieved with steroids does not allow for a reliable evaluation of drug efficacy. The second study was a randomized controlled trial on the efficacy and safety of 12 weeks' treatment with metronidazole plus ciprofloxacin vs. systemic steroids in 41 patients with active CD[30]. According to the CDAI, 10 of 22 antibiotics patients (45%) and 12 of 19 steroids patients (63%) reached clinical remission by the end of the study. The best results in terms of efficacy and side-effects were observed at six weeks. Six patients on antibiotics (27%) and two on steroids (11%) were withdrawn because of side-effects. The authors concluded that, despite the higher incidence of side-effects, this antibiotic combination could represent an alternative to steroids in the treatment of acute CD. The third trial, published as an abstract, showed that ciprofloxacin is as effective as mesalazine in treating mild to moderate CD flare-up[31].

The efficacy of combination therapy with metronidazole and ciprofloxacin in active CD has been confirmed in a recent retrospective analysis of 233 patients treated between 1984 and 1996. In this study, clinical remission was obtained in 54% of patients treated with two antibiotics for a period of 12 weeks. Metronidazole and ciprofloxacin were found to be more efficacious in Crohn's colitis and ileocolitis, whereas ciprofloxacin alone seemed to be less effective in colitis; in the operated patients, all the antibiotics were particularly efficacious[32].

Side-effects

The side-effect rates are different in the few published studies. One trial from Italy reported a 59% incidence of adverse events related to the two antibiotics[30]. In another controlled study, a 16% incidence of side-effects was observed but patients had also received other concomitant drugs[29]. The rate of side-effects depends on the dosage and the duration of treatment. Most side-effects are of gastrointestinal origin, but skin reactions, not-infrequent increases of transaminase levels, a case of high serum amylase, and a possibly related case of transitory ischaemic attack have all been described[27].

CONCLUSIONS

Although the hypothesis that CD is caused by a single pathogenic bacterium is not substantiated, at the present time antibiotics are essential in the armamentarium of CD therapies. A combination of metronidazole with ciprofloxacin seems to be useful in treating the CD active phase as an alternative to or in combination with steroids. These antibiotics seem to be more efficacious in Crohn's colitis and ileocolitis. At the present time, treatment with 1 g/day of each of these two antibiotics for a period of 6–12 weeks appear to be advisable. Side-effects and bacterial resistance are of concern in their long-term use.

References

1. Rutgeerts P, Ghoos Y, Van Trappen G, *et al.* Ileal dysfunction and bacterial overgrowth in patients with Crohn's disease. Eur J Clin Invest. 1981;11:199–206.
2. Burman JH, Thompson H, Cooke WT, *et al.* The effects of diversion of intestinal contents on the progress of Crohn's disease of the large bowel. Gut. 1971;12:11–15.
3. Rutgeerts P, Geboes K, Peeters M, *et al.* Effect of faecal stream diversion on recurrence of Crohn's disease in the neoterminal ileum. Lancet. 1991;338:771–4.
4. Marion JF, Lachman P, Greenstein AJ, *et al.* Rarity of fistulas in Crohn's disease of the jejunum. Inflamm Bowel Dis. 1995;1:34–6.
5. Brandt LJ, Bernstein LH, Boley SS, *et al.* Metronidazole therapy for perianal Crohn's disease: a follow up study. Gastroenterology. 1982;83:383–7.
6. Turunen U, Farkkila M, Valtonen V, *et al.* Long-term outcome of ciprofloxacin treatment in severe perianal or fistulous Crohn's disease. Gastroenterology. 1993;104:A793.
7. Chiodini RJ, Van Kruiningen HJ, Merkal RS, *et al.* Ruminant paratuberculosis (Johne's disease): the current status and future prospects. Cornell Vet. 1984;74:218–62.
8. Van Kruiningen HJ, Colombel JF, Cartun RW, *et al.* An in-depth study of Crohn's disease in two French families. Gastroenterology. 1993;104:351–60.
9. Allan RN, Pease P, Ibbotson JP. Clustering of Crohn's disease in a Cotswold village. Q J Med. 1986;59:473–8.
10. Chiodini RJ, Van Kruiningen HJ, Merkal RS, *et al.* Characteristics of an unclassified Mycobacterium species isolated from patients with Crohn's disease. J Clin Microbiol. 1984;20:966–71.
11. Thayer WR, Coutu JA, Chiodini RJ, *et al.* Possible role of mycobacteria in inflammatory bowel disease. II. Mycobacterial antibodies in Crohn's disease. Dig Dis Sci. 1984;29:1080–5.
12. Graham DY, Markesich DC, Yoshimura HH. Mycobacteria and inflammatory bowel disease. Results of culture. Gastroenterology. 1987;92:436–42.
13. Stainsby KL, Lowes JR, Allan RN, *et al.* Antibodies to Mycobacterium paratuberculosis and nine species of environmental mycobacteria in Crohn's disease and control subjects. Gut. 1993;34:371–4.
14. Wyatt J, Vogelsang H, Hubl W, *et al.* Intestinal permeability and the prediction of relapse in Crohn's disease. Lancet. 1993;341:1437–9.
15. Macpherson A, Khoo UY, Forgacs I, *et al.* Mucosal antibodies in inflammatory bowel disease are directed against intestinal bacteria. Gut. 1996;38:365–75.
16. Beeken WL, Kanich RE. Microbial flora of the upper small bowel in Crohn's disease. Gastroenterology. 1973;65:390–7.
17. Shaffer JL, Hughes S, Linaker BD, *et al.* Controlled trial of rifampicin and ethambutol in Crohn's disease. Gut. 1984;25:203–5.
18. Swift GL, Srivastava ED, Stone R, *et al.* Controlled trial of anti-tuberculous chemotherapy for two years in Crohn's disease. Gut. 1994;35:363–8.
19. Graham DY, Al-Assi MT, Robinson M. Prolonged remission in Crohn's disease following therapy for Mycobacterium paratuberculosis. Gastroenterology. 1995;108:A826.
20. Afdhal NH, Long A, Lennon J, *et al.* Controlled trial of antimycobacterial therapy in Crohn's disease. Clofazimine versus placebo. Dig Dis Sci. 1991;36:449–53.
21. Prantera C, Kohn A, Mangiarotti R, *et al.* Antimycobacterial therapy in Crohn's disease: results of a controlled, double-blind trial with a multiple antibiotic regimen. Am J Gastroenterol. 1994;89:513–18.
22. Ursing B, Alm T, Barany F, *et al.* A comparative study of metronidazole and sulfasalazine for active Crohn's disease: the Cooperative Crohn's Disease Study in Sweden. II. Result. Gastroenterology. 1982;83:550–62.
23. Ambrose NS, Allan RN, Keighley NW, *et al.* Antibiotic therapy for treatment in relapse of intestinal Crohn's disease: a prospective randomized study. Dis Colon Rectum. 1985;28:81–3.
24. Sutherland L, Singleton J, Sessions J, *et al.* Double blind, placebo controlled trial of metronidazole in Crohn's disease. Gut. 1991;32:1071–5.

25. Rutgeerts P, Hiele M, Geboes K, *et al.* Controlled trial of metronidazole treatment for prevention of Crohn's recurrence after ileal resection. Gastroenterology. 1995;108:1617–21.
26. Peppercorn MA. Is there a role for antibiotics as primary therapy in Crohn's ileitis? J Clin Gastroenterol. 1993;17:235–7.
27. Prantera C, Kohn A, Zannoni F, *et al.* Metronidazole plus ciprofloxacin in the treatment of active, refractory Crohn's disease: results of an open study. J Clin Gastroenterol. 1994;19(1):79–88.
28. Greenbloom SL, Steinhart AH, Greenwerg GR, *et al.* Ciprofloxacin and metronidazole: combination antibiotic therapy for ileocolonic Crohn's disease. Clin Invest Med. 1995;18(A):48.
29. Turunen U, Farkkila M, Hakala K, *et al.* Ciprofloxacin treatment combined with conventional therapy in Crohn's disease. A prospective, double blind, placebo controlled study. Gut. 1995;37(A):193.
30. Prantera C, Zannoni F, Scribano ML, *et al.* An antibiotic regimen for the treatment of active Crohn's disease: a randomized, controlled clinical trial of metronidazole plus ciprofloxacin. Am J Gastroenterol. 1996;91:328–32.
31. Colombel JF, Lemann M, Cassagnou M, *et al.* Ciprofloxacin vs mesalazine in the treatment of active Crohn's disease. Gut. 1996;39(suppl 3):A188.
32. Prantera C, Scribano ML, Berto E, Falasco G. Antibiotics in active Crohn's disease: a retrospective analysis of 233 patients treated with metronidazole and ciprofloxacin. Ital J Gastroenterol Hepatol. 1998;(in press).

37
Alternative therapeutic approaches in IBD

C. FOLWACZNY

INTRODUCTION

Conventional therapy for patients with inflammatory bowel disease (IBD) comprises treatment with corticosteroids, sulphasalazine, 5-aminosalicylic acid (5-ASA) compounds and various immunosuppressive agents. However, despite remarkable progress in the treatment of active disease, or in the maintenance of remission, during the past 50 years, conventional forms of therapy are still far from being satisfactory. Thus, similar to other chronic diseases, physicians have always searched for new and alternative forms of treatment. The aims of these attempts were to offer additional treatment options for patients who do not respond to standard therapy, to provide therapeutic alternatives with fewer side-effects and to gain new insights in the pathophysiology of IBD. In Table 1 the different treatment forms are listed.

NICOTINE

The association between cigarette smoking and a more favourable clinical course in ulcerative colitis remains the sole epidemiological feature that distinguishes it

Table 1   Alternative therapeutic approaches for IBD

Allopurinol*	Factor XIII
Boswellia serrata gum resin	Fish oil
Butyrate*	Heparin
Chloroquine	Nicotine
Clonidine	Short-chain fatty acids*
Cromoglycate*	Superoxide dismutase*
Dexpanthenol*	Ridogrel*
Escherichia coli Nissle	Xylocain*

* Denotes topical therapy.

from Crohn's disease[1]. Smokers are less likely to have ulcerative colitis, smoking may ameliorate its clinical manifestations, and the onset of colitis is often associated with the cessation of smoking. In contrast, there is a well-documented association between cigarette smoking and a less favourable clinical course in Crohn's disease[2].

The potential effects of smoking on the gastrointestinal tract include alterations in colonic mucus composition and in cellular and humoral immunity[2]. Moreover, increased intestinal permeability after cigarette smoking was reported[2]. Nicotine may be the mediator of these effects. It has favourable consequences on the balance of eicosanoid production, as it leads to inhibition of thromboxane synthase, cyclooxygenase and lipoxygenase[2]. Furthermore, nicotine stimulates the production of mucus in the colon[2].

In 1994 Pullan and co-workers evaluated the effect of transdermal nicotine patches on various parameters in 35 patients with ulcerative colitis and compared it with 37 patients who were receiving a placebo preparation over a duration of 6 weeks[3]. The dose of nicotine was adjusted to the tolerance of side-effects. The mean dose in the nicotine group was 17 ± 6 mg/day. (The average smoker absorbs about 1 mg of nicotine per cigarette smoked.) In addition, all patients had been taking mesalamine and 12 patients were receiving low-dose glucocorticosteroids. These medications were not changed during the study period. The clinical symptom score and the histological score improved significantly, whereas the change in the endoscopic score fell short of significance. Moreover, the authors reported complete resolution of symptoms in 17 of 35 patients in the nicotine group compared to nine out of 37 patients in the placebo group. However, the authors did not state the proportion of patients with an endoscopic or histological remission. This, and the fact that the study population was heterogeneous with respect to former smoking status, concurrent medication and the final dose of nicotine, justifies the conclusion that this paper does not provide convincing evidence in support of a biological effect of nicotine in the therapy of ulcerative colitis. It did, however, stimulate further studies.

In a subsequent study, by Sandborn and colleagues from the Mayo Clinic[4], patients were stratified on the basis of smoking history, extent of the disease, and concomitant medical therapy. After stratification a total of 64 patients were randomly assigned to daily treatment with transdermal nicotine or placebo. In this trial the daily nicotine dose was comparable to the dose used by Pullan and co-workers. In the nicotine group a significant improvement in the clinical disease activity index score was observed, whereas this was not the case in the placebo group. However, the rate of complete clinical remission in the nicotine group, which reached 6%, did not differ significantly from the rate which had been achieved in the placebo group. Thus, from these data it was concluded that transdermal nicotine, if administered together with conventional therapy, is capable of reducing clinical activity, but is not useful to induce remission.

Based on these studies, Thomas and colleagues investigated the effects of transdermal nicotine as maintenance therapy for ulcerative colitis[5]. In this 6-month trial the maximum dose of nicotine per day was 15 mg and, therefore, was lower than in the previous studies. Once the maximum dose which was tolerated by the patient was reached, the mesalamine preparations which had been administered before study entry were stopped. The relapse rate was defined by use of clinical, sigmoidoscopic and histological assessment. Between the two groups there were no significant differences concerning the number of relapses. Furthermore, as in the previous trials the number of patients with side-effects resulting in early withdrawal from the study was remarkably high in the nicotine group. Twenty-one out of 40 patients who had been treated with nicotine experienced side-effects such as nausea, light-headedness and itching.

In summary, nicotine appears to impair inflammatory activity in active ulcerative colitis, albeit the transdermal application did not induce remission. On the other hand, this treatment form is certainly not an option to maintain remission in ulcerative colitis. Furthermore, side-effects occur frequently when using nicotine patches. Hence, it appears unlikely that the transdermal application of nicotine will be a widely accepted alternative for the therapy of patients with ulcerative colitis.

FISH OIL

Omega-fatty acids are long-chain polyunsaturated fatty acids with a double bond between carbon atom 3 and 4 proximal to the methyl end of the fatty acid[6]. Species of this lipid class that naturally occur in appreciable amounts are eicosapentaenoic acid, docosahexaenoic acid and α-linolenic acid[6]. Of these eicosapentaenoic and docosahexaenoic acid are present at 10–100-fold higher concentrations in lipid sources of marine as compared to terrestrial origin[6]. Some common inflammatory pathways have been postulated for Crohn's disease and ulcerative colitis. Omega-3 fatty acids compete in the substrate pool of the lipoxygenase pathway, and thus reduce the production of inflammatory leukotrienes[6]. In mononuclear cells omega-3 fatty acids have also been shown to suppress effectively the synthesis of other inflammatory cytokines such as interleukin-1α and β and tumour necrosis factor[7-9]. Moreover, several studies have demonstrated a protective effect of eicosapentaenoic acid in rat models of colitis[6].

In 1989 Lorenz and co-workers evaluated the effect of dietary supplementation with fish oil, which provided 3.2 g omega-3 fatty acids per day in a 7-month placebo-controlled crossover trial, which comprised 29 patients with active Crohn's disease and 10 patients with active ulcerative colitis[10]. Twenty patients were receiving conventional therapy, which was kept constant during the study period. In patients with Crohn's disease clinical activity remained unchanged. In patients with ulcerative colitis clinical disease activity fell during fish oil supplementation and thereafter. However, the reduction in disease activity was not significant.

In a second placebo-controlled trial, which evaluated the effect of 4.2 g of omega-3 fatty acids on disease activity in 11 patients with active ulcerative colitis, a significant decrease of the disease activity index during the 8-month study period could be demonstrated[11]. In an additional study, by Hawthorne and colleagues[12], a trend towards faster achievement of remission was observed, albeit this difference was not significant. Lastly, during a 4 month dietary supplementation with fish oil, Stenson and co-workers[13] reported significant reductions in rectal dialysate leukotriene B_4 levels, improvements in histological findings and a significant weight gain. However, stool frequency did not change significantly.

Loeschke and co-workers evaluated the effect of 5.1 g of fish oil per day on the prevention of relapse in a placebo-controlled trial, involving 64 patients with ulcerative colitis, who did not use any corticosteroids[14]. In addition, 5-ASA compounds were stopped 3 months after randomization. Clinical disease activity was monitored over a period of 2 years. Actuarial relapse rate was improved by omega-3 fatty acids only during months 2 and 3, but cumulative relapse-free survival after 2 years was not significantly different in the placebo and the fish oil group.

In Table 2 the studies which evaluated the effect of fish oil therapy in patients with ulcerative colitis are listed. By summarizing these data it appears possible that fish oil supplementation might exert some beneficial short-term effects on active disease and on the maintenance of remission. However, the results of these trials certainly do not justify the general use of fish oil instead of 5-ASA compounds or sulphasalazine.

In a widely recognized study an Italian group was able to demonstrate the effectiveness of a novel enteric-coated fish oil preparation in the reduction of the relapse rate in 78 patients with Crohn's disease in remission during a 1-year placebo-controlled trial[15]. Following the author's statement this new enteric-coated preparation resulted in a higher rate of absorption of fish oil. Hence, the dose needed to achieve effective incorporation of fish oil in the phospholipid membranes was one-third of that used in previous studies. As a result the incidence of side-effects of the fish oil capsules (such as eructation with fishy odour) was expected to be lower. In this trial patients were receiving 2.7 g of omega-3 fatty acids per day. After 1 year 23 patients in the fish oil group remained in remission, as compared to 10 patients in the placebo group.

However, in an even larger multicentre trial from Germany, conducted by Lorenz-Meyer and co-workers[16], in which a conventional fish-oil preparation was used, these promising results could not be confirmed. After remission was attained by corticosteroid therapy during an 8-week period patients were receiving 5 g of omega-3 fatty acids per day over 1 year. The proportions of patients without relapse within 1 year were quite similar in the placebo and fish oil group.

Table 3 summarizes the trials which evaluated the effect of fish oil therapy in Crohn's disease. From the present findings it seems unlikely that fish oil treat-

Table 2 Trials which evaluated the effect of fish oil in ulcerative colitis

Reference	Year	Placebo-controlled	Dose	Duration	Effective
Active disease:					
Lorenz et al.[10]	1989	Yes	3.2 g	7 months	No
Aslan et al.[11]	1992	Yes	4.2 g	8 months	Yes
Hawthorne et al.[12]	1992	Yes	4.5 g	1 year	?
Stenson et al.[13]	1992	Yes	3.2 g	9 months	?
Maintenance of remission					
Loeschke et al.[14]	1996	Yes	5.1 g	1 year	No

Table 3 Trials which evaluated the effect of fish oil in Crohn's disease

Reference	Year	Placebo-controlled	Dose	Duration	Effective
Active disease					
Lorenz et al.[10]	1989	Yes	3.2 g	7 months	No
Maintenance of remission					
Belluzzi et al.[15]	1996	Yes	2.7 g	1 year	Yes
Lorenz-Meyer et al.[16]	1996	Yes	5 g	1 year	No

ment is justified in patients with active Crohn's disease. Furthermore, the data by Lorenz Meyer *et al.* argue strongly against the use of fish oil in order to maintain remission in patients with Crohn's disease. In the study by Belluzzi and colleagues the relapse rate in the placebo group was remarkably high. Studying patients in whom the rate of spontaneous relapse is high obviously facilitates the assessment of strategies for the maintenance of remission. Thus, it is possible that in this study fish oil acted by treating low-grade active inflammation, rather than by preventing reinitiation of the disease from a truly quiescent state. However, these data should be confirmed in subsequent trials.

SHORT-CHAIN FATTY ACIDS

The group of 'short-chain fatty acids' comprises mainly acetate, propionate and butyrate[17]. Short-chain fatty acids arise in the colon as end-products of bacterial carbohydrate fermentation[17,18]. They constitute important luminal fuels for colonocytes, in particular in the distal segments of the large bowel[17,19,20]. In diversion colitis a lack of luminal nutrients may lead to mucosal atrophy in the excluded segment and consecutively to inflammation[21]. In ulcerative colitis experimental data suggest an impaired utilization of short-chain fatty acids by colonocytes[22]. Based on these considerations short-chain fatty acids were administered topically in patients with distal ulcerative colitis[20,23].

In a placebo-controlled trial, Steinhart and co-workers investigated the effect of nightly-administered butyrate enemas in 38 patients with distal ulcerative colitis[24]. Clinical improvement was noted in 37% of butyrate-treated patients and in 47% of the placebo group. Moreover, clinical remission was achieved in three patients in each group. From these data an effect of butyrate enemas on distal ulcerative colitis could obviously not be concluded.

However, in the majority of studies a combination of short-chain fatty acids was used, as initially described by Harig and co-workers in patients with diversion colitis in 1989[21]. In an open-labelled trial Patz *et al.* evaluated the effects of short-chain fatty acid enemas, which were administered twice daily in 10 patients with ulcerative colitis, who had failed to respond to conventional oral therapy[25]. The authors demonstrated a significant decrease in the degree of bleeding after the 6-week study period. They also observed a significant improvement of endoscopic but not histological appearance. In five patients a clinical response was observed and in four patients remission was obtained.

Table 4 Trials which evaluated the effect of topical butyrate monotherapy in ulcerative colitis

Author/Reference	Year	Placebo-controlled	Effective
Scheppach et al.[20]	1992	Yes	Yes
Steinhart et al.[24]	1996	Yes	No
Scheppach et al.[26]	1996	Yes	No

Scheppach and co-workers compared the effect of short-chain fatty acids with butyrate monotherapy or placebo[26]. The study population comprised 47 patients with ulcerative colitis. The enemas were instilled twice daily. The disease activity index, which was chosen as the major endpoint after 8 weeks, decreased significantly in all three groups. The same was observed concerning histological and endoscopic scores. Hence there was no significant difference compared to the placebo group.

Table 4 summarizes the present studies which evaluated the effect of butyrate in ulcerative colitis. Due to the conflicting nature of these data the previous studies do not demonstrate consistent effectiveness of this treatment form. However, with regard to the well-documented safety and tolerability of this topical therapy, its use seems justified in patients with otherwise refractory distal colitis.

HEPARIN

Various epidemiological and clinical observations suggest a link between IBD and a disorder of coagulation. The increased risk of thromboembolic complications in patients with ulcerative colitis and Crohn's disease is well recognized[27]. In 1989 Wakefield and co-workers demonstrated occlusive fibrinoid lesions of arteries in the muscularis propria, compatible with multifocal gastrointestinal ischaemia[28]. A British group evaluated a reduced incidence of IBD in patients with haemophilia or von Willebrand Jürgens syndrome[29]. This observation suggests that the arteriolar lesions observed by Wakefield and co-workers are probably not just the consequence of an inflammatory process.

In 1994 Gaffney and his group presented a series of 10 patients with ulcerative colitis, who had successfully been treated with unfractioned heparin[30]. The same group had already reported three case reports about this effect in patients with ulcerative colitis in 1991[31]. In the larger series, from 1994, stool frequency, rectal bleeding and histology improved significantly under treatment with unfractioned heparin.

Stimulated by these promising results we used unfractioned heparin in 1995 for the first time. The first to receive this treatment were two female patients aged 18 and 21, who did not respond to high-dose corticosteroid treatment over a period of several weeks. In both patients we did achieve remission within 2 weeks. These experiences then resulted in the initiation of a prospective study. For this study patients with ulcerative colitis and Crohn's disease who did not respond to conventional high-dose corticosteroid treatment over a period of more than 4 weeks, or patients who refused to take corticosteroids, were eligible after they had given written and informed consent. Patients had to be older than 18 years, a surgical intervention should not be planned and osteopenia had to be ruled out by radiological measurement of bone density before study entry. The latter was required because long-term treatment with heparin can lead to bone demineralization. During the first 2 weeks patients received unfractioned heparin intravenously as a continuous infusion, aiming at a partial thromboplastin time above 60 s. In the following 6 weeks patients injected 12 500 units of heparin twice daily. According to the reports by Gaffney and co-workers the patients also received sulphasalazine in a standard dose during the study period. Corticosteroids were tapered when possible. A clinical and laboratory assessment was performed weekly during the first month of treatment, and thereafter patients were seen every other week.

So far 11 patients with ulcerative colitis and five patients with Crohn's disease have been enrolled in this pilot study. Two patients with ulcerative colitis had to be excluded due to osteopenia or because consent was withdrawn after the first week of treatment. In one patient with Crohn's disease a bowel perforation occurred after the initial endoscopy. The Colitis Activity Index showed a significant decrease during the study period in the remaining nine patients with ulcerative colitis (14.5 ± 1.1 vs 6.3 ± 1.9 points; $p = 0.0108$). This decrease was paralleled by a significant decline in the values for C-reactive protein (CRP) and erythrocyte sedimentation rate (ESR) (35 ± 9 vs 12 ± 5 mg/dl; $p = 0.0177$; 47 ± 11 vs 16 ± 6 mm/h; $p = 0.0357$). Moreover, the mean daily prednisolone dose could also be reduced significantly. In contrast to these findings we were not able to observe significant changes in the Crohn's Disease Activity Index (CDAI) (345 ± 31 vs 248 ± 44 points; $p = 0.729$) or CRP values (29 ± 13 vs 26 ± 14 mg/dl; $p = 0.0833$) and ESR values (37 ± 10 vs 37 ± 9 mm/h; $p = 0.1859$) in our patients with Crohn's disease.

In one male patient with ulcerative colitis we observed a dramatic increase in rectal bleeding at day 11 of the study, requiring several blood transfusions. Heparin therapy was interrupted immediately and the patients was admitted to the intensive-care unit. However, after a period of 12 h the stool frequency showed a remarkable decrease from 15 to three stools per day and rectal bleeding stopped quite suddenly. After a thorough discussion of the situation with the patient we continued the heparin treatment after 3 days and the patient later did well. Other observations we made include the improvement of arthralgia in two patients with Crohn's disease and a slight, reversible increase of alanine transaminase (ALT) activity in four patients with ulcerative colitis during the study.

Five out of nine patients with ulcerative colitis attained complete remission during treatment with heparin, whereas in none of the four patients with Crohn's disease did the CDAI drop below 150 points. Hence, from our limited experience we can conclude that heparin appears to be beneficial in patients with ulcerative colitis but not in patients with Crohn's disease. The latter finding contrasts with preliminary data from other groups, which showed efficacy also in Crohn's disease. However, our data were obtained in a prospective, albeit not placebo-controlled, randomized study. Moreover, four patients with ulcerative colitis did not attain remission, although in these patients the CDAI showed a mean decrease of five points. Hence, larger placebo-controlled series will be required to answer whether the positive effects of heparin therapy, which were observed in several pilot trials, will be preserved in placebo-controlled trials. Furthermore, future investigation should aim at defining possible predictors for response to therapy with heparin. Lastly, heparin might have a role as an adjunctive therapeutic agent in IBD.

If a beneficial effect of heparin, at least in patients with ulcerative colitis, is postulated, it remains to be elucidated how this effect is mediated. The thromboembolic complications and hypercoagulable state which associate flares of IBD suggest that heparin may produce a benefit by treating microthrombi in the intestinal circulation. However, recent research indicates that a broader endothelial dysfunction in regulation and coagulation, inflammation and vascular repair may be important events in the pathogenesis of these diseases. Heparin, with its well-known diverse immunomodulating effects, may be an ideal agent to reverse these defects. Hence, we investigated the possible effects of heparin on systemic values of L-selectin, an important mediator of leukocyte migration; tumour necrosis factor alpha (TNF-α), a proinflammatory cytokine of paramount importance; and on the values of TNF-binding proteins I and II, which act as anti-inflammatory proteins, in five patients with ulcerative colitis[32]. However, TNF-α and L-selectin concentrations did not change significantly during the 8-week study period; furthermore, TNF-binding proteins even decreased (Table 5). Thus, from these findings we cannot conclude that the anti-inflammatory effects of heparin contribute to the observed clinical effects.

ESCHERISCHIA COLI NISSLE

From various *in-vivo* data, obtained from animal and human studies, it has been hypothesized that the intestinal environment plays a significant role in the aetiology of IBD[33]. Large numbers of pathogenically adhesive and enterohaemorrhagic *E. coli* have been reported in ulcerative colitis[34]. The presence of these pathogenic strains is reciprocally related to the number of non-pathogenic *E. coli* bacteria[35]. Thus, therapeutic colonization with non-pathogenic *E. coli* may be beneficial in IBD.

Kruis and co-workers compared the effect of an oral *E. coli* preparation (*E. coli* Nissle) versus mesalazine in maintaining remission in ulcerative colitis[36].

Table 5 Laboratory values at study entry and after 8 weeks of treatment with unfractioned heparin in five patients with ulcerative colitis. Data are given as mean ± one standard error of mean.

	Week		
	0	*8*	*p-Value*
CRP (mg/dl)	6.1 ± 2.2	0.7 ± 0.3	0.021
L-selectin (mg/ml)	0.75 ± 0.08	0.99 ± 0.14	0.225
TNF-α (pg/ml)	33.2 ± 4.8	27.0 ± 3.2	0.819
TNF-BP-1 (ng/ml)	3.2 ± 0.6	2.0 ± 0.3	0.009
TNF-BP-ll (ng/ml)	6.3 ± 0.9	4.6 ± 0.9	0.074

Fifty patients received *E. coli* Nissle and 53 patients were treated with mesalazine over a period of 12 weeks. There were no significant differences between the two treatment modalities with regard to mean time until first relapse and mean relapse-free time. At the end of the study the histological findings in the two study groups did not reveal any significant differences, whereas the endoscopic appearance was slightly better in the mesalazine group.

Recently, Malchow demonstrated a shorter time before onset of remission in patients with active colonic Crohn's disease, if patients who were treated after a standard prednisolone protocol, with an initial dose of 60 mg prednisolone per day, additionally received *E. coli* Nissle as compared to patients who received prednisolone and placebo[37]. However, the rate of remission was even higher in the placebo group. In the same article Malchow further reported on a remarkable difference in the relapse rate of patients with Crohn's disease over a 12-month period. The patients had been treated with an oral *E. coli* formulation or placebo. The difference was observed, regardless of whether the patients additionally received prednisolone treatment or not.

BOSWELLIC ACIDS

Treatment with boswellic acids comprises a new approach which is currently being tested in various inflammatory conditions. The gum resin of *Boswellia serrata* acts as a specific non-redox inhibitor of leukotriene synthesis via the inhibition of 5-lipoxygenase[38,39]. In a pilot study by an Indish group 34 patients with active ulcerative colitis were administered *Boswellia serrata* gum resin over 6 weeks[40]. This treatment was compared with sulphasalazine therapy. According to the authors the rates of remission were identical in the two study groups.

CONCLUSION

In summary, for the majority of alternative therapeutic approaches the promising results of open-label trials could not be confirmed in subsequent controlled clinical investigations. Because of this, and the fact that 90% of patients presenting with IBD can be brought into remission with conventional therapy, the indication for alternative treatment options has to be considered carefully. However, in patients who do not respond to conventional therapy some of the treatment regimens discussed above may offer an alternative. If possible, these patients should be included in ongoing therapeutic trials.

References

1. Calkins BM. A meta-analysis of the role of smoking in inflammatory bowel disease. Dig Dis Sci. 1989;34:1841–54.
2. Osborn MJ, Stansby GP. Cigarette smoking and its relationship to inflammatory bowel disease: a review. J R Soc Med. 1992;85:214–16.
3. Pullan RD, Rhodes J, Ganesh S *et al.* Transdermal nicotine for ulcerative colitis. N Engl J Med. 1994,330.811–15.
4. Sandborn WJ, Tremaine WJ, Leighton JA *et al.* Nicotine tartrate liquid enemas for mildly to moderately active left-sided ulcerative colitis unresponsive to first-line therapy: a pilot study. Aliment Pharmacol Ther. 1997;11:663–7.

5. Thomas GAO, Rhodes J, Mani V *et al.* Transdermal nicotine as maintenance therapy for ulcerative colitis. N Engl J Med. 1995;332:988–92.
6. Endres S, De Caterina R, Schmidt EB, Kristensen SD. n-3 Polyunsaturated fatty acids: update 1995. Eur J Clin Invest. 1995;25:629–38.
7. Endres S, Sinha B, Eisenhut T. Omega 3 fatty acids in the regulation of cytokine synthesis. World Rev Nutr Diet. 1994;76:89–94.
8. Endres S, Meydani SN, Ghorbani R, Schindler R, Dinarello CA. Dietary supplementation with n-3 fatty acids suppresses interleukin-2 production and mononuclear cell proliferation. J Leukoc Biol. 1993;54:599–603.
9. Endres S, Eisenhut T, Sinha B. n-3 Polyunsaturated fatty acids in the regulation of human cytokine synthesis. Biochem Soc Trans. 1995;23:277–81.
10. Lorenz R, Weber PC, Szimnau P, Heldwein W, Strasser T, Loeschke K. Supplementation with n-3 fatty acids from fish oil in chronic inflammatory bowel disease – a randomized, placebo-controlled, double-blind cross-over trial. J Intern Med Suppl. 1989;225:225–32.
11. Aslan A, Triadafilopoulos G. Fish oil fatty acid supplementation in active ulcerative colitis: a double-blind, placebo-controlled, crossover study. Am J Gastroenterol. 1992;87:432–7.
12. Hawthorne AB, Daneshmend TK, Hawkey CJ *et al.* Treatment of ulcerative colitis with fish oil supplementation: a prospective 12 month randomised controlled trial. Gut. 1992;33:922–8.
13. Stenson WF, Cort D, Rodgers J *et al.* Dietary supplementation with fish oil in ulcerative colitis. Ann Intern Med. 1992;116:609–14.
14. Loeschke K, Ueberschaer B, Pietsch A *et al.* n-3 Fatty acids only delay early relapse of ulcerative colitis in remission. Dig Dis Sci. 1996;41:2087–94.
15. Belluzzi A, Brignola C, Campieri M, Pera A, Boschi S, Miglioli M. Effect of an enteric-coated fish-oil preparation on relapses in Crohn's disease. N Engl J Med. 1996;334:1557–60.
16. Lorenz-Meyer H, Bauer P, Nicolay C *et al.* Omega-3 fatty acids and low carbohydrate diet for maintenance of remission in Crohn's disease. A randomized controlled multicenter trial. Scand J Gastoenterol. 1996;31:778–85.
17. Scheppach W. Effects of short chain fatty acids on gut morphology and function. Gut. 1994;35:S35–8.
18. Cummings JH, MacFarlane GT. The control and consequences of bacterial fermentation in the colon. J Appl Bacteriol. 1991;70:443–59.
19. Roediger W. Metabolic basis of starvation diarrhoea: implications for treatment. Lancet. 1986;1:1082–4.
20. Scheppach W, Sommer H, Kirchner T *et al.* Effect of butyrate enemas on the colonic mucosa in distal ulcerative colitis. Gastroenterology. 1992;103:51–6.
21. Harig JM, Soergel KH, Komorowski RA, Wood CM. Treatment of diversion colitis with short-chain-fatty acid irrigation. N Engl J Med. 1989;320:23–8.
22. Roediger W. What sequence of pathogenic events leads to acute ulcerative colitis? Dis Colon Rectum. 1988;31:482–7.
23. Scheppach W, Christl SU, Bartram HP, Richter F, Kasper H. Effects of short-chain fatty acids on the inflamed colonic mucosa. Scand J Gastroenterol Suppl. 1997;222:53–7.
24. Steinhart AH, Hiruki T, Brzezinski A, Baker JP. Treatment of left-sided ulcerative colitis with butyrate enemas: a controlled trial. Aliment Pharmacol Ther. 1996;10:729–36.
25. Patz J, Jacobsohn WZ, Gottschalk Sabag S, Zeides S, Braverman DZ. Treatment of refractory distal ulcerative colitis with short chain fatty acid enemas. Am J Gastroenterol. 1996;91:731–4.
26. Scheppach W. Treatment of distal ulcerative colitis with short-chain fatty acid enemas. A placebo-controlled trial. German–Austrian SCFA Study Group. Dig Dis Sci. 1996;41:2254–9.
27. Folwaczny C, Fricke H, Spannagl M, Loeschke K. Heparin for therapy of ulcerative colitis: therapy of a concomitant phenomenon or indication of pathophysiology? Z Gastroenterol. 1995;33:723–4.
28. Wakefield AJ, Sawyerr AM, Dhillon AP *et al.* Pathogenesis of Crohn's disease: multifocal gastrointestinal infarction. Lancet. 1989;2:1057–62.
29. Thompson NP, Wakefield AJ, Pounder RE. Inherited disorders of coagulation appear to protect against inflammatory bowel disease. Gastroenterology. 1995;108:1011–15.
30. Gaffney PR, Doyle CT, Gaffney A, Hogan J, Hayes DP, Annis P. Paradoxical response to heparin in 10 patients with ulcerative colitis. Am J Gastroenterol. 1995;90:220–3.
31. Gaffney PR, O Leary JI, Doyle CT *et al.* Response to heparin in patients with ulcerative colitis. Lancet. 1991;337:238–9.

32. Folwaczny C, Fricke H, Endres S *et al.* Antiinflammatory properties of unfractioned heparin in patients with highly active ulcerative colitis: pilot study. Am J Gastroenterol. 1997;92:911–12.

33. Sartor RB. Current concepts of the aetiology and pathogenesis of Crohn's disease and ulcerative colitis. Gastroenterol Clin N Am. 1995;24:475–507.

34. Burke DA, Axon ATR. Ulcerative colitis and *E. coli* with adhesive properties. J Clin Pathol. 1987;40:782–6.

35. Sonnenborn U, Greinwald R. *Escherichia coli* im menschlichen Darm: nützlich, schädlich oder unbedeutend? Dtsch Med Wochenschr. 1990;115:906–12.

36. Kruis W, Schütz E, Fric B *et al.* Double-blind comparison of an oral *Escherichia coli* preparation and mesalazine in maintaining remission in ulcerative colitis. Aliment Pharmacol Ther. 1997;11:853–8.

37. Malchow HA. Crohn's disease and *Escherichia coli*. A new approach in therapy to maintain remission of colonic Crohn's disease? J Clin Gastroenterol. 1997;25:653–8.

38. Ammon HP, Mack T, Singh GB, Safayhi H. Inhibition of leukotriene B4 formation in rat peritoneal neutrophils by an ethanolic extract of the gum resin exudate of *Boswellia serrata*. Plant Med. 1991;57:203–7.

39. Ammon HP, Safayhi H, Mack T, Sabieraj J. Mechanism of antiinflammatory actions of curcumine and boswellic acids. J Ethnopharmacol. 1993;38:113–19.

40. Gupta I, Parihar A, Malhotra P *et al.* Effects of *Boswellia serrata* gum resin in patients with ulcerative colitis. Eur J Med Res. 1997;2:37–43.

38
Endoscopic therapy

W. KRUIS, C. POHL and M. BEHNKE

The introduction of endoscopy for the diagnosis of intestinal diseases was a landmark and endoscopy became the mainstay of diagnosis in inflammatory bowel disease (IBD). The development of endoscopic intervention techniques, among these polypectomy and haemostatic procedures, led to endoscopy being not only a diagnostic but also a therapeutic tool. Consequently, endoscopic intervention was also brought into focus in IBD.

ENDOSCOPIC TECHNIQUES USED FOR THE TREATMENT OF IBD

Table 1 depicts a list of interventional procedures reported for endoscopic treatment of patients with IBD. Most of these techniques are applied to patients with Crohn's disease (CD), while endoscopic therapy is used only infrequently in ulcerative colitis (UC). The data basis on which these methods are practised is relatively small. Many techniques are reported anecdotally or in small observational series, only a few are studied in a controlled fashion. Therefore, general

Table 1   List of interventional techniques for endoscopic therapy in IBD

	Technique	*Indication*
Crohn's Disease:		
	Balloon dilatation	Stenoses
	Stenting	Stenoses
	Percutaneous endoscopic gastrostomy	Nutrition
	Laser coagulation	Stenoses Bleeding
	Injection therapy	Bleeding Stenoses
	Fibrin sealing	Fistulae
Ulcerative Colitis:		
	Air suction/decompression	Megacolon

recommendations should be seen critically. By far the most experience exists in the endoscopic therapy of patients with CD and stenotic complications.

ENDOSCOPIC THERAPY IN CROHN'S DISEASE

Treatment of stenotic complications

With the introduction of the neodymium–YAG laser, therapeutic application of laser energy to the intestines became available. Soon, laser coagulation of haemorrhage and malignant stenosis emerged as routine methods. The successful reopening of a stenosis in a patient with CD was firstly reported by Sander *et al.* from Munich[1]. Though the same group expanded on this first experience[2], laser therapy is not commonly used in Crohn's stenoses as yet.

In contrast to laser therapy, balloon dilatation of Crohn's strictures is widely performed at present. Dilatation has been successfully applied to stenoses of the oesophagus[3], duodenum[4] and most often of the colon as well as of the ileocolonic junction. Table 2 summarizes results from the literature. Considering only larger series, success rates between 50% and 86% are reported. However, these numbers reflect short-term results only. In a recent prospective long-term analysis[15] the success rate dropped over time from 73% to 62%. Another restriction of balloon dilatation is that frequently the procedure has to be repeated until reopening of the

Table 2 Results of balloon dilatation in patients with Crohn's disease and strictures (modified according to ref. 13)

Reference	Patients (n)	Localization of stenosis	Success rate (%)	Complications (patients)
Alexander-Williams *et al.* 1986[5]	1	Duodenum	100	0
Bower, 1986[6]	1	Ileum	100	0
Kozarek, 1986[7]	3	Ileum/colon	33	0
Neufeld *et al.* 1987[8] Follow-up > 6 months	3	Ileum/colon	100	0
Kirtley *et al.* 1987[9]	1	Ileum	100	0
Dobson and Robertson, 1988[10]	1	Ileum/colon	0	0
Williams and Palmer, 1991[4] Follow-up > 6 months	7	Ileum/colon/ duodenum	71	0
Blomberg *et al.* 1992[11]	73	Ileum/colon	86	11
Breysen *et al.* 1992[12] Follow-up > 6 months	18	Ileum/colon	50	0
Junge and Züchner, 1994[13] Follow-up > 6 months	10	Ileum/colon	70	1
Mathis *et al.* 1994[3], Follow-up > 6 months, dilatation by Savary bougies	1	Oesophagus	100	0
Kelly and Hunter, 1995[14] Follow-up > 6 months	3	Duodenum	100	0
Couckuyt *et al.* 1995[15] Follow-up > 6 months	55	Ileum/colon	73	6

stricture occurs. Safety and complication rates of the procedure seem to be considerable but acceptable. The only prospective study[15] shows complications in 11% of the patients (all perforations) and no mortality which compares well to the numbers of the largest series[11], reporting complications in 15% of the patients.

Several attempts have been made to improve the long-term results of balloon dilatation. Two routes were followed: either combined local treatment or additive systemic therapy. Lavy from Haifa reported[16] a patient with a rectal stricture. After balloon dilatation they injected locally 40 mg of triamcinalone using a standard sclerotherapy needle. The patient stayed asymptomatic for a follow-up of 9 months. In a larger series of 13 patients a betamethasone preparation was applied locally[17]. It is stated that during the follow up period of 9 to 73 months all patients remained well and the authors concluded that a controlled study would be needed to confirm the results of this pilot study.

Another approach to maintaining open strictures after balloon dilatation was used by a group from Japan[18]. In two patients self-expanding metallic Z-stents (Gianturco Z-stent) were placed into dilated stenoses. In one patient the stent was discharged through the anus within one month. In the second patient after 5 months the stent migrated and was removed transanally. At control investigations more than one year after the stent implantation both patients showed a good passage through the formerly stenotic segments and both were free of symptoms. Our group also tried this approach in two patients using another type of stent (Endocoil). In one patient with a stenotic ileotransversostomy it was not possible to correctly place the stent. In a second patient with a stenosis and a fistula in the descending colon the stent could be placed correctly. Within one month the stent was spontaneously discharged. The passage stayed open but the fistula also remained open.

Recently, the results of balloon dilatation in combination with subsequent systemic therapy were reported[19]. After successful endoscopic therapy 30 patients with ileocolonic stenoses received either placebo or azathioprine 100 mg/day and budesonide 9 mg/day. After 6 months and 12 months the placebo group had significantly more symptoms associated with stenoses than verum patients. The rate of surgical interventions was significantly lower in the patient groups with azathioprine/budesonide than under placebo.

Treatment of fistulae

Formation of fistulae is a common problem in CD and, as yet, no ideal treatment exists. To accomplish closure of a fistula by sealing seems to be an intriguing idea and promising results were reported of successful treatment procedures using fibrin glue. But most of these reports concern non-CD patients. Fibrin glue must be injected via catheters which can be directly guided or through an endoscope. Eimiller *et al.* described[20] successful sealing of anal, rectovaginal and vesicorectal fistulae in CD. In a small series of 10 patients with rectovaginal and complex fistulae overall success rate of autologous fibrin glue, measured by fistulae closure, was 69%[21]. However, among these 10 patients only 3 had CD. In these 3 patients, treatment failed in 2 and was successful in the third patient after repeated treatment procedures. Active CD was felt to be the reason for unsuccessful fibrin sealing of an ischiorectal abscess caused by a fistula[22]. In contrast, an oesophagomediastinal fistula was successfully closed with fibrin sealant[3], but there was a recurrence 18 months later. Our own experiences are limited to two cases: one with perianal fistulae and one with a fistula between the ileum and the abdominal wall. Fibrin sealing failed in both patients to close their fistulae.

From the results of these anecdotal reports fibrin sealing of fistulae in patients with CD seems not to be a promising therapeutic option and cannot be recommended.

Nutritional therapy via percutaneous endoscopic gastrostomy (PEG)

Enteral nutrition with defined diets is an important mode of treatment for CD, particularly in malnourished children. Patients only very rarely accept these diets for an extended time period when given by mouth. Therefore, nutritional therapy is generally applied by chronic nasogastric tubes. In 20 children with CD, prolonged use of PEG or nasogastric tubes for enteral hyperalimentation was investigated[23]. PEG was found to be safe and well tolerated.

In a recent study of 10 children with CD PEG was better accepted than a nasogastric tube and was associated with only minor complications[24].

Thus, in appropriate patients PEG may offer a valuable alternative route for nutritional therapy in CD.

Management of bleeding

Significant bleeding from a single or circumscribed source is a very rare event in IBD. Well established endoscopic interventional techniques such as injection therapy or laser coagulation, especially with argon beamers, may be able to effectively stop focal as well as diffuse bleeding also in IBD. To our knowledge (Medline, Knowledge Finder), there exists no published experience in this area.

ENDOSCOPIC THERAPY IN ULCERATIVE COLITIS

Gaseous distension of the bowel causes considerable discomfort to patients with UC, increases transmural pressure and may, thus, lead to megacolon and subsequent perforation. In intestinal diseases other than UC some small studies show successful colonoscopic decompression of a megacolon. Few anecdotal reports in UC[25-27] indicate that this procedure may be helpful also in the management of toxic megacolon. Though no complications of colonoscopic decompression are known from the literature, the method has potential risks in this regard. These must be balanced against the benefits and risks of the so-called rolling technique[28] which works without any intervention.

References

1. Sander R, Poesl H. Treatment of non-neoplastic stenoses with the neodymium–YAG laser – indications and limitations. Endoscopy 1986;18 (Suppl 1):53–56.
2. Sander R. Lasertherapie bei Crohnstenosen. In: Jenss H, editor. Morbus Crohn, Neue Therapieansätze, Behandlungen von Komplikationen. Stuttgart: Schattauer, 1990:132–136.

3. Mathis G, Sutterlütti G, Dirschmid K, Feuerstein M, Zimmermann G. Crohn's disease of the esophagus: Dilatation of stricture and fibrin sealing of fistulas. Endoscopy 1994;26:508.
4. Williams AJ, Palmer KR. Endoscopic balloon dilatation as a therapeutic option in the management of intestinal strictures resulting from Crohn's disease. Br J Surg 1991;78:453–454.
5. Alexander-Williams J, Allan A, Morel P, Rohner A, Haynes JG. The therapeutic dilatation of enteric strictures due to Crohn's disease. Ann Roy Coll Surg 1986;68:95–97.
6. Brower RA. Hydrostatic balloon-dilatation of a terminal ileum stricture secondary to Crohn's disease. Gastrointest Endosc 1986;32:38–41.
7. Kozarek RA. Hydrostatic balloon-dilatation of gastrointestinal stenoses. A national survey. Gastrointest Endosc 1986;32:15–19.
8. Neufeld DM, Shemesh EI, Kodner IJ, Shatz BA. Endoscopic management of anastomotic colon strictures with electrocautery and balloon dilatation. Gastrointest Endosc 1987;33:24–26.
9. Kirtley DW, Willis M, Thomas E. Balloon-dilatation of recurrent terminal ileal Crohn's strictures. Gastrointest Endosc 1987;33:399–400.
10. Dobson HM, Robertson DAR. Balloon catheter dilatation of an ileocolonic stricture. Clin Radiol. 1988;39:202–204.
11. Blomberg B. Endoscopic balloon-dilatation of strictures due to inflammatory bowel disease. Bildgebung 1992;19(Suppl):12.
12. Breysen Y, Janssens JF, Coremans G, Vantrappen G, Hendrickx G, Rutgeerts P. Endoscopic balloon-dilatation of colonic and ileo-colonic Crohn's strictures. Long-term results. Gastrointest Endosc 1992;38:142–147.
13. Junge U, Züchner H. Endoskopische Ballondilatation symptomatischer Strikturen bei Morbus Crohn. Dtsch Med Wschr 1994;119:1377–1382.
14. Kelly SM, Hunter JO. Endoscopic balloon dilatation of duodenal strictures in Crohn's disease. Postgrad Med J 1995;71:623–634.
15. Couckuyt H, Gevers AM, Coremans G, Hiele M, Rutgeerts P. Efficacy and safety of hydrostatic balloon dilatation of ileocolonic Crohn's strictures: a prospective longterm analysis. Gut 1995;36:577–580.
16. Lavy A. Steroid injection improves outcome in Crohn's disease strictures. Endoscopy 1994;26:366.
17. Ramboer C, Verhamme M, Dhondt E, Huys S, Van Eygen K, Vermeire L. Endoscopic treatment of stenosis in recurrent Crohn's disease with balloon dilatation combined with local corticosteroid injection. Gastrointest Endosc 1995;42:252–255.
18. Masuhashi N, Nakajima A, Suzuki A, Akanuma M, Yazaki Y, Takazoe M. Non-surgical stricture plasty for intestinal strictures in Crohn's disease: preliminary report of two cases. Gastrointest Endosc 1997;45:176–178.
19. Raedler A, Peters I, Schreiber S. Treatment with azathioprin and budesonide prevents reoccurrence of ileocolonic stenoses after endoscopic dilatation in Crohn's disease. Gastroenterology 1997;112:A1067.
20. Eimiller A, Zellmer R, Neuhaus H, Paul F. Fibrin sealing of fistulae in Crohn's disease. Z Gastroenterol 1987;25:450.
21. Abel ME, Chiu YSY, Russell TR, Volpe PA. Autologous fibrin glue in the treatment of rectovaginal and complex fistulas. Dis Colon Rectum 1993;36:447–449.
22. Lange V, Meyer G, Wenk H et al. Fistuloscopy – an adjuvant technique for sealing gastrointestinal fistulae. Surg Endosc 1990;4:212–216.
23. Israel DM, Hassal E. Prolonged use of gastrostomy for enteral hyperalimentation in children with Crohn's disease. Am J Gastroenterol 1995;90:1084–1088.
24. Cosgrove M, Jenkins HR. Experience of percutaneous gastrostomy in children with Crohn's disease. Arch Dis Child 1997;76:141–143.
25. Banez AV, Yamanishi F, Crans CA. Endoscopic colonic decompression of toxic megacolon, placement of colonic tube, and steroid colonclysis. Am J Gastroenterol 1987;82:692–694.
26. Riedler L, Wohlgenannt D, Stoss F, Thaler W, Schmid KW. Endoscopic decompression in 'toxic megacolon'. Surg Endosc 1989;3:51–53.
27. Hoashi T, Tsuda S, Yao T et al. A case of ulcerative colitis with toxic megacolon, successfully treated with colonoscopic decompression. Nippon Shokakibyo Gakkai Zasshi 1991;88:91–95.
28. Present DH, Wolfson D, Gelernt IM, Rubin PH, Bauer J, Chapman ML. Medical decompression of toxic megacolon by "rolling". A new technique of decompression with favorable long-term follow-up. J Clin Gastroenterol 1988;10:485–490.

39
Surgical therapy of Crohn's disease

U. T. HOPT and U. ADAM

INTRODUCTION

The cause of Crohn's disease is unknown. Neither medical nor surgical therapy is curative. Thus, the goal of any therapy in these patients must be to alleviate symptoms and to prevent or treat complications. There is general agreement that medical therapy should be employed initially. On the other hand, however, there is ample evidence that the majority of patients with Crohn's disease will eventually need surgical therapy. The probability of surgical resection being required at some time during the course of illness ranges from 88% to 96%, and the average number of resections per patient has been reported to be 2.4[1-3]. Thus, it is obvious that Crohn's disease is also a surgical disease. There is considerable controversy, however, regarding timing and indication for surgery. The concern for early recurrence and the potential for multiple small bowel resections with the risk of short bowel syndrome has led to the admonition by some physicians that surgery should be avoided unless it is absolutely necessary. On the other hand, however, undue delay of surgery may unnecessarily prolong the patient's disease state and increase the risk for secondary complications due to the well-known side-effects of medical treatment, e.g. bone and soft tissue damage, increased risk of sepsis or growth retardation in children due to use of corticosteroids. In addition, it is obvious that the postoperative complication rate will be much higher when the patient has to be operated urgently because of preoperative septic complications[4]. Thus, the challenge for all clinicians caring for these patients is to select the appropriate indication and timing of surgery.

INDICATIONS FOR SURGERY

When looking for indication for surgery in a large cohort of patients with Crohn's disease there are a series of indications which will not be questioned, such as small bowel obstruction, symptomatic fistulas, an inflammatory, therapy-resistant mass, septic problems such as abscesses or peritonitis and haemorrhage[5]. Interestingly enough the majority of patients, however, are operated on because of failure of medical therapy. This type of indication for operation is obviously somewhat subjective. Persistence, progression or frequent recurrence of severe symptoms, as well as severe side-effects, must be regarded as failures in medical therapy. Hulten, for example, emphasizes that reappearance or persistence of symptoms (weight loss, anaemia, abdominal pain and diarrhoea) after a 2–3-month course of intensive medical therapy renders a patient a candidate for surgery[4]. Nevertheless, the definition of such situations remains controversial. Therefore good communication and close cooperation between gastroenterologist and surgeon is of the utmost importance.

Recently Nissan *et al.* have raised the question of whether quality of life should be an indication for surgery[6]. Parameters were pain, frequency of bowel movements, nutritional status, response to medication, side-effects of medication, growth retardation, impairment of family and social life and impairment of career. Their results of 'minimal surgery' were excellent. Although these results have to be confirmed by others, Fischer stated in his editorial comment that, if Nissan *et al.* are correct, these findings might represent a major contribution to the treatment of patients who are unhappy having a disease for which surgeons classically deny them surgical therapy.

SURGICAL TECHNIQUE

Surgical strategy in patients with Crohn's disease depends on a series of criteria. Most important certainly is the location of the disease[7,8]. Furthermore, disease activity, performance status of the patient, presence or absence of local complications and urgency of operation need to be considered[9]. There are a variety of surgical options such as resection, strictureplasty, primary anastomosis, staged procedures and temporary or permanent stoma. The indication and surgical technique of these different procedures are widely accepted.

Surgical therapy of ileocolic disease consists in a conservative ileocaecal resection. In contrast to oncological patients no safety margins at the bowel and no lymphadenectomy are necessary. It has clearly been shown that the recurrence rate is unrelated to microscopic disease at the resection margin[10]. Thus the proximal and distal margins of resection need only be in grossly normal-appearing bowel. Although recurrence cannot be prevented, in more than two-thirds of patients no further surgical intervention is necessary. Three and more reoperations are necessary in less than 5%. Thus, ileocaecal resection is a relatively successful therapy in patients with Crohn's disease of the distal ileum[11]. It is interesting that in the majority of patients recurrent disease in the preanastomotic ileum is the indication for reoperation. The postanastomotic colon, or other sites in the colon or small bowel, are seldom affected. Therefore a second ileum resection or a right hemicolectomy are the procedures most often performed after primary ileocaecal resection.

While limited resection is the procedure of choice in patients with the disease confined to the distal ileum, in case of multicentric disease in the small bowel strictureplasty has emerged as the better alternative to multiple resections. Often both bowel resection and strictureplasty are used to deal with a dominant site of obstruction and additional skip areas of stricture[12]. The results of strictureplasty are excellent[13]. Recurrence of stenosis in an area of former strictureplasty rarely occurs. If the patient has to be operated because of recurrent stricture the stenotic area is usually distal or proximal of the site of former strictureplasty. In spite of these excellent results it has to be kept in mind, however, that resection is still by far the most frequent surgical procedure used in patients with Crohn's disease.

ABSCESSES

Abscesses are common in patients with Crohn's disease. The main goal in these patients must be to drain the pus. This can be done interventionally[14]. The symptoms, such as pain, fever, etc., will disappear promptly after such a procedure. It should be kept in mind, however, that in the vast majority of patients external drainage results in the development of a fistula. Thus, external drainage is the procedure of choice if the patient has to be stabilized before operation. If the patient is in good condition drainage of pus and resection of the diseased bowel segment can be done simultaneously, thereby reducing for the patient the period of symptomatic disease.

FISTULAS

Fistulas are a frequent complication with which the surgeon is confronted. A fistula is an abnormal communication between two epithelialized structures. Fistulas typically originate from an area with active disease that is often proximal to a site of partial obstruction. Many such fistulas produce only minor symptoms, and some of them heal with conservative treatment. Thus, the presence of a fistula *per se* is not an absolute indication for surgery. In the majority of enteroenteral, enterovesical and enterocutaneous fistulas, however, surgical therapy is necessary. Criteria for operation are the development of a significant enteric bypass, septic complications and pain. In addition, however, social and personal embarrassment and significant reduction of quality of life are clear indications for operative intervention. Surgical strategy consists in resection of the diseased bowel segment from which the fistula originates. At the draining sites of the fistulas in the so-called 'victim organs' local excision of the fistula and local closure is sufficient[15]. This technique is performed almost exclusively in enterogastric, enteroduodenal, enterovesical and enterogenital fistulas and in the majority of patients with enterosigmoid fistulas. Sigmoid resection is indicated only in case of active Crohn's disease in the sigma itself, in case of a pericolic abscess or phlegmon, and if the defect in the sigma is large and located at the mesenteric site of the colon[16]. For enteroenteric fistulas, however, en-bloc resection of both parts of the small bowel is done in most cases.

CROHN'S COLITIS

About one-third of patients with Crohn's disease seen by the surgeon suffer from Crohn's colitis. In two-thirds of them the total colon is involved, while in one-third only segmental disease is found. Main symptoms in these patients are persistent, and there is often bloody diarrhoea and abdominal pain, despite medical therapy. Less common complications are inflammatory masses, intra-abdominal or retroperitoneal abscesses, fistulas, recurrent haemorrhage, obstruction, toxic megacolon and neoplastic transformation. Surgical options in patients with Crohn's colitis consist of segmental colonic resection, subtotal or total colectomy with Hartmann pouch and ileostomy or with ileorectal anastomosis, and proctocolectomy. It is generally accepted that the recurrence rate after surgery for Crohn's colitis is strongly dependent on the type of surgical procedure performed[17]. Segmental colonic resection may be indicated in a minority of patients with Crohn's disease confined to a segment of the large bowel. The advantage of this technique is that it preserves part of the colon. Recurrence rate after segmental colonic resection, however, is rapid and very frequent. Nevertheless, although most patients treated by segmental resection will ultimately require further surgery, segmental resection remains a good option in some patients, particularly the elderly.

Crohn's colitis with rectal sparing occurs in about 20% of patients. In these cases subtotal or total colectomy with an ileorectal anastomosis is the procedure of choice. Prerequisites of such an operation are a rectum free of active Crohn's disease, good distensibility of the rectum, an intact anal sphincter and the absence of severe perineal disease. It is clear that the recurrence rate after ileo-rectostomy is much higher than after total proctocolectomy. About one-half of patients will eventually have a permanent ileostomy. The frequency of recurrence and the final outcome in respect to a permanent stoma, however, are not the only criteria for choosing the most suitable surgical procedure for the individual patient. Avoidance of an ileostomy for a number of years might well be an important quality-of-life issue for certain patients. In addition, one has to take into account the risk of proctectomy, i.e. damage of the pelvic nerves with the well-known consequences for sexual life and the risk of delayed perineal wound healing. It is characteristic for Crohn's patients that one-third of them will suffer after proctectomy from delayed wound healing or persistent perineal sinuses. Thus, in order to reduce such complications after proctectomy abdominal dissection close to the rectal wall is mandatory, and intersphincteric dissection should be performed from the perineal site. In spite of these potential complications total proctocolectomy is indicated in patients with pancolitis, severe rectal disease, incompetent anal sphincter and severe perineal disease[9]. Although total proctocolectomy can be performed routinely as a one-stage procedure, in severe perineal sepsis a two-stage procedure might be the better choice. Preservation of the anal sphincter and creation of an ileoanal pouch is contraindicated in patients with Crohn's disease. In most series between 40% and 50% of pouches had to be removed because of local fistulas, recurrent disease in the pouch or other local complications[18,19].

About one-third of surgical patients with Crohn's disease will eventually have a temporary or permanent stoma. A loop ileostomy may be conveniently made with laparoscopic technique. Temporary faecal diversion may be indicated in case of sphincter repair, advancement flap or sleeve repair for perianal or rectovaginal fistulas. Closure can be performed after local healing. In many patients with severe perineal sepsis or severe rectal disease faecal diversion leads to prompt remission. Closure of the ileostomy, however, will be possible only in the minority of these patients; the majority will ultimately require proctectomy. In patients requiring a temporary or permanent stoma correct surgical technique is of utmost importance in respect to quality of life. The best location of the stoma at the abdominal wall has to be looked for in the standing and sitting patient before operation. The intraoperative formation of a prominent nipple is also essential.

PERINEAL DISEASE

More than 50% of patients with Crohn's disease suffer from perineal disease. Perianal manifestations include fissures, fistula-in-ano, skin tags, rectovaginal fistulas, strictures, ulcers and incontinence[20]. Occasionally perianal disease is the first manifestation of Crohn's disease. Surgery is required for pain and recurrent sepsis. Acute severe pain is usually caused by abscess formation. Drainage should always be done promptly; it relieves the pain and prevents extension and local destruction. Non-attendance to perineal infections often results finally in destruction of the perineum and anal sphincter. Fistulas which are asymptomatic or only intermittently symptomatic should be treated conservatively[21]. Medical therapy or seton placement are the preferred therapies. When the perineal disease has a significant impact on essential activities such as sitting, walking, defaecating, ability to work and participating in social and sexual life, a more aggressive approach is indicated. Therapeutic nihilism, due to the fear that perineal wounds will not heal and fistulas will recur in patients with Crohn's disease, is widespread, but certainly the wrong attitude[22]. Special experience, however, is necessary for surgical treatment in complicated cases. Low fistulas may be treated by the typical laying-open operation, provided that the tract is superficial. Every attempt should be made to preserve the sphincter mechanism. Jeopardizing the sphincter may be disastrous in these patients because of the voluminous watery stools due to intestinal disease and bowel resection. In high fistulas excision of the fistula and closure of the internal opening with a rectal or anal advancement flap may be of benefit[23].

Diversion of faecal stream will not heal the fistulas, but will make them asymptomatic. In addition it is a useful therapeutic procedure in those in whom severe pelvic sepsis or poor general health would make immediate proctectomy dangerous. It may also be considered in patients who are not yet psychologically prepared for proctectomy. Nevertheless, in patients with severe perineal disease in combination with severe rectal disease or extensive Crohn's colitis, and in those with severely impaired function of the anal sphincter, proctectomy or total coloproctectomy is the procedure of choice. More than 50% of patients with perineal disease and colonic involvement eventually have a permanent stoma. Rectovaginal fistulas should be treated only if they are symptomatic; if there is only minimal discharge through the vagina they should not be treated surgically. This is the case in about half of the patients. One-fourth suffer from anorectal and perineal disease so severe that proctectomy is clearly indicated. In the remaining one-fourth of patients local closure with different techniques such as sliding flap, interposition of the gracilis muscle and so on should be tried[24]. With this approach about 70% of rectovaginal fistulas operated on can be successfully closed.

References

1. Cook WT, Mallas E, Prior P, Allan RN. Crohn's disease: course, treatment and long-term prognosis. Q J Med. 1980;49:363–84.
2. Farmer RG, Whelan G, Fazio VW. Longterm follow up of patients with Crohn's disease: relationship between the clinical pattern and prognosis. Gastroenterology. 1985;88:1818–25.
3. Harper PH, Fazio VW, Lavery IC *et al*. The longterm outcome in Crohn's disease. Dis Colon Rectum. 1987;30:174–9.
4. Hulten L. Surgical management and strategy in classical Crohn's disease. Int Surg. 1992;77:2–8.
5. Hurst RD, Molinari M, Chung TP, Rubin M, Michelassi F. Prospective study of the features, indications, and surgical treatment in 513 consecutive patients affected by Crohn's disease. Surgery. 1997;122:661–8.
6. Nissan A, Zamir O, Spira RM *et al*. A more liberal approach to the surgical treatment of Crohn's disease. Am J Surg. 1997;174:339–41.
7. Michelassi F, Block GE. Surgical management of Crohn's disease. Adv Surg. 1993;26:307–22.
8. Makowiec F, Schmidtke C, Paczulla D, Lamberts R, Becker HD, Starlinger M. Progression and prognosis of Crohn's colitis. Z Gastroenterol. 1997;35:7–14.
9. Buhr HJ, Kroesen AJ, Herfarth Ch. Chirurgische Therapie beim Rezidiv des Morbus Crohn. Chirurg. 1995;66:764–73.
10. Fazio VW, Marchetti F, Church JM *et al*. Effect of resection margins on the recurrence of Crohn's disease in the small bowel. Ann Surg. 1996;224:563–73.
11. Kim NK, Senagore JA, Luchtefeld MA *et al*. Long-term outcome after ileocecal resection for Crohn's disease. Am J Surg. 1997;63:627–33.
12. Michelassi F. Side-to-side isoperistaltic strictureplasty for multiple Crohn's strictures. Dis Colon Rectum. 1996;39:345–9.
13. Ozuner G, Fazio VW, Lavery IC, Milsom JW, Strong SA. Reoperative rates for Crohn's disease following strictureplasty. Dis Colon Rectum. 1996;39:1199–203.
14. Fulcher AS, Turner MA. Percutaneous drainage of enteric-related abscesses. Gastroenterologist. 1996;4:276–85.
15. Saint-Marc O, Tiret E, Vaillant JC, Frileux P, Parc R. Surgical management of internal fistulas in Crohn's disease. J Am Coll Surg. 1996;183:97–100.
16. Young-Fadok TM, Wolff BG, Meagher A, Benn PL, Dozois RR. Surgical management of ileosigmoid fistulas in Crohn's disease. Dis Colon Rectum. 1997;40:558- 61.
17. Fazio VW, Wu JS. Surgical therapy for Crohn's disease of the colon and rectum. Surg Clin N Am. 1997;77:197–210.
18. Sagar PM, Dozois RR, Wolff BG. Long-term results of ileal pouch–anal anastomosis in patients with Crohn's disease. Dis Colon Rectum. 1996;39:893–8.
19. Panis Y, Poupard B, Nemeth J, Lavergne A. Hautefeuille P, Valleur P. Ileal pouch/anal anastomosis for Crohn's disease. Lancet. 1996;347:854–7.
20. Frizelle FA, Santoro GA, Pemberton JH. The management of perianal Crohn's disease. Int J Colorect Dis. 1996;11:227–37.
21. Scott H, Northover JMA. Evaluation of surgery for perianal Crohn's fisitulas. Dis Colon Rectum. 1996;39:1039–43.
22. McKee RF, Keenan ChM. Perianal Crohn's disease – is it all bad news? Dis Colon Rectum. 1996;39:136–42.
23. Köhler A, Athanasiadis S. Die anodermale Verschiebelappenplastik als alternative Behandlungsmethode zu den endorectalen Verschluβtechniken bei der Therapie hoher Analfisteln. Chirurg. 1996;67:1244–50.
24. Hull TL, Fazio VW. Surgical approaches to low anovaginal fistula in Crohn's disease. Am J Surg. 1997;173:95–8.

40
Surgical therapy in ulcerative colitis with special reference to restorative proctocolectomy

N. RUNKEL and H. J. BUHR

INTRODUCTION

Until the 1980s, proctocolectomy with a permanent terminal ileostoma was the only curative therapeutic option for patients with ulcerative colitis. The restorative continence-preserving resection first described by Parks and Nicholls in 1978[1] was a milestone in the treatment of ulcerative colitis and became accepted as the operation of choice for ulcerative colitis within a few years. Large series with over 1000 patients have since been published[2]. The ileal J-pouch has proven to be technically and functionally superior to the S- and W-pouch contruction[3]. The type of pouch–anal anastomosis, stapled or hand-sewn, has been controversially discussed[4,5]. It is also debatable whether a protective ileostoma can be omitted to lower costs and hospitalization times. This chapter discusses the surgical therapy and especially the standard procedure with colectomy, proctomucosectomy and J-pouch construction.

INDICATION FOR SURGERY

Surgical alternatives to the ileoanal pouch operations include ileorectostomy and permanent ileostomy. Colectomy and ileorectostomy result in an excellent quality of life if the inflammation of the rectal mucosa is mild. The number of bowel movements is comparable to that after restorative proctocolectomy, but continence is generally better. The main disadvantage is, however, that the rectum is left in place and may be the origin of new episodes of acute inflammation. Thus, we consider ileorectal anastomosis only for exceptional cases such as young men with minimal rectal involvement, who do not want to take the risk of potency (maximum 5%) and ejaculation disorders (maximum 10%), and who are willing to be under regular postoperative surveillance. The carcinoma risk is estimated to be 5%[6,7].

Table 1   Indication for restorative proctocolectomy in ulcerative colitis

Failure of medical therapy
Side-effects of drugs
Local complications: bleeding, stenosis, perforation
Frequent recurrences with reduction of life quality
Toxic course
Dysplasia
Cancer

Proctocolectomy with a terminal ileostoma results in a markedly poorer quality of life than restorative pouches; therefore it is performed only if pouch surgery is contraindicated or fails. With a Kock pouch a continent ileostomy is created via a valve mechanism constructed from the small intestine with a prestomal reservoir. This method has a very high complication rate, due to its technical complexity, and thus has never become a routine procedure, although good results were obtained by the Swedish originator Nils G. Kock[8].

The diagnosis, timing and surgical strategy are decisive for the success of restorative proctocolectomy. The indications for surgery are the failure of conservative therapy, considerable side-effects of drug therapy, local complications (toxic megacolon, perforation, stenosis, bleeding), and restricted quality of life due to frequent recurrences (Table 1). Furthermore, ulcerative colitis is considered to be a precancerous condition. The risk is 1.7 times higher in proctitis alone, and about 15 times higher in pancolitis after 30 years[9–12]. The risk increases with disease duration and appears highest with an onset in childhood. Rather than performing prophylactic proctocolectomy at fixed intervals, regular endoscopic screening with multiple biopsies from the entire colon is now recommended for patients with more than 10 years of pancolitis. It is our view that the detection of any dysplasia is a clear indication for resection regardless of its grade. This opinion is based on a meta-analysis of 1225 patients in which concomitant colorectal carcinoma was found in 19% of cases with low-grade dysplasia, 42% of cases with high-grade dysplasia and in 43% of cases with dysplasia associated with a lesion or mass (DALM), according to ref. 13.

CONTRAINDICATIONS FOR SURGERY

Contraindications for restorative proctocolectomy include Crohn's disease because of pouch involvement and possible fistula formation, advanced rectal carcinomas in the middle and lower rectal third with a high risk of local recurrence, pronounced anal sphincter insufficiency and perianal septic processes (Table 2). There is a relative contraindication for patients over 70 years with moderate anal sphincter insufficiency.

SURGICAL STRATEGY

Restorative proctocolectomy is generally performed in two steps: first step: coloproctomucosectomy, ileoanal pouch, loop ileostomy; second step: take-down of ileostomy after 8–12 weeks.

Table 2 Contraindication of ileoanal pouch construction

Contraindication	Cause
Absolute	
Crohn's disease	Crohn's disease of pouch, pelvic fistula formation
Rectal cancer of lower third	Local recurrence
Anal sphincter insufficiency	Incontinence
Perianal septic process	High risk of postoperative recurrence
Relative	
Asymptomatic anal sphincter weakness	Improvement by sphincter training
Age > 70 years	Anal sphincter weakness

Indications for a three-step procedure include emergency interventions, severe secondary Cushing's disease, cortisone therapy with marked adiposity and a considerably reduced general condition: first step: Hartmann's colectomy or sigmoid mucosal fistula, loop ileostomy; second step: residual proctomucosectomy, ileoanal pouch; third step: take-down of ileostomy.

PREOPERATIVE DIAGNOSTICS AND PREPARATION

The main goal of preoperative diagnostics is to macroscopically and histologically confirm ulcerative colitis, since restorative proctocolectomy is contraindicated in Crohn's colitis. Specific diagnostic measures include:

1. Colonoscopy to substantiate the diagnosis and to document the extent and intensity of the inflammatory disease with histological confirmation.
2. Rectoscopy to evaluate the rectal mucosa and to exclude fistulas or tumours.
3. Abdominal ultrasound to assess the liver (primary sclerosing cholangitis, cholecystolithiasis, liver metastases).
4. Anal manometry to qualify and document sufficient anal sphincter function.
5. Sellink examination of the small intestine to exclude Crohn's disease.

Special surgical preparation consists of clarifying the possibility of autologous blood donation. Orthograde intestinal rinsing is not required, since a colon anastomosis is not performed; a high enema is sufficient. All patients are preoperatively instructed in stoma care, familiarized with the systems and informed about possible problems. Stoma location must be selected in such a way that the care system is not visible through clothing and is comfortable when sitting, lying and standing. The stoma position is marked before surgery and, in the ideal case, is slightly medial to an imaginary line between the navel and anterior superior iliac spine in the lower right abdomen.

TECHNIQUE OF RESTORATIVE PROCTOCOLETOMY (Table 3)

Surgery is performed under general anaesthesia. The patient is placed in a modified Trendelenburg position. The legs can be lifted during surgery for better

Table 3 Technique of restorative proctocolectomy

Resection

Dissection of omentum from transverse colon

Colectomy and supra-anal proctectomy; preservation of ileocolic artery

Peranal distal mucosectomy of rectum (2–3 cm)

Reconstruction

Mobilization of mesenteric root

J-pouch construction (15 cm) using stapler

Pouch–anal anastomosis hand-sewn

---

access to the perineum. The standard incision is a generous median laparotomy, which extends from about 5 cm above the navel to the symphysis.

First step: colon resection

The surgeon stands on the right side. After exploring the abdomen and excluding secondary diseases, the left colon is detached from the retroperitoneum. After severing the fetal adhesions to the lateral abdominal wall, the peritoneal duplicature is entered and the avascular plane split. The left colonic flexure is carefully pulled in the caudal direction for dissection of the phrenicocolic ligament, which is vascularized; thus, it must be electrocoagulated or clamped and ligated. The traction on the omentum or colon must be applied carefully under visual control to avoid serosal spleen injuries. The omentum is dissected from the transverse colon in such a way as to leave the omentum fully vascularized. This can also be easily done in a colon strongly altered by inflammation. The ligamentary suspension of the right colonic flexure is also vascularized and must therefore be electrocoagulated or ligated. After incision of the peritoneal duplicature of the right hemicolon, the avascular layer becomes visible when the colon is carefully pulled in the medial direction. It is important to preserve the ileocolic artery with the ileal branch. The distal ascending mesocolon is dissected close to the intestine, in which only the colonic branch of the ileocolic artery is cut. The line of dissection in the remaining mesocolon is about a hand-width away from the large intestine. Using diaphanoscopy the main vessels can be visualized, isolated and ligated. The remaining avascular fatty tissue of the mesocolon is cut with the electrocauter. The terminal ileum is separated close to Bauhin's valve.

Second step: proctectomy

The surgeon changes to the left side. The rectum is mobilized by an adjacent lyre-shaped incision of the peritoneum on both sides. The superior rectal artery is divided distal to the promotory. In this way it is ensured that the pelvic plexus cannot be injured. From this point one proceeds dorsally and vertically into the depth with further exposure in the presacral separating layer in front of Waldayer's fascia. Along this embryonic border the pelvic floor muscles are reached using large curved scissors. The separating layer between the rectum and vagina or seminal vesicle and prostate gland is visible on the ventral side. In men, exposure must be done dorsal to Denonvielle's fascia in order to avoid injuring the underlying autonomous nerves. In contrast to carcinoma surgery, the lateral mesorectum is divided close to the intestine. Abdominal mobilization of the rectum is completed when its entire circumference is dissected down to the pelvic floor.

Third step: construction of the ileum pouch (J-pouch)

An essential step is the mobilization of the small-bowel mesentery in order to later shift the pouch to the lesser pelvis without tension. After detaching the embryonic adhesions the mesenteric root is exposed. Over the mesenterium, multiple transverse incisions are made into the peritoneum to achieve the maximal length. The pouch apex is located 15 cm before the end of the small intestine and should be as mobile as to be able to reach up to two finger-breadths over the symphysis. For this the division of a main vessel is usually necessary. Blood is then supplied to the distal ileum via arcades from the ileocolic artery. The terminal ileum is J-folded, the apex is incised, the stapler (GIA 90) is inserted, and fired antimesenterically (Figure 1). Two GIA rounds are required for the entire pouch length. The open end of the J-pouch is closed with interrupted sutures or a TEA stapler.

Fourth step: transanal mucosectomy

The legs are now elevated and the surgeon changes to the perineal position. It is best to be in a sitting position with an additional forehead lamp. The anus is held open with special circular retractors enabling good visibility of the dentate line and the rectal mucosa. Ornipressin solution (1:100 000) is then submucosally injected. The mucosectomy starts at the dentate line and moves cranially forward for 2–3 cm. At this level the rectal wall is divided from perianally or abdominally. It is imperative that the mucosectomy is complete. The sutures for the anal pouch anastomosis (3/O vicryl) are circularly placed in the area of the dentate line. The anocutaneous border and a part of the sphincter muscle serve as the suture bed (Figure 2). Frequent nocturnal incontinence is observed if the sutures are too deep.

Fifth step: ileoanal pouch anastomosis

Two Ellis clamps are transanally inserted into the pelvis. In this way the pouch can be grasped and pulled in the caudal direction. Care should be taken that the mesenteric root is not torqued. The preinserted sutures are passed through the ileum as full transmural stitches and also circularly placed. Thereafter they are individually knotted. An easy-flow drainage is inserted into the pouch for postoperative drainage of secretion and mucus. This drainage is left in place for 8–10 days.

Sixth step: creation of an ileostoma

The surgeon returns to the left position. The patient's legs are lowered. Two easy-flow drainages are transabdominally inserted into the area of the anastomosis. The skin is circularly incised at the previously marked ileostomy position and the rectus abdominis is split. The small intestine can usually be pulled through without tension 20–30 cm before the pouch. The afferent loop of the

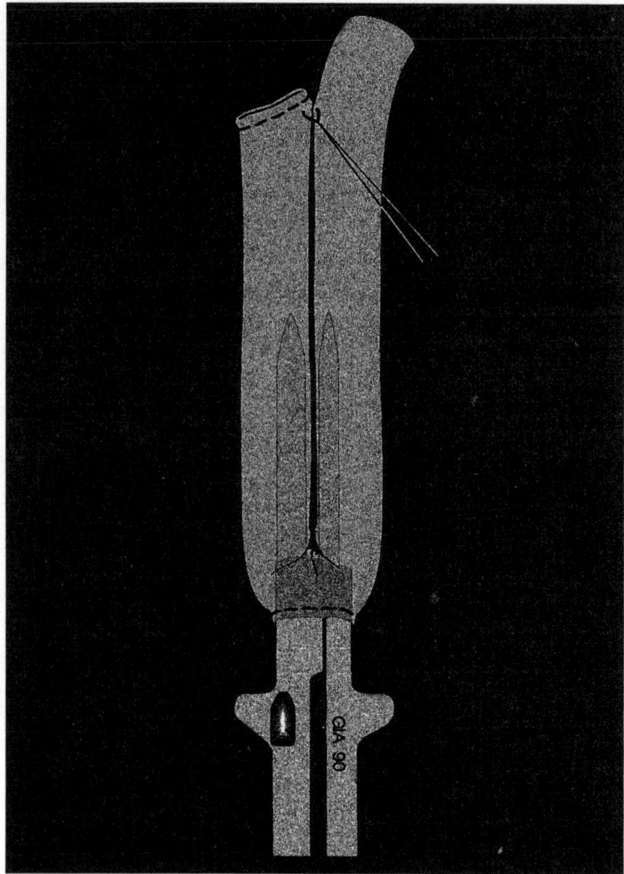

Figure 1 Pouch construction: via an opening in the area of the pouch tip the staple gun (GIA 90) is initially fired in such a way that the suture lies in the antimesenterial direction. The procedure is repeated to achieve a length of 15 cm and a volume of about 160 ml

small intestine is placed caudally and the efferent cranially. The abdominal cavity and presacral space is subsequently rinsed and the abdomen closed. After sterile dressing the ileostoma is opened near the aboral part of the loop at skin level and folded in the caudal direction, so that the oral part of the loop is everted and prominent. The edge is fixed to the skin with interrupted sutures.

SPECIAL SITUATIONS

Indeterminate colitis

Crohn's colitis is a general contraindication for restorative proctocolectomy with pouch reconstruction because there is a very high rate of septic or fistulous complication in the small pelvis, and over 50% of the pouches must be removed in the

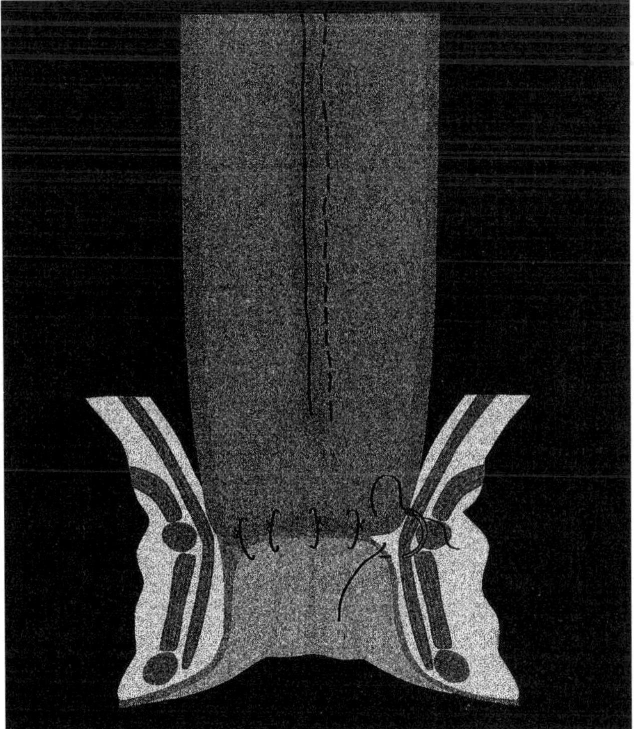

Figure 2 Pouch–anal anastomosis as a three-point suture (hand-sewn): about 14–16 interrupted sutures are needed

further course. In about 15% of cases the clinical and histopathological parameters of colitis are not conclusive[14]. Almost 50% of these cases with indeterminate colitis will later prove to have Crohn's disease[2]. The outcome of restorative proctocolectomy for indeterminate colitis is worse than for ulcerative colitis[15]. The frequency of pouch loss ranges between 1.9%[2] and 90%[16]. Restorative proctocolectomy is thus not the ideal procedure for indeterminate colitis. The operation of choice would be a colectomy with ileorectostomy or, in cases with a highly acute course, a discontinuity resection with creation of a sigmoid fistula. After a definitive diagnosis of ulcerative colitis, residual proctectomy with pouch reconstruction can be performed in a second step. The long-term results of an ileoanal pouch are surprisingly good when typical histological signs of Crohn's disease are absent. Hyman *et al.*[17] from the Cleveland Hospital reported a functional pouch in 15 of 16 patients with indeterminate colitis. These results were recently confirmed in a larger patient population ($n = 44$)[2] and also by the Mayo Clinic[18].

Technical complications in pouch reconstruction

In about 5% of cases the pouch construction fails due to technical problems such as pouch ischaemia or severely uncontrollable presacral bleeding. More important, however, is a short mesentery not enabling the mobilization of the small intestine to the anus. This situation occurs especially in cases of very adipose patients, previous surgery with dissection of the ileocolic artery, or intestinal malrotation. An associated right colon carcinoma represents a particular challenge to the surgical strategy because the ileocolic artery must be sacrificed during lymphadenectomy.

Children

The course of ulcerative colitis is generally more severe in children than in adults. The percentage of emergency operations in children is higher than in adults. The children are frequently retarded by the medication and the disease. Proctocolectomy offers a chance for normal development and should thus be performed before closure of the epiphyseal bones. The surgical technique for children is the same as in adults, but is often easier to carry out. A protective ileostomy should also be created in children[19,20]. Experience from the 1980s shows that the best results are achieved with a 8–12 cm J-pouch. In children, hand-sewn anastomoses are preferred because of the usually strong rectal involvement and lower traumatization compared to stapling. There are only a few series on restorative proctocolectomy in children[19,21,22]. In Fonkalsrud's series, from the UCLA, 36 of 94 children required resurgery[19]. Six children, three of whom were later diagnosed with Crohn's disease, required a permanent ileostoma. The incidence of pouchitis after proctocolectomy was about twice as high in children as in adults.

Colitis-associated carcinomas

Dissemination and prognosis are the same in colitis-associated and 'normal' colorectal carcinomas. The aim of curative tumour resection is the complete eradication of the tumour with locoregional lymphadenectomy. In colon carcinomas, radical resection with central ligation of the supplying vessels can usually be combined with ileoanal pouch construction without difficulty. However, ascending colon carcinomas can be problematic because the ileocolic artery must be sacrificed. Continence can be preserved in rectal carcinomas if anterior rectal resection with total mesorectal excision is curative. There is controversy regarding the value of postoperative adjuvant radiotherapy of the lesser pelvis as recommended for stage II and III rectal carcinomas. Due to the high risk of radiogenic pouchitis with a loss of function, we dispense with radiotherapy in favour of systemic adjuvant chemotherapy. Moreover, the pouch procedure should not be performed in cases with a high risk of local recurrence (T4 or lymphogenic metastasis) to enable high-dose postoperative radiotherapy.

POSTOPERATIVE COMPLICATIONS AND THEIR MANAGEMENT

Coloproctectomy with an ileoanal pouch is a difficult and complicated procedure. In a large series from Cleveland, with 1005 pouch operations, the early complication rate was 28% and the late complication rate 50%[2]. The frequency of non-specific postoperative complications such as bleeding or ileus is the same

Table 4 Postoperative early and late complications following restorative proctocolectomy for ulcerative colitis (244 patients; according to ref. 31)

Complications	Early	Late
Rebleeding	6 (2.5%)	0
Ileus	4 (1.6%)	9 (3.7%)
Local septic complications	27 (11.1%)	8 (3.3%)
Anastomotic stenosis	4 (1.6%)	10 (4.1%)
Pouchitis	0	35 (14.3%)
Mortality	0	0

as after other major abdominal operations (Table 4). Specific complications after restorative proctocolectomy include local septic processes in the lesser pelvis, which usually start at the pouch–anal anastomosis and less often from the pouch itself. The incidence is about 10%. Even after healing of these fistulas long-term pouch function may be compromised by fibrous secondary healing. In addition to reduced pouch capacity there is also a risk of stenosis and loss of sphincter strength. The reasons for secondary surgery are given in Table 5.

After pouch–anal reconstruction a reduction in sphincter function is regularly observed. Manometrically there is a mean reduction of resting tone from 60 to 45 mmHg and squeezing pressure from 144 to 120 mmHg[23]. This is most probably caused by complex neurological damage and not by direct injury of the sphincter during surgery. With normal preoperative function this decrease in sphincter strength is asymptomatic; however, it may be manifest in cases with pre-existing sphincter weakness. Thus, it is important to measure sphincter function before the take-down of the ileostomy. Special sphincter training has a very high success rate[23].

Pouchitis is a specific late complication after restorative proctocolectomy. The cause is still unknown. Pouchitis is related to pouch construction, since similar

Table 5 Functional results of restorative proctocolectomy

Variable	Runkel et al., 1998[31]	Sagar et al., 1993[29]	Fazio et al., 1995[2]	Fonkalsrud, 1996[19]
No. of patients	244	103	521	116 children
Stool frequency per day (median, range)	5.4 (3–10)	5 (4–7)	6 (1–20)	3.6
Urgency	14%	12%	13%	
Seepage		24%		
Night	31%		29%	6%
Day and night	10%		17%	<10%
Antidiarrhoeal medications		52%		
Always	11%		15%	
Sometimes	40%		47%	
Pads	31%	18%		

inflammation has been observed in the Kock pouch and in neo-bladders after cystectomy, and to the underlying disease occurring more frequently in ulcerative colitis than familial polyposis. Inflammatory changes of the pouch mucosa are endoscopically evident in 50% and histologically in almost all. However, pouchitis becomes symptomatic in only a quarter of patients. Symptoms include lower abdominal and defaecation pain, perianal bleeding, an increase in stool frequency and new incontinence complaints. It is decisive for the further management to exclude secondary pouchitis due to ischaemia or sepsis in the lesser pelvis. Diagnostic measures include pouchography, pouchoscopy with biopsy, endosonography and magnetic resonance imaging (MRI). Idiopathic pouchitis is treated according to a stepwise pattern. Metronidazole (alternative: ciprofloxacin) is given initially. Cortisone is then topically applied. In severe cases cortisone is systemically applied or an ileostoma is even connected. It is extremely rare that chronic pouchitis leads to pouch extirpation.

FUNCTIONAL RESULTS

In the great majority of patients (> 90%), the ileostomy can be taken down within 6 months. Due to local septic complications, anastomotic stenosis, pouchitis or anal sphincter insufficiency, the ileostomy has either been left in place or reopened in the remainder. Definitive pouch extirpation is required in less than 3%[2]. The main causes are ischaemic and local septic processes as well as a false diagnosis of Crohn's disease. The number of bowel movements is five (four to seven) during the day and one (none to two) at night[24] (Table 5). More than a quarter of patients regularly take antidiarrhoeal drugs. However, some patients complain of more than 10 stools during the day and more than three at night. Ninety per cent of patients are completely continent during the day and 25% need a diaper at night. Discrimination for faeces/air is adequate in 80% of patients. The majority of patients regularly apply ointment. A later pregnancy is no problem and vaginal delivery is also possible[25].

QUALITY OF LIFE

The quality of life is an important criterion for deciding on a certain surgical procedure. Functional pouch results are, however, only a part of the quality of life, which also includes social, cultural, psychological and disease-related aspects as well as the patient's subjective disease experience. The study by Irvine[26] demonstrates the extent to which patients suffer from ulcerative colitis; it showed that even patients in remission have a 25% poorer quality of life index than healthy controls. Köhler et al.[27] examined the subjective estimation of surgical success after Brooke stoma ($n = 406$), Kock pouch ($n = 313$) and ileoanal pouch ($n = 298$). The subjective evaluation of the surgical results was the same in all groups. The percentage of patients' general satisfaction was also identical (93–96%). In contrast, patients gave very different answers to the question of whether they would have preferred another operation: 39% after ileostoma, 14% after Kock pouch and 4% after ileoanal pouch. The ileostoma, especially in women, lowers self-esteem, which negatively affects social activities and partnership. A quarter of the men and almost all of the women find that it limits their sexuality. The positive results of the Kock pouch from the early 1980s were not reproducible later[28]. In contrast, ileoanal pouch results are markedly better in many life-quality aspects than the ileostoma[27]. Sagar *et al.*[29] compared the quality of life after pouch with non-operated patients in remission. The social limitation rate is lower with than without a pouch (21% vs 46%). Potency and ejaculation disorders occur in 8% of cases after the pouch and in 26% with drug therapy. Anxiety and depression are found more frequently in the remission group. The positive pouch effect on the quality of life continues for many years[30].

CONCLUSION

Restorative proctocolectomy is the operation of choice in ulcerative colitis. Many technical aspects of ileoanal pouch construction have been standardized, such as the J-pouch design. It is currently discussed whether to perform the pouch–anal anastomosis manually or by stapler, and when to omit the protective ileostomy. Sphincter weakness can usually be improved by sphincter training. Septic complications in the lesser pelvis occur in up to 10% of patients and require experience to treat. Pouchitis is an important late complication but can be managed conservatively in most cases. The functional results after pouch–anal anastomosis are excellent in more than 80% of patients (stool frequency four to six per day; full continence). The ileoanal reconstruction is a complex procedure and should be performed only in experienced centres.

References

1. Parks AG, Nicholls RJ. Procotocolectomy without ileostomy for ulcerative colitis. Br Med J. 1978;2:85–8.
2. Fazio VW, Ziv Y, Church JM *et al.* Ileal pouch–anal anastomoses complications and function in 1005 patients. Ann Surg. 1995;222:120–7.
3. Sagar PM, Taylor BA. Pelvic ileal reservoirs: the options. Br J Surg. 1994;81:325–32.
4. Luukkonen P, Jarvinen H. Stapled vs hand-sutured ileoanal anastomosis in restorative proctocolectomy. A prospective, randomized study. Arch Surg. 1993;128:437–40.
5. Ziv Y, Fazio VW, Church JM, Lavery IC, King TM, Ambrosetti P. Stapled ileal pouch–anal anastomoses are safer than handsewn anastomoses in patients with ulcerative colitis. Am J Surg. 1996;171:320–3.
6. Oakley JR, Jagelman DG, Fazio VW *et al.* Complications and quality of life after ileorectal anastomosis for ulcerative colitis. Am J Surg. 1985;149:23–30.
7. Johnson WR, Hughes ES, McDermott FT, Pihl EA, Katrivessis H. The outcome of patients with ulcerative colitis managed by subtotal colectomy. Surg Gynecol Obstet. 1986;162:421–5.
8. Kock NG, Myrvold HE, Nilsson LO, Philipson BM. Achtzehn Jahre Erfahrung mit der kontinenten Ileostomie. Chirurg. 1985;56:299–304.
9. Ekbom A, Helmick C, Zack M, Adami HO. The epidemiology of inflammatory bowel disease: a large, population-based study in Sweden. Gastroenterology. 1991;100:350–8.
10. Gilat T, Fireman Z, Grossman A *et al.* Colorectal cancer in patients with ulcerative colitis. A population study in central Israel. Gastroenterology. 1988;94:870–7.
11. Gyde SN, Prior P, Allan RN *et al.* Colorectal cancer in ulcerative colitis: a cohort study of primary referrals from three centres. Gut. 1988;29:206–17.
12. Kvist N, Jacobsen O, Kvist HK *et al.* Malignancy in ulcerative colitis. Scand J Gastroenterol. 1989;24:497–506.
13. Bernstein CN, Shanahan F, Weinstein WM. Are we telling patients the truth about surveillance colonoscopy in ulcerative colitis? Lancet. 1994;343:71–4.
14. Corman ML. Colon and Rectal Surgery, 2nd edn. Philadelphia: Lippincott; 1989:741.

15. Atkinson KG, Owen DA, Wankling G. Restorative proctocolectomy and indeterminate colitis. Am J Surg. 1994;167:516–18.
16. Bodzin JH, Klein SN, Priest SG. Ileoproctostomy is preferred over ileoanal pull-through in patients with indeterminate colitis. Am Surg. 1995;61:590–3.
17. Hyman NH, Fazio VW, Tuckson WB, Lavery IC. Consequences of ileal pouch–anal anastomosis for Crohn's colitis. Dis Colon Rectum. 1991;34:653–7.
18. Pezim ME, Pemberton JH, Beart RW Jr *et al.* Outcome of 'indeterminant' colitis following ileal pouch–anal anastomosis. Dis Colon Rectum. 1989;32:653–8.
19. Fonkalsrud EW. Long-term results after colectomy and ileoanal pull-through procedure in children. Arch Surg. 1996;131:881–5.
20. Cohen Z, McLeod RS, Stephen W, Stern HS, O'Connor B, Reznick R. Continuing evolution of the pelvic pouch procedure. Ann Surg. 1992;216:506–11.
21. Orkin BA, Telander RL, Wolff BG, Perrault J, Ilstrup DM. The surgical management of children with ulcerative colitis. The old vs. the new. Dis Colon Rectum. 1990;33:947–55.
22. Coran AG. A personal experience with 100 consecutive total colectomies and straight ileoanal endorectal pull-throughs for benign disease of the colon and rectum in children and adults. Ann Surg. 1990;212:242–7.
23. Kroesen AJ, Stern J, Buhr HJ, Herfarth C. Kontinenzstörungen nach ileoanaler Pouchanlage – diagnostische kriterien und therapeutische Folgerungen. Chirurg. 1995;66:385–91.
24. Buhr HJ, Heuschen UA, Stern J, Herfarth C. Kontinenzerhaltende Operation nach Proktokolektomie. Indikation, Technik und Ergebnisse. Chirurg. 1993;64:601–13.
25. Scott HJ, McLeod RS, Blair J, O'Connor B, Cohen Z. Ileal pouch–anal anastomosis: pregnancy, delivery and pouch function. Int J Colorectal Dis. 1996;11:84–7.
26. Irvine EJ. Quality of life – measurement in inflammatory bowel disease. Scand J Gastroenterol Suppl. 1993;199:36–9.
27. Köhler LW, Pemberton JH, Zinsmeister AR, Kelly KA. Quality of life after proctocolectomy. A comparison of Brooke ileostomy, Kock pouch, and ileal pouch–anal anastomosis. Gastroenterology. 1991;101:679–84.
28. Gerber A, Apt MK, Craig PH. The improved quality of life with the Kock continent ileostomy. J Clin Gastroenterol. 1984;6:513–17.
29. Sagar PM, Lewis W, Holdsworth PJ, Johnston D, Mitchell C, MacFie J. Quality of life after restorative proctocolectomy with a pelvic ileal reservoir compares favorably with that of patients with medically treated colitis. Dis Colon Rectum. 1993;36:584–92.
30. Köhler LW, Pemberton JH, Hodge DO, Zinsmeister AR, Kelly KA. Long-term functional results and quality of life after ileal pouch–anal anastomosis and cholecystectomy. World J Surg. 1992;16:1126–31.
31. Runkel N, Kroesen A, Buhr HJ. Technik und Ergebnisse des ileoanalen Pouches bei Colitis ulcerosa nach Colektomie und Proctomukosektomie. Zentralbl Chir. 1998;123:375–80.

Index

Note. There are main entries for Crohn's disease and ulcerative colitis which give page references to large sections of text or whole chapters containing material specific to only one of the two diseases. Abbreviation used: CD, Crohn's disease; ECM, extracellular matrix; LPS, lipopolysaccharide; MAb, monoclonal antibody; UC, ulcerative colitis.

Falk Symposium Series

43. Reutter W, Popper H, Arias IM, Heinrich PC, Keppler D, Landmann L, eds.: *Modulation of Liver Cell Expression*. Falk Symposium No. 43. 1987   ISBN: 0-85200-677-2*

44. Boyer JL, Bianchi L, eds.: *Liver Cirrhosis*. Falk Symposium No. 44. 1987   ISBN: 0-85200-993-3*

45. Paumgartner G, Stiehl A, Gerok W, eds.: *Bile Acids and the Liver*. Falk Symposium No. 45. 1987   ISBN: 0-85200-675-6*

46. Goebell H, Peskar BM, Malchow H, eds.: *Inflammatory Bowel Diseases – Basic Research & Clinical Implications*. Falk Symposium No. 46. 1988   ISBN: 0-7462-0067-6*

47. Bianchi L, Holt P, James OFW, Butler RN, eds.: *Aging in Liver and Gastrointestinal Tract*. Falk Symposium No. 47. 1988   ISBN: 0-7462-0066-8*

48. Heilmann C, ed.: *Calcium-Dependent Processes in the Liver*. Falk Symposium No. 48. 1988   ISBN: 0-7462-0075-7*

50. Singer MV, Goebell H, eds.: *Nerves and the Gastrointestinal Tract*. Falk Symposium No. 50. 1989   ISBN: 0-7462-0114-1

51. Bannasch P, Keppler D, Weber G, eds.: *Liver Cell Carcinoma*. Falk Symposium No. 51. 1989   ISBN: 0-7462-0111-7

52. Paumgartner G, Stiehl A, Gerok W, eds.: *Trends in Bile Acid Research*. Falk Symposium No. 52. 1989   ISBN: 0-7462-0112-5

53. Paumgartner G, Stiehl A, Barbara L, Roda E, eds.: *Strategies for the Treatment of Hepatobiliary Diseases*. Falk Symposium No. 53. 1990   ISBN: 0-7923-8903-4

54. Bianchi L, Gerok W, Maier K-P, Deinhardt F, eds.: *Infectious Diseases of the Liver*. Falk Symposium No. 54. 1990   ISBN: 0-7923-8902-6

55. Falk Symposium No. 55 not published

55B. Hadziselimovic F, Herzog B, Bürgin-Wolff A, eds.: *Inflammatory Bowel Disease and Coeliac Disease in Children*. International Falk Symposium. 1990 ISBN 0-7462-0125-7

56. Williams CN, eds.: *Trends in Inflammatory Bowel Disease Therapy*. Falk Symposium No. 56. 1990   ISBN: 0-7923-8952-2

57. Bock KW, Gerok W, Matern S, Schmid R, eds.: *Hepatic Metabolism and Disposition of Endo- and Xenobiotics*. Falk Symposium No. 57. 1991   ISBN: 0-7923-8953-0

58. Paumgartner G, Stiehl A, Gerok W, eds.: *Bile Acids as Therapeutic Agents: From Basic Science to Clinical Practice*. Falk Symposium No. 58. 1991   ISBN: 0-7923-8954-9

59. Halter F, Garner A, Tytgat GNJ, eds.: *Mechanisms of Peptic Ulcer Healing*. Falk Symposium No. 59. 1991   ISBN: 0-7923-8955-7

60. Goebell H, Ewe K, Malchow H, Koelbel Ch, eds.: *Inflammatory Bowel Diseases – Progress in Basic Research and Clinical Implications*. Falk Symposium No. 60. 1991   ISBN: 0-7923-8956-5

61. Falk Symposium No. 61 not published

62. Dowling RH, Folsch UR, Löser Ch, eds.: *Polyamines in the Gastrointestinal Tract*. Falk Symposium No. 62. 1992   ISBN: 0-7923-8976-X

63. Lentze MJ, Reichen J, eds.: *Paediatric Cholestasis: Novel Approaches to Treatment*. Falk Symposium No. 63. 1992   ISBN: 0-7923-8977-8

64. Demling L, Frühmorgen P, eds.: *Non-Neoplastic Diseases of the Anorectum*. Falk Symposium No. 64. 1992   ISBN: 0-7923-8979-4

64B. Gressner AM, Ramadori G, eds.: *Molecular and Cell Biology of Liver Fibrogenesis*. International Falk Symposium. 1992   ISBN: 0-7923-8980-8

*These titles were published under the MTP Press imprint.

Falk Symposium Series

65. Hadziselimovic F, Herzog B, eds.: *Inflammatory Bowel Diseases and Morbus Hirschprung*. Falk Symposium No. 65. 1992   ISBN: 0-7923-8995-6

66. Martin F, McLeod RS, Sutherland LR, Williams CN, eds.: *Trends in Inflammatory Bowel Disease Therapy*. Falk Symposium No. 66. 1993   ISBN: 0-7923-8827-5

67. Schölmerich J, Kruis W, Goebell H, Hohenberger W, Gross V, eds.: *Inflammatory Bowel Diseases – Pathophysiology as Basis of Treatment*. Falk Symposium No. 67. 1993   ISBN: 0-7923-8996-4

68. Paumgartner G, Stiehl A, Gerok W, eds.: *Bile Acids and The Hepatobiliary System: From Basic Science to Clinical Practice*. Falk Symposium No. 68. 1993   ISBN: 0-7923-8829-1

69. Schmid R, Bianchi L, Gerok W, Maier K-P, eds.: *Extrahepatic Manifestations in Liver Diseases*. Falk Symposium No. 69. 1993   ISBN: 0-7923-8821-6

70. Meyer zum Büschenfelde K-H, Hoofnagle J, Manns M, eds.: *Immunology and Liver*. Falk Symposium No. 70. 1993   ISBN: 0-7923-8830-5

71. Surrenti C, Casini A, Milani S, Pinzani M , eds.: *Fat-Storing Cells and Liver Fibrosis*. Falk Symposium No. 71. 1994   ISBN: 0-7923-8842-9

72. Rachmilewitz D, ed.: *Inflammatory Bowel Diseases – 1994*. Falk Symposium No. 72. 1994   ISBN: 0-7923-8845-3

73. Binder HJ, Cummings J, Soergel KH, eds.: *Short Chain Fatty Acids*. Falk Symposium No. 73. 1994   ISBN: 0-7923-8849-6

73B. Möllmann HW, May B, eds.: *Glucocorticoid Therapy in Chronic Inflammatory Bowel Disease: from basic principles to rational therapy*. International Falk Workshop. 1996   ISBN 0-7923-8708-2

74. Keppler D, Jungermann K, eds.: *Transport in the Liver*. Falk Symposium No. 74. 1994   ISBN: 0-7923-8858-5

74B. Stange EF, ed.: *Chronic Inflammatory Bowel Disease*. Falk Symposium. 1995   ISBN: 0-7923-8876-3

75. van Berge Henegouwen GP, van Hoek B, De Groote J, Matern S, Stockbrügger RW, eds.: *Cholestatic Liver Diseases: New Strategies for Prevention and Treatment of Hepatobiliary and Cholestatic Liver Diseases*. Falk Symposium 75. 1994.   ISBN: 0-7923-8867-4

76. Monteiro E, Tavarela Veloso F, eds.: *Inflammatory Bowel Diseases: New Insights into Mechanisms of Inflammation and Challenges in Diagnosis and Treatment*. Falk Symposium 76. 1995.   ISBN 0-7923-8884-4

77. Singer MV, Ziegler R, Rohr G, eds.: *Gastrointestinal Tract and Endocrine System*. Falk Symposium 77. 1995.   ISBN 0-7923-8877-1

78. Decker K, Gerok W, Andus T, Gross V, eds.: *Cytokines and the Liver*. Falk Symposium 78. 1995.   ISBN 0-7923-8878-X

79. Holstege A, Schölmerich J, Hahn EG, eds.: *Portal Hypertension*. Falk Symposium 79. 1995.   ISBN 0-7923-8879-8

80. Hofmann AF, Paumgartner G, Stiehl A, eds.: *Bile Acids in Gastroenterology: Basic and Clinical Aspects*. Falk Symposium 80. 1995   ISBN 0-7923-8880-1

81. Riecken EO, Stallmach A, Zeitz M, Heise W, eds.: *Malignancy and Chronic Inflammation in the Gastrointestinal Tract – New Concepts*. Falk Symposium 81. 1995   ISBN 0-7923-8889-5

82. Fleig WE, ed.: *Inflammatory Bowel Diseases: New Developments and Standards*. Falk Symposium 82. 1995   ISBN 0-7923-8890-6

82B.Paumgartner G, Beuers U, eds.: *Bile Acids in Liver Diseases*. International Falk Workshop. 1995 ISBN 0-7923-8891-7

83. Dobrilla G, Felder M, de Pretis G, eds.: *Advances in Hepatobiliary and Pancreatic Diseases: Special Clinical Topics*. Falk Symposium 83. 1995. ISBN 0-7923-8892-5

84. Fromm H, Leuschner U, eds.: *Bile Acids – Cholestasis – Gallstones: Advances in Basic and Clinical Bile Acid Research*. Falk Symposium 84. 1995 ISBN 0-7923-8893-3

85. Tytgat GNJ, Bartelsman JFWM, van Deventer SJH, eds.: *Inflammatory Bowel Diseases*. Falk Symposium 85. 1995 ISBN 0-7923-8894-1

86. Berg PA, Leuschner U, eds.: *Bile Acids and Immunology*. Falk Symposium 86. 1996 ISBN 0-7923-8700-7

87. Schmid R, Bianchi L, Blum HE, Gerok W, Maier KP, Stalder GA, eds.: *Acute and Chronic Liver Diseases: Molecular Biology and Clinics*. Falk Symposium 87. 1996 ISBN 0-7923-8701-5

88. Blum HE, Wu GY, Wu CH, eds.: *Molecular Diagnosis and Gene Therapy*. Falk Symposium 88. 1996 ISBN 0-7923-8702-3

88B.Poupon RE, Reichen J, eds.: *Surrogate Markers to Assess Efficacy of TReatment in Chronic Liver Diseases*. International Falk Workshop. 1996 ISBN 0-7923-8705-8

89. Reyes HB, Leuschner U, Arias IM, eds.: *Pregnancy, Sex Hormones and the Liver*. Falk Symposium 89. 1996 ISBN 0-7923-8704-X

89B.Broelsch CE, Burdelski M, Rogiers X, eds.: *Cholestatic Liver Diseases in Children and Adults*. International Falk Workshop. 1996 ISBN 0-7923-8710-4

90. Lam S-K, Paumgartner P, Wang B, eds.: *Update on Hepatobiliary Diseases 1996*. Falk Symposium 90. 1996 ISBN 0-7923-8715-5

91. Hadziselimovic F, Herzog B, eds.: *Inflammatory Bowel Diseases and Chronic Recurrent Abdominal Pain*. Falk Symposium 91. 1996 ISBN 0-7923-8722-8

91B.Alvaro D, Benedetti A, Strazzabosco M, eds.: *Vanishing Bile Duct Syndrome – Pathophysiology and Treatment*. International Falk Workshop. 1996 ISBN 0-7923-8721-X

92. Gerok W, Loginov AS, Pokrowskij VI, eds.: *New Trends in Hepatology 1996*. Falk Symposium 92. 1997 ISBN 0-7923-8723-6

93. Paumgartner G, Stiehl A, Gerok W, eds.: *Bile Acids in Hepatobiliary Diseases – Basic Research and Clinical Application*. Falk Symposium 93. 1997 ISBN 0-7923-8725-2

94. Halter F, Winton D, Wright NA, eds.: *The Gut as a Model in Cell and Molecular Biology*. Falk Symposium 94. 1997 ISBN 0-7923-8726-0

94B.Kruse-Jarres JD, Schölmerich J, eds.: *Zinc and Diseases of the Digestive Tract*. International Falk Workshop. 1997 ISBN 0-7923-8724-4

95. Ewe K, Eckardt VF, Enck P, eds.: *Constipation and Anorectal Insufficiency*. Falk Symposium 95. 1997 ISBN 0-7923-8727-9

96. Andus T, Goebell H, Layer P, Schölmerich J, eds.: *Inflammatory Bowel Disease – from Bench to Bedside*. Falk Symposium 96. 1997 ISBN 0-7923-8728-7

97. Campieri M, Bianchi-Porro G, Fiocchi C, Schölmerich J, eds. *Clinical Challenges in Inflammatory Bowel Diseases: Diagnosis, Prognosis and Treatment*. Falk Symposium 97. 1998 ISBN 0-7923-8733-3

98. Lembcke B, Kruis W, Sartor RB, eds. *Systemic Manifestations of IBD. The Pending Challenge for Subtle Diagnosis and Treatment*. Falk Symposium 98. 1998 ISBN 0-7923-8734-1

Falk Symposium Series

99.   Goebell H, Holtmann G, Talley NJ, eds. *Functional Dyspepsia and Irritable Bowel Syndrome: Concepts and Controversies.* Falk Symposium 99. 1998
ISBN 0-7923-8735-X

100.   Blum HE, Bode Ch, Bode JCh, Sartor RB, eds. *Gut and the Liver.* Falk Symposium 100. 1998
ISBN 0-7923-8736-8

101.   Rachmilewitz D, ed. *V International Symposium on Inflammatory Bowel Diseases.* Falk Symposium 101. 1998
ISBN 0-7923-8743-0

102.   Manns MP, Boyer JL, Jansen PLM, Reichen J, eds. *Cholestatic Liver Diseases.* Falk Symposium 102. 1998
ISBN 0-7923-8746-5

102B. Manns MP, Chapman RW, Stiehl A, Wiesner R, eds. *Primary Sclerosing Cholangitis.* International Falk Workshop. 1998.
ISBN 0-7923-8745-7

103.   Häussinger D, Jungermann K, eds. *Liver and Nervous System.* Falk Symposium 102. 1998
ISBN 0-7924-8742-2

103B. Häussinger D, Heinrich PC, eds. *Signalling in the Liver.* International Falk Workshop. 1998
ISBN 0-7923-8744-9

103C. Fleig W, ed. *Normal and Malignant Liver Cell Growth.* International Falk Workshop. 1998
ISBN 0-7923-8748-1

104.   Stallmach A, Zeitz M, Strober W, MacDonald TT, Lochs H, eds. *Induction and Modulation of Gastrointestinal Inflammation.* Falk Symposium 104. 1998
ISBN 0-7923-8747-3

105.   Emmrich J, Liebe S, Stange EF, eds. *Innovative Concepts in Inflammatory Bowel Diseases.* Falk Symposium 105. 1999
ISBN 0-7923-8749-X

106.   Rutgeerts P, Colombel J-F, Hanauer SB, Schölmerich J, Tytgat GNJ, van Gossum A, eds. *Advances in Inflammatory Bowel Diseases.* Falk Symposium 106. 1999
ISBN 0-7923-8750-3